Nursing Your Baby, Fourth Edition

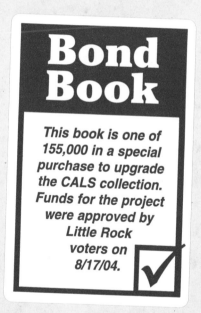

ALSO BY KAREN PRYOR

Don't Shoot the Dog:
The New Art of Teaching and Training

ALSO BY GALE PRYOR

Nursing Mother, Working Mother:
The Essential Guide for Breastfeeding
and Staying Close to Your Baby
After You Return to Work

Fourth Edition

Nursing Your
BABY

Karen Pryor and Gale Pryor

HarperResource
An Imprint of HarperCollins*Publishers*

HarperCollins books may be purchased for educational, business, or sales promotional use. For information please write: Special Markets Department, HarperCollins Publishers, 10 East 53rd Street, New York, NY 10022.

Designed by Ellen Cipriano

The Library of Congress Cataloging-in-Publication Data

Pryor, Karen.
  Nursing your baby / Karen Pryor and Gale Pryor.— 4th ed.
    p. cm.
  Includes bibliographical references and index.
  ISBN 0-06-056069-X
    I. Pryor, Gale. II. Title.

RJ216.P77 2005
649'.33—dc22   2004060908

---

05 06 07 08 09 WBC/RRD 10 9 8 7 6 5 4 3 2 1

To
Max, Gwen, Wylie, Ellie,
Micaela, Nathaniel, and Maile,
all breastfed babies

Acknowledgments

An extraordinary expansion of knowledge has taken place in recent years in the areas of human lactation and the practical management of breastfeeding. In every edition of *Nursing Your Baby* we have turned to many specialists for information and insight in order to summarize this huge body of knowledge for nursing mothers.

For many years, Kathleen Auerbach, PhD, has guided and reviewed our understanding of the research. The author, with Jan Riordan, of *Breastfeeding and Human Lactation*, Second Edition, a guide for lactation consultants and other medical professionals, a founder of the International Lactation Consultants Association, and past assistant professor of Clinical Pediatrics at the University of Chicago School of Medicine, has an encyclopedic knowledge of the breastfeeding research literature. We are grateful for her contributions.

We also thank Armond Goldman, MD, of the University of Houston, Allan Cunningham, MD, at Columbia University Medical School, the late Niles Newton, PhD, Lewis Lipsitt, PhD, Edward Cerutti, MD, Marvin Eiger, MD, Kittie Frantz, PNP, Carl and Muchnick, MD, and also Boston area lactation consultants Jackie Shina, Janet Repucci, Dot Norcross, and Sandra Corsetti, for their assistance in keeping us up to date on research in lactation and breastfeeding management.

Toni Sciarra, executive editor at HarperCollins Publishers, took time and care to be sure that every word of the fourth edition was clear, while Nick Darrell, associate editor, kept us on track and on schedule. Illustrator Alexis Seabrooke refreshed the book with charming illustrations of Katharine and Maggie MacPhail, our patient and willing mother and nursing newborn, and Ruthanne and Willa Rudel, our mother and nursing toddler models. Katharine MacPhail not only modeled for our illustrations, but read every chapter of the fourth edition in the last weeks of her pregnancy, at the hospital where Maggie was born, and in the early weeks of nursing. Her comments and reflections on life as a nursing mother were invaluable. Miranda Helin, Gale's partner at Pen and Press, encouraged and applauded every completed chapter of the revision.

Finally, we would like to thank Kolya Leabo, Gale's husband, who cheerfully puts up with the many drawbacks of being married to a writer. We also thank Max, Wylie, and Nathaniel Leabo for their patience with a mother and grandmother who have the tiresome habit of carrying on long conversations about breastfeeding (and clicker training) in their presence.

Karen Pryor
Gale Pryor

Contents

Nursing Your Baby, Fourth Edition

This book contains advice and information relating to health care. It is not intended to replace medical advice and should be used to supplement rather than replace regular care by your doctor. It is recommended that you seek your physician's advice before embarking on any medical program or treatment.

All efforts have been made to ensure the accuracy of the information contained in this book as of the date published. The authors and the publisher expressly disclaim responsibility for any adverse effects arising from the use or application of the information contained herein.

Preface to the Fourth Edition

I have grown up with this book. At eight, I read *Nursing Your Baby* cover to cover, not because I was fascinated by breastfeeding, but because so much of my mother, Karen Pryor, could be found in its pages. The mother herself was right there beside me, driving me and my brothers to school, getting dinner on the table, managing a busy household and career. But her mind—her unique blending of biology, anthropology, sociology, and everyday mothering—was explained to me in her readable writer's voice on the pages of *Nursing Your Baby*. It shaped, in turn, my mind, my writing, and my mothering.

Her ability to communicate the value of breastfeeding to her peers in her writing and lectures was one of the lifelines that saved breastfeeding. Nearly eradicated in the United States by the 1960s when just 18 percent of babies were breastfed, a few dedicated women, my mother among them, coaxed the art of breastfeeding back into our culture. For nursing is an art, and one best taught woman to woman, one mother and baby at a time. Perhaps that is why *Nursing Your Baby*, written by a mother for other mothers, has endured for more than forty years. This book's gift is the confidence it instills in women that they can nurse their babies. It has assured two generations of women that not only does breastfeeding matter a great deal, but so do they.

With confidence gained through successfully breastfeeding their babies against the odds, thousands of women have gone on to devote their lives to helping other mothers do the same. They formed La Leche League International and established the new medical profession of certified lactation consultants. They've organized, legislated, protested, campaigned, and written articles and more books. Thanks to their work, and that of the research scientists drawn by the fascination of lactation, it is at last well known and widely accepted that "breast is best."

Even so, the majority of American babies are weaned within a few months. Why? The United States is still not a very friendly place for mothers and babies. Breastfeeding beyond the newborn period requires more than knowing how to put a baby to the breast; it asks for a culture that supports a mother and baby as a couple. Culture is a pervasive thing, and we are not always aware of its influence in our individual lives. It can be found in a neighbor's advice, a medical opinion, a television commercial, a human resources department, a magazine article, or a Hollywood movie. Despite the resurgence of breastfeeding in recent decades, the overwhelming majority of cultural messages given new mothers are that bottlefeeding is the rule and breastfeeding the exception, that mothers who work (as most do) cannot also breastfeed, and that nursing, at least for a few weeks, is an obligation rather than a source of satisfaction and joy. None of these beliefs is true, and all interfere with successful breastfeeding.

With each new edition of *Nursing Your Baby*, my mother and I are surprised by how much work still needs to be done to support mothers and babies, how many obstacles remain for women who wish to blend the pleasure of mothering, beginning with breastfeeding, with the rest of their active twenty-first-century lives. Now, with the fourth edition, we are gratified to witness the progress of breastfeeding over the last decade. So much has changed for the better. In many ways, however, our increased understanding of the mechanisms and benefits of breastfeeding has also broadened our mission in giving mothers and babies the best start possible. Now we know that we need to take better care of mothers, so that they may take better care of their babies.

Since the last edition of *Nursing Your Baby*, Karen has moved on to new adventures, including writing and lecturing about the art of positive reinforcement teaching, called clicker training or TAG teaching, to groups as various as animal trainers, gymnastics instructors, and special education teachers. Once in a while, someone will come up to her at a conference to ask if she is the same Karen Pryor who wrote *Nursing Your Baby*. The question always comes from a nursing mother, another woman for whom breastfeeding was the blueprint for a new positive, mutually beneficial way of interacting with others, whether a child, a dog, or a student, without punishment or coercion. They see immediately that the mission Karen is on now is not very different from her work as a breastfeeding advocate.

A science writer by trade, I too find the lessons of nursing my three sons have lasted long past the day my youngest weaned himself. A fascination with the biology and behavior of parenting and the amazing capabilities of infants was sparked by breastfeeding, and has developed into a writing specialty. It has been a privilege to replenish *Nursing Your Baby* with the rich research and new knowledge about lactation that has emerged since the last edition—and to provide a new generation of mothers with its unique blend of science and warmth, and its gift of confidence and joy.

Gale Pryor
Belmont, Massachusetts
January 2005

Part One

The Science and History of Breastfeeding

The Nursing Couple

The oneness of the nursing mother and her baby has always fascinated mankind. Like lovers, they are united both physically and spiritually. Unlike lovers, their union lacks the ambivalence and tensions of sexuality. The Egyptians portrayed their chief goddess, Isis, with the infant Horus at her breast. Christianity reveres the Madonna, the image of mother and infant, as a symbol of pure love. The Dalai Lama, spiritual leader of Tibetan Buddhism, speaks of compassion and altruism as first learned at a mother's breast, as the mother gives of herself to her child. Artists through history and across geography have been inspired by the nursing couple to convey, in stone and clay and paint, two souls who are one.

It is brief, this unity. In most cultures, the baby is weaned in a year or two—or much less—and his world expands beyond his mother's arms. She then becomes a part of her child's life, sharing its center more each day with other people, other interests, eventually yielding her place of primacy entirely. Yet for all its brevity, the nursing couple is an intense relationship. Mother and child share a rapport so complete that it can exert a profound effect on both. Without this rapport, this mutuality, breastfeeding may cease. Nursing a baby is as much about the giving and taking of self as it is about the giving and taking of milk.

Nursing a baby is an art; a domestic art, perhaps, but one that, like cooking and gardening, brings to a woman the release and satisfaction only creative work can give. The author Anne Morrow Lindbergh wrote, "When I cannot write a poem, I bake biscuits and feel just as pleased." Nursing gives the same sort of satisfaction and joy. Successful nursing mothers tend to feel that breastfeeding is special, and are thankful for the experience.

Breastfeeding is special for the baby, too. While drinking from a bottle is a passive experience, nursing at the breast is a participation sport. Babies can throw themselves into it with an endearing, almost comical gusto. British novelist Angela Thirkell offers an observation of a grandmother watching her daughter nursing her new baby: "Edith was sitting in a low chair, her baby in her arms, while the said baby imbibed from nature's fount with quite horrible greed. Her face became bright red, a few dark hairs were dank with perspiration, one starfish hand was clenched on a bit of her nightgown . . . she was victualling herself as far as her adoring grandmother could make out for a six weeks' siege at least." Nobody ever felt that way about a plastic bottle.

THE REWARDS OF NURSING

Before a woman nurses a baby, she may assume that the chief reward of doing so is a sense of virtue, the knowledge that by choosing to breastfeed, she is doing the right thing for her baby's health. The evidence of the long- and short-term benefits of breastfeeding to both mother and baby's health and development is indisputable. In fact, for many reasons detailed in the following chapters, breastfed babies in the United States are 20 percent less likely to die before their first birthday; the longer a baby nurses, the lower the risk. If all babies in the United States were breastfed, reports a large study published in the May 2004 issue of *Pediatrics*, the journal of the American Academy of Pediatrics, approximately 720 infant deaths could be prevented each year.

And yet enduring good health is just one of the gifts of breast-feeding. The nursing mother may be proud that her baby thrives, but her daily reward lies in the peace, even the bliss, of the nursing experience. Nursing feels good. It brings physical comfort to both mother and baby, as it eases the baby's hunger and floods his mother with oxytocin, the hormone for peaceful and loving feelings, and prolactin, the milk-making hormone that also seems to induce a sense of calm in the mother.

The obvious and lavish love a nursing baby displays for his mother is a special sort of joy. Being in close contact with each other is tremendously rewarding. Nursing babies love to gaze at and touch their mothers. Mothers are gratified that they are just what their babies want. A nursing mother tends to feel that her baby is not a job or a chore, but her little friend, a member of the team. This partnership is the essence of the nursing relationship, an equal exchange of effort and satisfaction.

As any nursing mother would tell you, another tremendous reward is that breastfeeding, once learned, is a lot less trouble than the chores involved in feeding a baby with formula and bottles. A breast is always warm, ready, and available, at home or away, while formula must be bought and mixed, and bottles washed and prepared, packed and carried.

As any working nursing mother knows, breastfeeding comforts with the assurance that no matter how much of each day her baby is with a substitute caregiver and no matter how much her baby adores that caregiver, only Mama can nurse the baby; only Mama has the warm breast full of milk.

Breastfeeding is the fastest way to lose weight and get back in shape after pregnancy, as nursing a baby devours as much as 600 calories a day, the equivalent calorie expenditure of thirty laps in a pool. Nursing your baby causes your uterus to contract after birth, flattening your stomach far sooner than if you were bottlefeeding. During pregnancy the body stores special fat reserves in the hips and abdomen that are intended to be used up during milk production. Lactation draws on these energy supplies. If breastfeeding does not occur, however, these special fat deposits can be difficult to reduce. Losing weight gained during pregnancy is welcomed by most women, but of critical importance for those with gestational diabetes in order to decrease their risk of developing lifelong diabetes. (And for women who do have prepregnancy Type 1 diabetes, breastfeeding tends to lower their sugar levels and they therefore may require less insulin as long as lactation continues.)

Breastfeeding benefits mothers long after nursing is done. Nursing reduces the risk of breast and ovarian cancer. The longer you nurse, the lower the risk. A woman who nurses two babies for a year each reduces her risk of premenopausal breast cancer by 28 to 61 percent. Every additional year of breastfeeding lowers a woman's lifetime risk of breast cancer by 4.3 percent. Women who have never breastfed not only have higher rates of breast and ovarian cancer, but endometrial cancer as well. Breastfeeding also strengthens a woman's bones, reducing her vulnerability to osteoporosis and hip fractures. In fact, women over sixty-five who have breastfed their babies have half the risk of fracturing a hip.

Women who breastfeed are one-third less likely to experience depression. Research has not yet explained why this should be so, although the relaxing, peace-giving hormones of lactation are strongly suspected. Experienced breastfeeding mothers might offer this additional explanation: The simple, pleasurable act of putting their baby to the breast, and the knowledge that doing so can keep both baby and mother safer from many risks for years to come, is a deep well of joy.

BEST FOR THE PLANET

Breastfeeding benefits more than the nursing mother and baby; it also contributes to the health of our planet. The most ecologically sound food available, it is produced and delivered and used without pollution or wasteful by-products. It requires no paper, plastic, or tin packaging, or all of the fibers, bleaches, and fuels used in manufacturing and distributing packaged products. It asks for no forests of lumber to be felled or herds of cows to overgraze the land. It does not contaminate water, or require water that may be contaminated to prepare. To breastfeed a baby is to step into our ecosystem, to play a role in a process as old and natural as falling rain and growing green leaves.

THE START OF THE NURSING RELATIONSHIP

The relationship between the nursing mother and her baby begins with a gentle give-and-take. When the mother's milk starts to flow easily, and the baby's suck becomes consistent and strong, they become partners in the process, or what psychiatrist M. P. Middlemore named the "nursing couple." This partnership can spring up at the very first feeding a few minutes after birth, or a few days or even weeks later. If nursing begins slowly, the way it can if the first feeding is delayed for medical reasons or, as happens sometimes, a baby does not develop a gusto for nursing until a few days after birth, a mother may be surprised and dismayed. Our assumption about a behavior as natural as nursing is that it should come to us, well, naturally.

Breastfeeding, however, is a learned skill. In cultures where all babies are nursed, mothers have learned the art of feeding their babies since they were little more than babies themselves. Like all primates, we learn much of what we know as social animals through observation. If a woman grows up watching mothers put their babies to the breast, seeing how they're held, how nursing is at the beginning and how it changes as the weeks go by, she is likely to pick up, hold, and feed even her first baby as if she's done it all her life.

In Western industrialized cultures, however, young girls rarely have the opportunity to observe nursing mothers and babies. They and their younger siblings may not have been nursed. The lady next door may not nurse her baby, and when they go shopping with their mothers, girls are even less likely to see a nursing couple. Until recently, nursing in public was on the fringe of legality; many breastfeeding mothers have been ushered out of shopping malls by security guards or scolded by restaurant maitre d's. Women still endure disapproving stares if they nurse in the presence of strangers. While nursing in public is certainly legal, and even explicitly protected by law in some states, the sight of a breastfed baby is still far from a daily experience for little girls in our culture. Mothers in nations where breastfeeding is not the cultural norm, therefore, must learn to do it on the job, without the learning-by-observation that nature expected.

A LEARNED MUTUAL SKILL

Under these biologically bizarre circumstances, a new mother may misperceive breastfeeding. We behave as if breastfeeding, like giving a bath, were something you do to a baby. In reality, breastfeeding is something you do with a baby, something you learn together. Some babies are born experts, other require time and help.

The baby must learn that milk is what he needs and that his mother's breast is the place to get it. He must learn how to get a hold on the breast. If the milk is slow to flow, he may have to acquire patience and perseverance. If it flows too quickly, he may have to learn to adjust, to sputter and swallow without falling apart, and to return to the breast for the rest of his meal. Babies are individuals right from the beginning, and their responses to the experience of learning to nurse vary as much as the color of their eyes and the pitch of their cry.

The baby is, of course, amply rewarded for his efforts. The sweet taste of human milk is a nice payoff, as is the easing of hunger—but his mother's enveloping scent, eyes, voice, touch, and presence reinforce and encourage his nursing skills, too.

His mother, meanwhile, must learn how to be comfortable with her baby, how to read his signals of need, to know when he is hungry, when he is sleepy, and when he would just like to be held. This takes time, too. Breastfeeding, however, provides an introductory course of sorts for reading a baby's wide range of signals. In the course of one feeding, a baby may signal frantic hunger as he opens his mouth wide and turns his head, followed by sociability as he gazes and gazes at his mother's face while calmly nursing, and soon enough, fatigue, as his sucking slows and his intense gaze softens and fades to sleep. His mother learns these signs of her baby's changing needs and moods, developing a sensitivity to his cues even when they are not nursing.

LEARNING TO MOTHER

The sensitivity acquired through nursing lasts long past weaning as a mother reads her toddler's signs of fatigue, her preschooler's shyness, and even her teenager's desire to talk with equal fluency and sensitivity. The breastfeeding relationship becomes the blueprint for a lifelong relationship between mother and child based on give-and-take, mutual satisfaction, and keen sensitivity for each other's needs and emotions.

When researchers have explored the question of whether breastfeeding creates happier or more well-adjusted children, the complexities of human life have resisted clear data. When evidence in favor of such a result shows up, it is usually challenged on the ground that the breastfed children are happier because they had mothers with more affectionate natures, who were thus more apt to breastfeed. The critics, however, may have it backward. It is not necessarily a mother's affectionate nature that motivates breastfeeding. It is the breastfeeding experience itself that teaches mothers to be generously affectionate and skilled in showing affection. The learning is built into the system.

CONTAGIOUS EMOTIONS

As Sibylle Escalona, MD, has pointed out, emotions are contagious. Even tiny babies can "catch" emotions from their mothers, and as parents of highly sensitive, highly reactive babies can testify, upset infants have upset parents. Sometimes this can lead to a cycle of difficulties, but the contagion of emotions can also work in favor of mother and baby. The calmed baby is a soothing armful for the mother. The father's enjoyment of the baby and pride in his partner as she dons motherhood can soothe mother and baby, too. An experienced, relaxed person can sometimes calm a frantic baby simply by holding him. And so when a baby settles down and begins nursing well, his evident enjoyment and relief convey themselves to the mother, so that she, too, begins to enjoy the feeding.

Some care providers—nurses, midwives, physicians, lactation counselors—spread calm; everyone around them, mothers and babies alike, absorbs their peace and cheer. Such a person often has remarkable success in helping mothers and babies become happy nursing couples. Sometimes a grandmother or sister or friend provides the confidence-giving aura of calm; sometimes the baby's father is the soothing presence. Once lactation is well established, the tranquil joy of mother and baby spreads back to the rest of the household—an extremely valuable contagious emotion.

THE BONDS OF LOVE

An established nursing relationship is not lightly broken. Mother and baby need each other both physically and emotionally. The baby, of course, has a physical need for milk. His emotional need is also great: a need for contact with his mother, and for the love and reassurance he receives through all his senses while nursing, but especially through his highly sensitive mouth.

The mother also has a physical need for the baby to take the milk from her breasts. Moderate fullness is not a discomfort; nevertheless, the letdown reflex that makes the milk flow is relieving, satisfying, like a drink of water when one is thirsty. Mothers' fondness for nursing comes in part from the rush of hormones associated with the first flow of milk, but also because nursing provides a legitimate excuse to sit down and do nothing for a while. A nursing mother yearns for the satisfaction of feeding her baby, for the break in her busy day it provides, but most of all, she yearns for her baby.

Mothers, like babies, need to be shown that they are loved.

The behavior of even a tiny baby at the breast is proof positive of that. His greed flatters, his bliss contagious, and his drunken satiety a comic compliment. As he grows older, his love of his mother becomes conscious and intense. The baby of three months stares and stares at his mother's face as he nurses, looking into her eyes—loving her with all his soul. At five or six months he plays at the breast, fiddling with a ribbon or button on his mother's blouse, patting her lovingly. He smiles out of the corner of his mouth, or puts a hand up to her lips to be kissed, showing her at every feeding how much he loves her. It is quite an experience. Life is not so full of true love that one regards it as commonplace in any circumstances.

Of course, the mother and baby who do not breastfeed love each other intensely as well. But a nursing couple has a different sort of intensity; mothers who have bottlefed one child and breastfed a subsequent baby are poignantly aware of the difference. The physical intimacy of breastfeeding dispels the barriers that always exist between individuals who do not have daily skin-to-skin contact, who do not breathe in each other's scent, knowing its uniqueness the way they know the difference between salt and sweet.

Mothers who have both bottlefed and breastfed infants often say the nursing baby was "easier." The ease lies not only in being free of the chores of bottlefeeding and the drawbacks of formula, but in feeling consistently companionable with their baby. The nursing baby tends to go along with his mother wherever she goes, not only because he needs his mother's milk, but because he is so little trouble, and she misses him when they are apart. And the easy rapport of the nursing couple endures long past weaning into the busy years of childhood, when it is often needed most.

THE HAPPY NURSING BABY

A baby whose physical and emotional needs are being met through nursing is a happy baby, and a happy baby is easier on the whole household. He is always around, but seldom in the way. Siblings who have every right to be jealous of any new baby soon become accustomed to the new baby, as for the first six weeks or so the baby is simply an extension of the mother. The nursing couple fits into the family as a unit. The baby nurses as his mother reads to the other children, nurses while she talks over the day with her partner, or while she naps, talks on the phone, or sits down to her own dinner. When nursing becomes this casual, the breastfed baby automatically receives so much physical contact that he demands less attention through fussiness. His smoothly running insides contribute to his cheerful demeanor. The baby may be the least demanding, least troublesome member of the family, and receives in return ample love and approval from all. The social learning fostered by breastfeeding also lasts long past weaning.

The mother who is returning to a job or school within a few weeks after birth will have an added appreciation for her even-tempered baby. Her pleasant baby will enjoy the admiration of his babysitter, and their relationship is likely to become warm and loving. Yet, he reserves his deepest adoration for his mother during breastfeeding. The intimacy of the nursing relationship bridges the hours of separation. Nursing illuminates their daily reunions, and replenishes both their physical and emotional strength. No matter that someone other than Mom cares for the baby during her working hours; breastfeeding is the one thing no one else but she can do for the baby. In preserving this privilege for herself, a mother also preserves the closeness that breastfeeding brings.

THE BRIDGE TO MATURITY

What effect, if any, does the nursing relationship have on the emotions and personality of a child as he grows? The attachment theorists, a body of research established by John Bowlby and Mary Ainsworth, suggest that a high-quality, keenly sensitive, and responsive maternal-infant relationship, epitomized by the nursing couple, is essential to the healthy emotional growth of a baby, and possibly to that of the mother as well. Ashley Montagu, the late anthropologist, suggested that the human infant is born after nine months of gestation because the rapidly growing brain cannot pass through the birth canal much later than that. The newborn, however, is not a "mature" infant until another nine months have passed, when it has teeth and a fair amount of mobility. In this view, our species requires a nine-month period of extrauterine gestation, during which the infant's needs must be met as fully as they were within the womb during pregnancy. A mother's breasts and arms become that postbirth womb. Perhaps this perspective helps to explain why some babies wean themselves spontaneously at or around the age of nine months, from breast or bottle. While nursing is often continued far beyond nine months of age, this seems to be the earliest point at which weaning occurs naturally.

The separation of mother and child at birth is a physical and emotional shock to both. Lactation eases their separation, permitting it to occur gradually over months rather than in the instant of birth. When the mother feeds her baby long and often at her breast, his world is still composed mainly of her warmth, motion, sound, and scent. The baby acquires his understanding of his new world of fluctuating temperatures, textures, lights, sounds, and people from the familiar home base of her body. His mother, in turn, is allowed a gradual, sweet separation from this small fruit of her body.

Nursing, if unhindered by cultural interference, usually does continue long past nine months for many good reasons. Throughout most of the world, babies nurse for at least one year, and often two or more. The older baby derives obvious and perhaps important reassurance from being able to nurse. This is true of other species as well. Cornell University scientists point out that when a person enters a field of goats or sheep, all the babies run in fear to their mothers and immediately begin to nurse. Anthropologists note the same behavior in villages in developing nations when a stranger enters a remote community; even children of five or six calm their anxiety with a reassuring moment at their mother's breast. The experienced nursing mother knows that while a toddler may cease to need the breast for nourishment, he still wants it very much when he is frightened or has hurt himself. The older bottlefed baby may derive this comfort from a blanket, bottle, or thumb. The breastfed toddler prefers his mother's lap and bosom.

WHAT ABOUT THE MOTHER?

How are mothers affected by becoming half of a nursing couple? Lactation is the final chapter in a woman's reproductive functioning. Men have only one biological function related to their gender: intercourse. Women, however, have five: the ovarian cycle, intercourse, pregnancy, childbirth, and lactation. Each of these events has a powerful effect on a woman's life.

We are quite aware of the physical and emotional changes that take place when a girl reaches puberty and begins the ovarian cycle. The emotional significance of intercourse is reasonably well understood. Pregnancy has become a field of considerable interest to students of human emotions. The emotional repercussions of a poorly managed childbirth versus the mental and physical rewards of a well-conducted labor and birth are sufficiently recognized for childbirth association and education programs to have sprung up across the country. Yet we are still generally unaware of the psychological effects on women of experiencing a normal lactation. The questions have not even begun to be asked.

Observing nursing mothers, however, we can propose some lines of inquiry. When a woman breastfeeds, she must give herself to the baby. She learns to let the baby set the pace, and allow herself to be guided by her baby. Many mothers find it difficult to surrender their control in this way, especially if they have been discouraged from doing so by a fixed set of rules for baby care and feeding. Most often, however, a woman eventually relaxes into a more flexible approach. She forgets to look at the clock, she doesn't interrupt the baby for her own reasons, she doesn't worry about when or why the baby wants to eat. She just accepts that he does. She actively and generously gives the baby milk, time, and love whenever he seems to want it. She lets him move around, start and stop, nurse at his own rate, interrupt his meals or prolong them. The mother learns to participate in feedings without dominating them. She becomes deeply interested in but quite relaxed about the whole matter. How does this transition change a woman's approach to other people, problems, and life in general? If she applies what she has learned through successful breastfeeding, a great deal.

The woman who doesn't develop this relaxed but attentive behavior pattern with her first baby often adopts it with her second. That may be why many nursing mothers "have more milk" the second time around. The casual yet involved attitude toward ourselves and others is rather foreign to our culture. More commonly we see the laid back as uninvolved and disinterested, and the involved as intensely focused, even controlling. For many American women, successful breastfeeding is their first experience of the happy balance of relaxed focus, one that may guide their parenting style for years to come.

The experience of breastfeeding can teach a mother how to go about being steady, wise, and balanced: in short, womanly and grown up. Her relationship with her partner may deepen, her interactions with co-workers more productive and less stressful. The sustained two-way caregiving and caretaking relationship with her baby is a powerful sort of education.

WHAT ABOUT THE FATHER?

A man usually derives deep satisfaction from the sight of his partner nursing his child. Dr. Hugh Smith, the Dr. Spock of eighteenth-century London, urging mothers to nurse their own babies (rather than employ a wet nurse), wrote: "Oh, that I could prevail upon my fair country-women to become still more lovely in the sight of men. I speak from the feelings of a man . . . rest assured, when he beholds the object of his soul cherishing and supporting in her arms the propitious reward of wedlock . . . it recalls a thousand delicate sensations to a generous mind." For a mother, then or now, one happy reward of nursing is the glow on her mate's face when he first sees the baby at her breast.

While a father here or there may fear he has been sidelined in his partner's affections, his support and contribution to the success of the nursing couple is essential. Many a mother attributes her ability to nurse her baby through a rough spot to her mate, who thought she should and knew she could, whatever the rest of the world said or did.

Not only are fathers able to care for new mothers, keeping them hydrated and well fed, ensuring their rest by entertaining other children and managing the household, but they can be vital when it comes to defending the nursing couple. In a large metropolitan hospital, one father supported his wife through delivery of a baby girl, who in due course was taken to the hospital nursery for "observation." When several hours passed and the baby had not been returned to their room, the father went to the nursery to fetch the baby. There he found a staff member ordering a bottle of sugar water for his baby, a practice he had learned along with his wife can interfere with breastfeeding. "We're breastfeeding," he said, "and this baby needs to be taken to my wife immediately." Which she was, and that baby never saw the inside of the nursery again. The father later said of the showdown in the nursery, "It was fun."

Large hospitals, brief stays, and harried staffs mean that a mother may not always get the start-up help she needs. Fathers and other partners can ensure that she gets what she needs, shield her from interference, and defend their baby's inalienable right to his mother's milk.

BREASTFEEDING IN A BOTTLEFED CULTURE

Despite the championship of breastfeeding in the medical community and the widespread agreement that "breast is best," it is still common for babies to be weaned after a few weeks of nursing for a variety of reasons that have little to do with breastfeeding.

Culture is a powerful influencer of behavior, and cultural prejudice against breastfeeding still permeates Western society. When outright prejudice does not interfere with breastfeeding, many seemingly unrelated cultural practices do. Despite the resurgence of breastfeeding after decades in which the mother who chose to nurse her baby was considered eccentric and foolhardy, regardless of the untiring efforts of thousands of breastfeeding advocates in both the lay and medical communities, we continue to live in a bottlefeeding culture.

While few children see babies being breastfed, all are familiar with the sight of a baby bottles in advertising, on television, in children's books, and as part of baby dolls' play sets. Even when the rare breastfed baby is shown in the media, never is that baby older than three or four months. In 1997, the American Academy of Pediatrics stated that all babies, with rare exceptions, be exclusively breastfed for the first six months of life, and that breastfeeding continue, with complementary foods, through the first year and beyond "as mutually desired." Yet, without access to images of other six-month-old and one-year-old nursing babies—or, heavens, nursing toddlers—most mothers inevitably feel out of step and isolated if their nursing baby is no longer a newborn. Feeling as though one is doing something that should not be done erodes a mother's confidence and leads directly to weaning.

No one speaks of bottlefeeding "discreetly" in public, yet nursing mothers practice breastfeeding invisibly in public with the skill of a magician rehearsing sleight-of-hand maneuvers. Mothers are advised to breastfeed, and yet simultaneously are prescribed numerous baby-care practices, from letting a newborn cry to training a three-month-old to sleep from 8:00 p.m. to 8:00 a.m., that interfere with nursing. Our society prizes independence, and so we encourage it in our children from the beginning. Parents read books on creating a "self-calmed" baby and purchase baby carriages, automated swings, and other devices that keep our infants on their own, at a distance, and soon weaned. Most influential of all, in our society, breasts are primarily sexual objects, their obscure function for feeding babies simply forgotten by a large majority of our population.

The result is that less than half of the nearly four million babies born each year in the United States are exclusively breastfed, others receiving bottled formula along with breast milk. Less than 30 percent are still breastfed at all by six months. By their first birthday, just 16 percent of American babies are still nursing.

Yet the health benefits and emotional pleasures of breastfeeding are astonishing and undeniable. Nursing is a straightforward business in many other countries. When breastfeeding is the cultural norm, no baby goes without because his mother does not "have enough milk" or must contribute to the family income while nursing. The complications of breastfeeding in the United States can too often be traced to a cultural element, whether it is lack of sufficient support for new mothers or rigid child-care practices or other "improvements" invented in recent decades.

The woman who learns all she can about breastfeeding and who seeks support and receives it when she asks, even in the midst of a culture that tells her otherwise, can nurse her baby.

How the Breasts Function

MAKING MILK: THE MAMMALIAN GIFT

We are mammals because we make milk. The remarkable ability of mammary glands to secrete ample and excellent nourishment for the newborn young separates mammals from lower creatures.

Lactation probably arose early in the evolution of species. In a sense, it is older than pregnancy. The monotremes, those ancient but still-living forms such as the duckbilled platypus, lay eggs like reptiles. But the young, once hatched, drink their mother's milk. The platypus has no nipples. Milk simply oozes through the pores of the skin on the abdomen, and the baby licks it off. The next step, as shown in marsupials such as the opossum, was the development of the nipple, which serves to collect the milk in one spot, giving the embryo-sized young something to grab, and reducing the chance of accidental separation from the milk supply. Pregnancy—internal gestation—in mammals was the final step in protecting and nourishing the young, long preceded by the giving of milk.

HOW THE BREASTS DEVELOP

The mammary glands, from which the word "mammal" is taken, appear early in the development of the embryo in the form of two thickened bands, the mammary ridges or milk lines, running down the center of the body. In the human species, these milk lines are discernible when the embryo is six weeks old. By the time it is five months along in utero, the nipple and the areola, or darkened area around the nipple, are all developed. In humans the mammary glands develop relatively high on the embryonic milk lines, in the chest region. In some other species, the glands may develop low on the milk lines, as in hoofed animals, or in serial pairs, as in dogs and cats. The existence of auxiliary pairs of nipples in human beings, either below or above the usual pair, is not uncommon, occurring about twice as often as the birth of triplets. These supernumerary nipples usually, but not always, are nonfunctioning during lactation. Mammary tissue may also exist along the milk lines, without a nipple. Once in a while, such tissue swells during the early lactation, but since the milk is not removed, the functioning soon ceases.

When a human baby is born, its breast tissue is usually enlarged, due to the presence of lactation hormones received from the placenta. Regardless of the sex of the child, the glands may actually secrete drops of milk during the first days after birth—what nurses and midwives sometimes call "witches' milk." Once this activity ceases, the mammary glands remain inactive, simply growing along with the rest of the body until a year or two before puberty. Then, in girls, the ovaries begin to release increasing quantities of estrogen into the bloodstream, causing the nipples and areolas to enlarge, and the glandular and duct tissue to grow and proliferate.

When menstrual cycles begin, the ovaries give off increased estrogen in amounts that wax and wane cyclically. When estrogen levels are highest, around the midpoint of each menstrual cycle, the major part of breast development takes place. The ducts continue to ramify and branch away from the nipples like tributaries of a river or branches of a tree, and fat is laid down around the duct system, giving the breasts their size and shape. (Buxomness, or lack of it, is not a good indication of potential ability to lactate; it is mostly a result of the quantity of nonfunctional fatty tissue in the breasts.) The development of the breasts depends not only upon estrogen, but also upon hormones secreted by the pituitary gland at the base of the *brain* which govern growth and sexual development. Once the body is mature and growth has ceased, in the late teens, breast growth is not noticeable until and unless the individual becomes pregnant.

BREAST CHANGES IN PREGNANCY

The changes that pregnancy produces in the breasts are noticeable in the very first weeks. Full and tender breasts are often a familiar sensation for a day or two before each menstrual period. When her breasts continue to feel full and tender day after day, however, the experienced mother flies to her calendar to calculate when the new baby might be expected.

By the time a mother's period is overdue, the glands of Montgomery, which lie in the areola in a ring around the nipple, have become prominent. These glands secrete special lubricants that make the areola elastic and flexible, so it can accommodate itself to being drawn into the infant's mouth. (Montgomery described these glands in a famous medical hyperbole as "a constellation of miniature nipples scattered over a milky way.") By the fifth month, the mother may need to buy larger bras as her breast tissue increases. Her nipples and areolas have become larger and darker. By the ninth month, even the new bras may seem tight, partly because her rib cage has expanded to make room for the baby.

All these changes prepare the breasts for lactation, and are brought about by hormones circulating in the maternal bloodstream. With elegant economy, nature borrows hormones for milk production from the same set that is used to govern the menstrual cycle. The menstrual cycle is maintained by a sort of hormonal round robin, in which the pituitary gland and the ovaries stimulate each other to produce a series of hormones that in the first half of the cycle develop and release an egg, and in the second half of the cycle prepare the uterus for possible pregnancy, should that egg become fertilized.

The ovarian hormone progesterone, which predominates in the second half of the cycle, causes the uterine lining to thicken. Progesterone also produces premenstrual changes in the breasts: the feeling of tenderness and fullness, and sometimes an actual increase in size. If no pregnancy takes place, progesterone production ceases, and the uterine lining is sloughed away in the menstrual flow. If conception takes place, however, the fertilized egg itself produces a hormone that keeps the ovaries producing progesterone, and the uterine lining remains to support the embryo.

About six weeks after conception, the placenta develops and begins to take over the hormone production job. The placenta releases very high levels of estrogen, as well as some of the progesterone and other hormones, into the body. This combination stimulates tremendous changes in the breasts. Up to now, growth has taken place only in the duct system, which will transport the milk down to the nipples.

Once the placenta has developed, a whole new system is added: the secretory system makes the milk to nourish the baby after birth, just as the placenta nourishes the baby before birth. The end of every duct branches and rebranches and buds off into little sacs, called the alveoli, lined with milk-secreting cells. The alveoli form clusters on their ducts, rather like bunches of grapes on their stems. The increase in breast size during pregnancy is a result mainly of the addition of alveoli to the mammary structure.

In the second half of pregnancy, the placenta begins producing prolactin, the lactation hormone, which stimulates further growth of the alveoli and also causes them to secrete milk. There is milk in the breasts from the fourth or fifth month of pregnancy; if miscarriage or premature delivery takes place from this time forward, it is followed by lactation.

If prolactin, which causes milk secretion, is present and the alveoli are capable of producing milk, why don't pregnant women lactate? This hormone does a lot more than just make milk—it is in men's bodies, too. However, another placental product, a prolactin-inhibiting factor, prevents, the secretion of milk until the placenta leaves the body.

Lactation researcher Marianne Neifert, MD, has reported a case of a new mother who could not give milk and also was bleeding a lot; on examination, her uterus proved to have retained a piece of the placenta—enough to stop the breasts from lactating. When that was removed, an ample milk supply developed within twenty-four hours.

PHYSICAL BENEFITS OF LACTATION
TO THE MOTHER

The physical benefits that breastfeeding can give to the mother begin in the hour her child is born. The oxytocin released at each feeding causes uterine contractions. At first, these can be uncomfortable; however, nursing in the hour of birth contracts the still-active uterus so effectively that it prevents the spasmodic cramping of the contractions or afterpains that are common when the first nursing is delayed. A nursing mother's uterus contracts during and after each feeding. Thus it involutes, or returns to normal size, more rapidly than that of the mother who doesn't nurse.

Breast tissue that has functioned in lactation is said to retain its shape over a longer period of years than that which has not. Some doctors think that breasts that have never lactated may be subject to atrophy and are more likely to be prematurely pendulous or shapeless. If lactation is ended abruptly, the breasts may seem soft or flat for a few weeks. By six months after weaning, however, the breasts have usually regained their former shape, but may have somewhat less fatty tissue. This makes little difference to the small-breasted woman, since she didn't have much fatty tissue to begin with. The woman with very large breasts may prefer her figure after lactation.

Lactation is good for the mother's body. Among many other benefits, it combats the cumulative effects on the figure of several pregnancies. Some of the weight gained in the pregnancy represents nutrients such as calcium, which are stored in the mother's body for use during lactation. Special fat deposits are laid down in pregnancy, to be drawn on during lactation; this is why a nursing mother need not eat as many calories as she is putting out to stay healthy while breastfeeding. When lactation is suppressed, it is possible that these stored nutrients remain in the body; each pregnancy therefore tends to make the mother a little heavier.

Finally, there is good evidence that lactation protects against some forms of breast cancer, especially among women who carry the BRCA1 genetic mutations, and that prolonged lactation (lasting two years or more) offers striking protection against ovarian cancer. There is evidence also that lactation offers significant protection, through mechanisms not yet understood, against the bone-thinning disease of osteoporosis.

HOW LACTATION BEGINS

Birth often leads swiftly to lactation. A mother who has just delivered a new baby is often overcome by the urge to pick up her baby right away and put it to the breast. In many hospitals, when mother and newborn are both doing well in the moments after birth, mothers are encouraged to nurse immediately, sometimes even before the placenta is delivered and the cord cut. Newborns are usually extremely alert and active during the first hour of life, and gaze into their mothers' eyes, ready to "latch on" to the breast for their first meal. A vigorous sucking reflex is often in evidence during this receptive period. The baby's sucking, through sensory and hormonal responses in the mother's body, causes the uterus to contract, facilitating delivery of the placenta, if that has not already occurred, and reducing postpartum bleeding.

The first milk present in the breasts at birth is colostrum, a creamy yellow fluid crammed with nourishment and vital antibodies as well as other protective agents. Even one feeding of colostrum provides the baby with important benefits. Colostrum also has a slightly laxative effect and helps to rinse the baby's intestines of waste products accumulated during its uterine life.

After an uncomplicated birth, a mother may rest with her new baby in her bed or very close by, so that they can nurse whenever she wishes to cuddle the baby, or whenever the baby peeps. A newborn may want to nurse in spurts, sometimes every hour or two; its stomach, after all, is no bigger than a walnut, quickly filling and easily emptying. When allowed to nurse frequently, they can take in considerable quantities of high-calorie colostrum. Many newborns spend their first couple of days dozing; yet, given support and patience, they too will begin to ingest quantities of this special first milk.

Whether the mother nurses sitting up or lying down, she holds the baby flat against her body, facing her, so that he does not have to reach or twist his neck to latch on. Whether the areola is large or small, the milk sinuses lie about the same distance behind the nipple, a distance matching the size of a newborn baby's mouth. While the baby is on the breast, his tongue and jaws apply pressure to the sinuses, not to the nipple itself. The nipple's well back in the baby's mouth, where it is virtually untouched during nursing. While a mother's nipples may be tender for a few hours or days, proper positioning and frequent, unrestricted nursing enable her breasts to adjust to their new task quickly.

Sometimes people unfamiliar with breastfeeding assume mothers need sleep that nursing a baby denies them, and that keeping the baby in the hospital nursery will allow a new mother to rest. In fact, a mother can doze and nurse as she could never do while holding a bottle. The production of milk depends upon prolactin secretion stimulated by suckling. Frequent and unrestricted nursings are important for a good start, benefit the mother physically, and are comforting to her and the baby. Many a mother feels fretful and depressed if her baby is away from her, and actually gets less rest if the baby is taken out of the room for even a brief period.

Within twenty-four to thirty-six hours, the colostrum changes to more mature milk, tailored to the needs of the newborn. Milk production may be overabundant at first. As one pediatrician tells his patients, "Nature doesn't know you didn't have twins." The breasts may feel full as the body discovers the level of production this baby, or these babies, require. Unrestricted nursing helps to keep the mother comfortable, and informs her body how much milk this particular baby needs. In breastfeeding, demand determines supply.

Babies almost always lose a little weight in the first days after birth. A breastfed baby may lose up to 7 percent of his birth weight in the first week, or as much as 12 percent if nursing is limited. With frequent, unrestricted nursings, a baby will regain his birth weight by the tenth day. Babies nursed frequently from birth on, however, experience less initial weight loss and more rapid weight gain. Babies born at home, or kept with their mothers and allowed to nurse without restriction, tend to regain their weight within a day or two.

As the mother gradually resumes her normal activities, she continues to keep the baby near her or with her day and night and to nurse him as long and as often as he wants. During the first month, a baby usually nurses an average of ten or twelve times in a twenty-four-hour period. This implies an average of two hours or more between feedings, but in real life the baby may sometimes want to nurse every hour—in the early or late evening, typically— and at other times will go for longer periods—three to four hours, perhaps—without nursing. As the baby grows and becomes more efficient, nursing sessions become shorter and fewer, occurring at longer intervals.

HUMAN PRODUCTION CAPACITY

The power of natural selection has made all female mammals efficient producers of milk. The amount of milk produced is a direct result of the amount removed. Ruth Lawrence, MD, professor of pediatrics at the University of Rochester Medical School, points out that the mammary gland is not a bladder, and the breast is not a storage tank. The breast is a production device; it is never truly empty as production is continuous. When the baby is hungrier, perhaps during a few days of rapid growth, he nurses longer or more frequently. Milk production then increases until the breasts are again meeting his needs, and in all likelihood producing a surplus. When he is less hungry for milk, perhaps once sampling solid foods at five or six months, production correspondingly slows down.

Peak production capacity is well above normal peak demand. Hospital milk banks, which collect and store human milk for premature and sick babies, have found that almost any woman who cares to be a donor can produce surplus milk beyond her own baby's needs. Some milk bank donors produce a few ounces of surplus milk a day, others donate a pint or more. Such individual variations seem to be entirely with the mammalian safety margin that ensures that every baby has more than enough milk. Some women can produce at least twice as much milk as is needed by the average baby; most can nurse twins.

Some mothers have successfully nursed triplets. A woman with a supernormal ability to lactate might be able to nurse more. In previous centuries, such women were valued staff members of foundling hospitals. (There is a record of a woman in a French orphanage who for a short time maintained seven babies on her own milk.) A woman with an inherited potential at the low end of the normal scale can still produce enough milk for one baby.

The existence of the hypogalactic woman, that is, the woman whose body cannot make sufficient milk to maintain one baby, has been postulated but never clearly demonstrated. What has been clearly demonstrated is that, in the presence of prolactin and possibly other lactation hormones, alveoli can be developed by the sucking stimulus alone. This fact means that mothers who start out producing just a few ounces of milk per day may yet be able to produce a quart or more daily after a few months of lactation.

It has been suggested that because we in the United States raise so many babies on the bottle, allowing the survival of offspring of mothers who have subnormal lactating ability, we are becoming in truth what the Russians call us in jest: a nation of milkless women. Fortunately, evolution does not work that quickly. The ancient mammalian equipment cannot be rendered nonfunctional in the random breeding of a few generations. Unsuccessful lactation in our society is usually due to misinformation and a multitude of cultural interferences in the lactation process, not to physical incapacity.

THE LETDOWN REFLEX

Certainly, despite normal equipment, a great many women "cannot" nurse a baby. They just don't seem to have enough milk. If prolactin causes milk secretion, why can't we solve the problem of the woman who "doesn't have enough milk" by giving her prolactin injections? This has been tried, but it is generally not a success. Almost always, the factor that is limiting the amount of milk a mother has for her baby is not prolactin production;

in fact, the hormone does not govern how much milk she is making.

Making milk, so simple and automatic a process when enough sucking stimulation is provided and enough milk removed, is only half of lactation. Giving milk is the other, equally important half. The nursing baby cannot get his mother's milk by himself. Even the powerful mechanical suction of a breast pump can remove no more than about a third of the milk, that milk which lies in the large collecting ducts or milk sinuses directly behind the nipple. The milk in the smaller ducts and alveoli cannot be withdrawn by outside forces; it must be delivered by actions within the breast itself.

This held-back milk is made available to the baby by a reflex within the breast called the letdown reflex. In England, this is sometimes termed the "the draught." The term "milk ejection reflex" is also used. In the milk-secreting lobes of the breast and along the walls of the ducts lie octopus-shaped cells called basket cells, which reach their threadlike arms around the alveoli and along the duct walls. As the baby starts to nurse, the tactile sensations received by the mother trigger the release of the hormone oxytocin, which causes the basket cells to contract. The alveoli are compressed and duct passages are widened. Fluid rushes from the bloodstream into the sinuses to mix with the milk constituents from the alveoli. The resulting milk is quickly pushed down into the sinuses under the nipple. In early lactation, it may even be pushed out of the duct openings to drip or spray from the nipples.

The baby does not actually remove milk by suction. His suction is merely sufficient to keep the nipple in place in the back of his mouth. Then with tongue and jaws he compresses the areola and the large milk sinuses beneath, pressing the milk in the sinuses into his mouth. In this way, he milks the breast, and this is the way all mammals (except, as mentioned, the platypus) get their milk.

The letdown reflex functions repeatedly during a single nursing. The baby need hardly make the effort to milk the breast; the milk is pumped into his throat of its own accord. Even a tiny premature baby can thus get plenty of milk almost effortlessly.

In fact, a newborn can be quite overcome by the sudden abundance from a strong letdown reflex. He may choke, gasp, sputter, get milk up his nose, and have to let go to catch his breath while the milk sprays all over the bedclothes and his face. Fortunately, most babies are excited rather than upset by this misadventure, and return to the breast with avid glee.

A functioning letdown reflex is crucial to the nourishment of the baby, not only because the baby receives just a third of the milk without the letdown action, but because he can receive the fat content of the milk only if the milk is let down. It has long been known that the last few swallows of milk are the richest; dairymen distinguish between the thin "fore milk" and the fat-filled "hind milk." F. E. Hytten, MD, of the University of Aberdeen in Scotland, has shown that the sticky fat particles tend to cling to the walls of the alveoli and ducts and to be drawn off last. While the fat mixes more evenly on "the second side," the breast that the baby is not nursing on, some gradation remains. British researcher Michael Woolwich, MD, identified several babies who were doing poorly because their mothers had been told to nurse only ten minutes on each breast at every feeding. By obediently following that rule, the women inadvertently fed their babies only the fore milk from each breast. The babies were rapidly losing weight because they were, in effect, being fed skim milk rather than whole, and no cream at all.

In human milk, 50 percent of the calories come from the fat content, the cream portion of the milk. Even if the baby nurses unrestrictedly, the fat globules will not reach the baby if the letdown reflex does not occur. An inhibited letdown reflex therefore can result in a hungry baby, even if a fair amount of fluid is being taken in. The letdown reflex is a straightforward physical response to a physical stimulus. It is supposed to work like clockwork. An insufficient letdown reflex, however, often leads to weaning. Why?

The letdown reflex can be conditioned to occur within moments after the baby begins suckling. It can even become conditioned (in the early days) to the scent of the baby or the sound of the baby's cry. Many a new mother has thought about her baby, who may be sound asleep in the next room, and discovered that her milk has suddenly begun to flow.

The process of conditioning the reflex to occur during suckling, however, can be interfered with by environmental and emotional factors. Until and unless the letdown reflex is firmly associated with nursing, it can be inhibited by embarrassment, irritation, or anxiety. Adrenaline, the hormone released during these and other stresses, negates the effects of oxytocin, the hormone governing letdown. Stress, often produced by the influences that work against breastfeeding in the United States, can prevent letdown. Physical problems such as sore nipples and engorgement, issues too often created by misinformation about breastfeeding, can cause discomfort that can interfere with letdown.

All too often, the first days at the hospital with a new baby can be stressful and emotional. Fatigue; interruptions; embarrassment; fear and pain; anxiety about the baby, work, children at home, about breastfeeding itself; separation from the baby; brusque doctors and nurses are all deleterious to development of a well-conditioned letdown reflex. Some mothers do not experience a real letdown until they leave the hospital and bring their new baby home. By that time, there may be some concern about the baby because he is not regaining his birth weight at a sufficient rate, or because he is "jaundiced," a condition that can develop with inadequate intake of mother's milk. Other mothers manage well in the hospital, but "lose their milk" on going home, when household responsibilities and family stresses inhibit the letdown reflex.

When the letdown reflex is functioning but weakly established, an otherwise minor disturbance—houseguests, a late evening, a cold, a quarrel—may be enough to tip the balance, to inhibit the reflex so that fatty hind milk is left in the breast, and the baby receives fewer calories than he would have otherwise. Consequently, the baby gets hungry again sooner than usual. His mother, worried that she does not have enough milk, gives him a bottle. Soon milk production and secretion are diminished because less milk is being removed from the breast. Unfortunately, this is usually regarded by the mother, her family, and all too often her health-care provider as the beginning of the end of lactation, rather than as a temporary and remediable situation.

At the opposite end of the spectrum is the mother with what has been called an overactive letdown reflex; her letdown is very efficient, the milk supply is abundant, and the baby, while gaining extremely well, chokes and sputters through each feeding, and is gassy and flatulent afterward. The baby, usually a powerful nurser, can rarely nurse just for comfort; once at the breast he must gulp the gushing flow. Early self-weaning can be the result. An overabundance of milk, however, can usually be brought into balance in a week or less by nursing on one breast only at each feeding, and by changing nursing positions with regularity.

The first and most important step in establishing strong letdown reflex is to reduce environmental stresses. New mothers are vulnerable, and all too ready to assume that they are simply imperfect people who can't lactate readily. In reality, too often their circumstances would make it hard for even an experienced breastfeeding mother to let down her milk. In addition to avoiding fatigue by cutting back on her own activities temporarily, a new nursing mother needs to consider other stresses she may be under: a chaotic household, worries about work or money, her partner's anxieties, visiting relatives, and any of the other day-to-day fusses that can disrupt our equilibrium. For now, a new mother would do well to distance herself from these external stresses as much as possible. In traditional societies, new mothers are allowed several weeks, and even months, of empty time in which to rest and nurse their babies. This protected period seems to be biologically important to establishing a strong letdown reflex and ensuring that both the baby and the mother rise up from birth strong and healthy.

After stress-load reduction, the easiest tool for encouraging a good letdown reflex is the nature of the reflex itself. It is a conditioned reflex; that is, its occurrence is associated with separate events: the sensation of a suckling baby, a baby's scent or cry, sitting down in the rocking chair in which the baby is nursed. Any one of these or similar events can set off the letdown reflex.

It can be helpful to choose a "stimulus" or signal to alert the reflex to operate. Any routine that is customarily followed before nursing, such as drinking a glass of water, bathing the breasts with a warm washcloth, turning on favorite music, or simply sitting down and unbuttoning your blouse, can become a conditioned signal, or stimulus, for the letdown reflex. Follow the routine consistently before nursing, and the association between the routine and nursing will become stronger and stronger, making the letdown reflex more and more reliable no matter the circumstances.

The scent of a baby may be the most powerful stimulus after actual suckling. Breastfed babies have a sweet fragrance that permeates their clothing. Mothers who pump their milk when separated from their baby often bring along a T-shirt or nightie the baby has recently worn, so that the scent of the baby the garment holds will help trigger their letdown.

The letdown reflex can also be conditioned to a time interval. Some babies settle down to a fairly predictable feeding pattern after the first few weeks. Their mothers' milk may then let down automatically when mealtime rolls around. It's often quite a surprise for a new mother, out at a party for the first time since the baby arrived, to find herself suddenly drenched with milk at 10:00 p.m.

As the reflex begins to be conditioned, the milk may let down when the mother sees the baby, or hears it cry, or even when she simply thinks of the baby. It can become conditioned to her emotion as she starts to nurse, therefore letting down whenever she feels a sense of pleasurable anticipation. One mother's milk let down in the early days whenever she sat down to a good dinner, another's when she stepped into a hot bath. One mother who had returned to work eight weeks after her baby arrived found that her milk always let down at the moment the elevator that began her trip home to her baby started to descend. In fact, any downward motion in any elevator could set off her letdown reflex.

This readiness to be conditioned to a variety of events is characteristic of the early days. Irregular events—leaking, surprise letdowns, hesitant letdowns, and fluctuations in milk production—are all signs that the letdown reflex is in the process of becoming reliable. The new mother's body is learning how to breastfeed. The more nursing it does, the quicker it will learn.

The milk lets down several times in one feeding, even though only the first letdown may be felt. When lactation is well established, the initial letdown in a feeding is very effective. For some mothers, this occurs from the first week or, especially with experienced mothers, the first feeding. For some women, letdown is accompanied by a pins-and-needles or pressured sensation; others never feel a thing.

Letdown can be recognized by the visible and sometimes audible gulps of the baby swallowing the free-flowing milk. The reflexive rush of fluid from the mother's bloodstream into the breast occurs rapidly, and may cause a mother to feel acutely thirsty when her milk lets down.

As lactation continues, sphincter muscles in the nipples begin to function, putting a stop to untimely leaking and spraying. Like a closed drawstring, these hold the milk in the breast until the baby relaxes the nipple by suckling. Once these muscles learn their job, the filled milk sinuses may stand out in visible ridges under the areola after the milk lets down, but no dripping or leaking occurs.

The well-conditioned letdown reflex of the experienced nursing mother is the secret of her ample, steady milk production, day in and day out, and of her satisfied, growing baby. She hardly thinks of it; she may not even be aware of it. Her baby wants to nurse, she gives him the breast, and the milk comes. It is infallible. Only when the baby begins to lose interest in the breast, which will not occur for at least nine or ten months (and usually not until after the first birthday), does her milk supply diminish and her letdown reflex operate later in the feeding and finally fade away. If the baby were to catch a cold or feel the need for extra comfort for a few days at this point and want the breast more often, both the milk secretion and the letdown reflex would return.

When the letdown reflex is truly secure, even a serious emotional shock may not inhibit it. And the normal extra efforts that occur in every woman's life—sitting up all night with a sick child, giving a dinner party or a speech, taking a night class or a trip, or catching the flu—can be withstood, and breastfeeding will remain unaffected.

BREASTFEEDING AND THE MOTHER'S NUTRITION

A nursing mother may produce from 600 to 1,000 milliliters (20 to 34 ounces) of milk per day, depending on the size and age of the baby. A mother nursing triplets may produce 3,000 milliliters of milk a day, or about 3 quarts. Each 1,000 milliliters of milk requires about 1,000 calories for the energy in the milk and the energy it takes to manufacture the milk. Not all of this comes from the diet; some of it is drawn from fat reserves laid down in the mother's body during pregnancy.

With anything approaching an adequate diet, most women produce plenty of milk without risking their body's own stores and intake of nutrients. A study of forty-five well-nourished nursing mothers in Texas showed that on a diet of about 2,200 calories a day these mothers gradually returned to their prepregnancy weights, while their babies all grew steadily. The amount or kinds of food they ate had no effect on the amount of milk they produced (the amount of milk, as we have seen, depends on the individual baby's needs).

During lactation the mother's body adapts to this new demand in several ways. Her gastrointestinal tract actually grows and elaborates, developing more intestinal surface for absorbing food, so that less of what she eats is wasted. She can also more easily absorb foods to which she may be allergic, thus making potential allergens available in the milk, a consideration for families with a history of allergies. Her metabolism lowers somewhat to save calories.

Unless the mother is actually starving, her body can provide adequate calories and fat even on a substandard diet. As for vitamins, calcium, and other minerals, nature will see to it that the baby's needs are met first. If these nutritional elements are missing in the mother's diet, her own body stores will inevitably be raided. Inadequate or restrictive diets take their toll; in one study in Nepal, the nursing babies of mothers on very marginal diets were small and growing slowly, but they were healthy nursing babies. The mothers, on the other hand, had urinary tract infections, parasites, B-vitamin deficiencies, and were susceptible to other illnesses.

The diet of Western women, though it may be ample in calories, may be inadequate in other ways. It is difficult to eat a truly whole-food diet in twenty-first-century North America. Nearly everything we buy in our supermarkets has been processed to some degree, sapping vitamins and trace minerals along the way. Prenatal vitamins should continue to be taken, therefore, through lactation to ensure that a nursing mother does not drain her own stores of nutrients while feeding her baby. More important, she needs to pay attention to the quality of her nutrition. Many American mothers try to diet by eating as little as possible; others subsist on precooked fast food; some are too busy or tired to bother to feed themselves, and some go on rigidly subscribed diets. All of these eating patterns put a woman at risk of mineral and vitamin deficiencies. Adding lactation on top of already poor nutrition drains the mother's reserves, from B-complex vitamins in her liver, to calcium and phosphorus in her bony skeleton. It may be that American nursing mothers' complaints of fatigue and barely adequate milk supply are sometimes due to unsuitable diets as much as overly demanding lives. Eating well does not mean eating expensively, but it does require real food: whole grains, fresh fruit and vegetables, beans, and other foods as close to their original state as possible.

An old superstition that mothers "lose a tooth for every baby" reflected a time when dental care was nonexistent and in which most people lost a tooth a year, baby or no baby. The bones of nursing mothers do lose calcium during lactation. It has long been assumed therefore that breastfeeding weakens women's bones, and that lactating women need to take calcium supplements. Recent research has revealed the surprising fact that, through a process still not understand, the calcium lost during lactation is replenished at weaning. Indeed, the amount of calcium in a woman's bones after weaning is higher than it was before lactation began. Breastfeeding, in some yet-to-be discovered way, strengthens bones, and women who have lactated are at lower risk of osteoporosis later in life.

Vitamin supplements can help to make up most deficiencies in the nursing mother's diet, and health-care providers generally recommend that nursing mothers continue taking their prenatal vitamins daily. Vitamin D, necessary for calcium metabolism, is especially important for women who do not go outdoors on a regular basis, or who have darkly pigmented skin, as sunlight is our primary source of vitamin D. You cannot better the norm by taking megadoses of vitamins; vitamin levels in the milk will stop climbing when the optimum is reached.

The best way to ensure an adequate supply of minerals, especially trace elements, to the mammary gland is to eat a varied diet of low- or unprocessed foods. Many plants, for example, pick up specific trace elements. That whiff of garlic in the salad or onions on the hamburger may seem like a frill, but it brings with it a few sulfur molecules, a crucial element in the oniony flavor and an essential component of some human enzymes. Lactation researcher Niles Newton, PhD, pointed out that the action of oxytocin, which governs the letdown reflex, depends on adequate supplies of calcium and also magnesium, both in short supply in the average American diet. A mother having trouble letting down her milk might increase her magnesium intake; leafy greens are one good source.

A nursing mother who complains of fatigue or exhaustion may be suffering from inadequate supplies of B-complex vitamins, which appear to be important in milk production especially at high levels, as when nursing a totally breastfed baby of fifteen pounds or more. (Researchers have found that a woman is even more likely to be deficient in B-complex vitamins if she was taking oral contraceptives before her pregnancy.) Although most vitamin supplements contain some parts of the B-vitamin group, individual needs vary, and the complete spectrum is more likely to be found in natural sources; mothers have reported dramatic recovery from feelings of exhaustion upon taking brewer's yeast or drinking fenugreek tea, an herbal source of B-complex vitamins.

In general, we all need the same nutritional elements, but some of us need more of one component or can thrive on less of another. An woman of Inuit heritage, for example, may tolerate a high-fat, low-starch diet. The mother of a Swiss family may get most of her protein from cow's milk and cheese, while a mother of Chinese descent can't digest dairy products at all. Although the government obligingly publishes RDA lists—Recommended Daily Allowances for dietary needs—it's important to remember that humans, like all other living things, come from various genetic backgrounds that have adapted to different environments, and biochemical needs are highly individual. Nursing mothers, like every other human being, need to meet their own individual needs.

There are no particular foods that will help or harm the milk supply. One often hears that chocolate is "binding" or that fruit has a laxative effect on the baby. In moderation, this is rarely the case. Excessive intake, however, of even the healthiest item can upset mother and baby both. A baby might develop a touch of diarrhea if his mother drank eight to ten glasses of orange juice a day. Also, there seems to be no dietary element that increases the milk supply in a mother who is not dietarily deficient, although every culture has its own pet lactagogue, ranging from powdered earthworms prescribed by Avicenna to innumerable herbal remedies. In the United States, the herb fenugreek is often recommended to nursing mothers to increase their milk supply, although controlled studies on its effectiveness have not been done.

Babies usually don't mind what their mothers eat. Volatile oils, which give most spices their characteristic odor and flavor, pass through the milk unchanged. Nature seems to have prepared babies to relish the dominant flavors of their mother's diet—whether garlic and onions, chilies, or curry—as these flavors permeate the amniotic fluid in which the baby bathes before birth. During the third trimester of pregnancy, a fetus may drink as much as a quart of amniotic fluid a day. All human babies do seem to be born with a sweet tooth, so it is no surprise that breast milk's dominant flavor is lightly sweet.

CHANGES IN MILK PRODUCTION AND COMPOSITION AS THE BABY GROWS

The initial fluid in the lactating breast, colostrum, looks different from real milk and is much higher in some nutrients and in protective components. Some ingredients of colostrum are manufactured in the breast, others are transferred through the cell membranes. Researcher Margaret Neville, PhD, has found that some constituents of colostrum pass between cells of breast tissues though intracellular gaps. This "leakiness" is very high during the first few days after birth, when large antibody molecules can pass directly from the mother's bloodstream into the milk. After the fifth day, this "leakiness" seals up. Within one to four days of frequent nursing, the thick, golden colostrum gives way to white "mature milk." Colostrum usually is no longer present by the end of the second week.

We used to believe that once colostrum gave way to mature milk, the milk remained the same for the rest of lactation. Now researchers have found that the milk of a nursing mother changes gradually as her baby grows. Although the quantity of milk will increase substantially, some of the initial components increase and others level off or decrease. Living white cells, for example, which protect the baby against disease, become less abundant after the first few weeks. Meanwhile, however, the enzyme lysozyme, which is also antibacterial (and possibly metabolically "cheaper" for the mother's body to produce), increases a hundredfold in the first three months, and stays at that level as long as lactation continues.

In the first six months, breast milk contains high levels of minerals and trace elements such as zinc, necessary for optimum muscle growth. But by the time the baby is six or seven months old, trace elements dwindle in the milk when the baby is sampling foods other than breast milk. "The mammary gland is a marvelous machine," says researcher Michael Hambidge, MD. As the baby begins to get some of its trace elements from other sources, the mammary gland gradually reserves the mother's supply once again for her own needs.

That marvelous machinery of the breast even produces specialized milk for premature babies. Researchers have found that the milk from mothers whose babies were born one to three months preterm has twice as many fatty acids necessary for nerve and brain growth as the milk of mothers of full-term babies, and 70 percent more of certain easily digested lipids for energy and general growth. Preterm milk also contains more protein and higher levels of some vitamins and minerals than full-term milk. In the past, research had seemed to indicate that preterm babies gain faster on formula than on mother's milk; but apart from other flaws, these studies were usually based on pooled milk from full-term mothers. Preterm babies who are fed their own mother's milk tend to grow well.

It was also once thought that preemies were unable to nurse at the breast and must be bottlefed or tube-fed their milk. Research in the 1980s and '90s, however, revealed that nursing at the breast requires less energy and coordination from a preemie than does feeding from a bottle. Studies of preemies as they grow reveal the lasting impact of breast milk during these important and vulnerable early weeks. In one significant study, preemies fed breast milk via a tube, even for a few short weeks, showed an eight-point increase in their IQ years later over preemies who had been fed formula via a tube.

As nursing intensity dwindles, the milk reduces in quantity and changes in content to "weaning milk." Weaning milk is lower in sugar and thus in calories, and higher in salt content, than the mature milk of full lactation. Some babies lose interest in the breast and wean themselves when this change occurs. In other cases, lactation may continue long after this transition in the milk begins. Many mother and baby couples enjoy bedtime nursings, early morning nursings, and occasional "comfort nursings" when a toe is stubbed or other bumps and bruises of childhood occur for months and even years before weaning.

BREASTFEEDING AND MENSTRUATION

In ancient times, breast milk was thought to be "white blood." When a woman became pregnant, it was believed, her monthly blood flow was redirected to nourish the embryo. While she lactated, the blood rose to the breasts, where it was turned to milk. As we shall see in Chapter 3, the ancients were not so very far from the truth.

The basis for the lack of menstruation during breastfeeding, however, is more hormonal than hematologic. Throughout pregnancy, the menstrual cycle can be thought of as being suspended at a point just before menstruation would have taken place, had conception not occurred. If a mother does not begin breastfeeding at birth, when the baby is born and the hormone-producing placenta are removed, the menstrual cycle takes up at the point where it left off.

The frequent and strong suckling of a healthy newborn, however, maintains the pause in the menstrual cycle in what is called "lactation amenorrhea." A variety of hormones, including prolactin and estrogen, seem to be responsible, although the physiologic mechanism is not entirely clear. What is clear is the link between natural, temporary infertility and breastfeeding frequency. When a baby is breastfed at least every four hours in the day and every six hours at night, no supplementary formula or solids are given, and a pacifier is not used, ovulation is very unlikely for the first six months postpartum. Thus exclusive breastfeeding provides natural contraception. As long as a mother has a fully breastfed infant under the age of six months, she is 98 percent less likely to conceive another. In many countries, breastfeeding is the primary method of contraception; it has been estimated that without breastfeeding there would be a 20 to 30 percent increase in the birthrate worldwide. The natural child-spacing effect of lactation in developing nations can be essential for the survival of both mother and baby.

As a contraceptive system, however, lactation is by no means impervious. If for any reason, breastfeeds become less frequent, nighttime feeds cease, or supplements are added, ovulation may take place even without menses occurring. The longer a woman breastfeeds exclusively, the more likely she is to ovulate before she menstruates, and to be taken unawares by the return of her fertility. More than once a nursing mother has gone through an unusually strenuous week—cooking Thanksgiving dinner or working overtime to meet a deadline—and, a few weeks later, found herself pregnant again.

Lactation amenorrhea is also dependent on a woman's individual physiology. About half of all women who breastfeed exclusively menstruate by six months postpartum. A small percentage resume as early as six to twelve weeks, while others may not until their babies are weaned entirely. If a woman wants to avoid becoming pregnant by surprise, she and her partner should practice an additional form of birth control throughout lactation.

When menstruation does resume, it does not change breast milk composition. There are some reports of babies becoming fussy at the breast while their mothers are menstruating. It is possible that the hormonal changes that accompany resumption of the cycle change the taste of the milk slightly or that the hormonal changes can make a mother tense, which a baby is almost certain to notice.

CONTRACEPTIVES AND BREASTFEEDING

Nursing mothers have a wide range of options for contraception to protect against unplanned pregnancies. All the barrier methods—diaphragms, condoms, and IUDs—are considered safe and effective during lactation, including those that require the use of a spermicide. (In one study, breastfeeding women were found to have a lower incidence of pain when their IUDs were inserted, and had fewer removals for bleeding and pain than other women, probably due to the hormonal effect of lactation.)

Oral contraceptives (OCs) can also be used during lactation, with selective care. OC pills that contain progestin only, without estrogen, have been shown in some studies actually to increase milk production and breastfeeding duration. The progesterone hormone does appear in the breast milk, but is not well absorbed by the baby during digestion and is therefore considered safe. Contraceptives containing estrogen, however, have been shown to decrease milk production by 20 to 40 percent, although newer lower doses seem to have less of an effect. In all cases, it is generally recommended that oral contraceptives not be begun, and IUDs not inserted, until six weeks postpartum.

BREASTFEEDING AND SEX

Since Roman times, and for hundreds of years afterward, doctors advised women that sex during lactation would curdle their milk, and forbade them from participating in it until their babies were weaned. Hence the rise of a thriving wet-nurse industry in previous centuries.

Sex, however, is more than compatible with breastfeeding;

indeed, the activities are hormonally quite similar. Oxytocin, the hormone responsible for milk ejection, also underlies intense feelings of love and tenderness, and is produced during both breastfeeding and sex. This similarity has given rise to another misconception: that breastfeeding is a source of sexual satisfaction to nursing mothers. In reality, although nursing is physically enjoyable, sexual pleasure is not the usual experience. Although the nipple itself is erogenous, during lactation it does not respond with the same sensations as during sex play. Furthermore, when the baby is latched on properly, the nipple itself receives no sustained physical stimulation; most contact falls upon the areola, which is relatively insensitive to the touch. A few women have reported finding nursing sexually stimulating, but this is usually transitory and may in fact indicate poor positioning of the baby, with a risk of developing nipple soreness.

Many mothers report diminished sexual desire in the months following their babies' birth. The adjustment to new motherhood can be enormous. Breastfeeding or not, a new mother is likely to feel fatigued and, if her baby is easily stimulated and hard to soothe, she may be at her wits' end on many days and nights. Her hormones may cause mild or more severe cases of the "baby blues." After a day of holding and comforting her baby, she may find that she's had more than her fill of physical contact; she's "touched out." Her relationship with her partner may be in transition as they both adjust to being parents as well as a couple.

During these early months, the breastfeeding mother benefits from the soothing, calming effects of prolactin and oxytocin, the lactation hormones. They flood her bloodstream repeatedly and daily. No wonder some women always remember their nursing months as a happy, tranquil period: Not only do these hormones produce and propel milk, but they help the mother withstand the intensity of caring for a new baby. Some women report that their general good mood and relaxed state intensify their interest in sex during this period.

Prolactin and oxytocin, being the hormones of lovemaking as well as milk-making, not only stimulate affectionate behavior, but are abundantly present during intimacy in men as well as women. Oxytocin is released during orgasm in both sexes; many men are aware of and enjoy the sense of peace and ease, at least partly oxytocin produced, that follows sexual climax.

A nursing mother may find in the early months that her letdown reflex, also stimulated by oxytocin, functions so strongly during orgasm that it sends sprays of milk into her surprised partner's face. Whether her partner enjoys this added frill to their lovemaking or not, there is no harm in it or any other involvement of the breasts during sex. Any milk that comes into the picture will not be missed by the baby. If a couple is bothered by a generous letdown, expressing milk before making love can minimize the effects. Keeping a small towel handy isn't a bad idea, either.

Other hormones, of course, also affect sexual functioning. Lower estrogen levels during lactation, as long as the menstrual cycle is paused, may lead to vaginal dryness. Added lubrication or extra foreplay may be needed for comfort during intercourse, until the menstrual cycle begins again.

BREASTFEEDING AND PREGNANCY

What happens to the nursing mother and her milk if she becomes pregnant while still nursing? For the first few weeks, very little. Then, as the placenta develops and produces high estrogen levels, milk production is suppressed. A mother's nipples become tender during pregnancy and may progress to true soreness if nursing continues. The taste of the milk changes to the saltier weaning milk as the mother approaches her due date. The pregnant mother may feel restless or irritated while nursing, especially in the second and third trimesters. If other nutritious food is available, the baby may spontaneously wean himself as the breast becomes less productive and the milk changes in taste.

It is possible, however, to continue nursing through a pregnancy and even to nurse both babies, the newborn and its older sibling, after birth. Some mothers feel that "tandem nursing" gives essential emotional reassurance to their older baby when a new baby arrives. To be sure that no one—baby, developing fetus or newborn, or mother—is shortchanged physiologically by doing so, it is crucial that the mother eats nutritiously and gets lots of rest. She must increase her daily calorie intake beyond what she would ingest if she were pregnant and not nursing, or beyond what she would if she were nursing one baby. If her nursing baby is younger than six months when she becomes pregnant, the decrease in her milk supply that comes with pregnancy may require that the baby receive supplementary formula after each nursing. When the new baby arrives, she must allow the newborn to nurse first to ensure that he receives the valuable colostrum he needs in the first days after birth, and all the milk he needs for steady growth afterward.

Two studies have shown that there is no significant difference in babies' birth weight when mothers nurse through pregnancy, as long as the mother is well nourished. If a mother does not have a nutritious diet and is underweight, the new baby's birth weight is likely to be low and the growth rate of the older sibling slowed. Nursing during pregnancy is not recommended if a mother experiences uterine pain or bleeding, has a history of preterm labor, or has difficulty gaining weight during pregnancy.

WEANING

The process of breast involution (the breast returning to its former condition) and the cessation of milk production begins, imperceptibly, when the baby starts taking in nourishment other than breast milk, at six months or later; but milk may continue to be produced according to the baby's needs for another year or two or three.

In unrestricted breastfeeding, weaning occurs gradually and is largely initiated and governed by the baby, a process called "baby-led weaning." Typically, nursing sessions become fewer, until the baby is nursing only at bedtime or when in need of comforting. A day, or two, may go by in which the baby doesn't nurse. Eventually, the mother realizes the baby has not nursed at all lately, and is in fact weaned. A weaned toddler will occasionally, playfully return to the breast to discover, sometimes with a ready laugh, that the milk is "all gone!" There is no regret or sense of loss, in baby-led weaning, by mother or child. Nursing was grand, but life holds many more pleasures. In cultures where breastfeeding is not socially restricted, complete weaning usually takes place somewhere between eighteen months and three years, but never before the end of the first year.

Mothers who plan to return to work may expect that they will need to wean their babies suddenly. Knowing that doing so can be traumatic for a baby, some working mothers may decide not to nurse at all. In fact, after breastfeeding has been established, lactation is a flexible process. A nursing baby readily adapts to schedule changes, including an eight-hour gap in meals at the breast, taking a cup or a bottle from a caregiver while his mother is gone.

If a mother begins to feel, after the first nine to twelve months, that she is ready to bring breastfeeding to a close, she can encourage the gradual weaning that would happen eventually on its own. Introducing a cup or a bottle of water or pumped breast milk for a meal here and there can begin the process gently. *The Nursing Mother's Guide to Weaning,* by Kathleen Huggins and Linda Ziedrich, explores all the ways of weaning when the time is right for both mother and baby.

RELACTATION AND INDUCED LACTATION

Relactation is the term for reestablishing the milk supply in a mother who for some reason has stopped nursing. Perhaps the mother and baby are separated because the mother must be hospitalized, or a mother must return to breastfeeding because her baby turns out to be allergic to formula.

It was once thought that if a woman "lost her milk," that was that. A milk supply, however, can almost always be redeveloped with frequent nursing and good management: rest and nutrition for the mother, and emotional support and encouragement from a lactation consultant or experienced nursing mother. A hospital-grade electric breast pump can make the process relatively straightforward.

The baby, however, makes all the difference. Sucking stimulation is needed to bring in the milk, and how much and how avidly a baby sucks will speed or slow the process. Kathleen Auerbach, PhD, points out that it is hard to predict which baby will "enthusiastically embrace" the reestablishment of breastfeeding. Some babies are lackadaisical, waiting contentedly for a long time between nursings, and playing at the breast during them, while others, as Dr. Auerbach says, "would get milk out of doorknobs."

Sometimes a woman will want to relactate or induce lactation because she has adopted a baby and would like to nurse him.

Induced lactation, the establishment of a milk supply in women who have never given birth, is possible if a woman has carried a pregnancy in the past to the fourth or fifth month. An adopted baby can be nursed with the help of a mechanical device that trickles formula into the baby's mouth as he nurses from the breast, thus feeding the baby as he learns to suck at the breast, thereby stimulating the production of breast milk. Marketed variously as the Lactaid or the Supplemental Nutrition System, the device is available through many lactation consultants. (See Resources.)

BREASTFEEDING UNDER SPECIAL CIRCUMSTANCES

There are many conditions under which mothers are sometimes told they cannot breastfeed, when in fact breastfeeding not only is possible but can be of real benefit to the mother. The blind mother, for example, usually finds breastfeeding infinitely easier than preparing bottles and formula. The skin-to-skin contact and enveloping scent of one another more than makes up for the interactions made through vision alone. Other physically challenged mothers also find that breastfeeding simplifies at least that aspect of life. Adolescent mothers are sometimes discouraged from breastfeeding on the grounds that they, themselves, are still growing. As long as the very young mother is well nourished, she can lactate without diminishing her own growth. In fact, the calming and maturing effects of breastfeeding may be just what she needs.

Many mothers successfully and even easily nurse their babies despite having diabetes, heart disease, epilepsy, and other chronic conditions. The joy of the experience provides a balance to the challenges of living with a chronic disease. Breastfeeding saves energy, dispensing with the effort of buying and preparing formula, and reducing trips to the pediatrician's office to treat ear infections and other illnesses more common among formula-fed babies. Unlike bottlefeeding, nursing can be done while lying down, enabling a mother to rest as she feeds the baby. Indeed, there is some evidence that lactation alters a mother's metabolism, providing more energy with less physical cost, a goal sought by every woman living with a chronic condition.

The hormones of lactation flood a mother with calm and reduce stress. In diabetes this reduction of stress can directly affect the amount of insulin a mother requires. When the relaxing effect of nursing is combined with the extra energy expended to produce milk, a diabetic mother may need less insulin as long as she breastfeeds. Women with cardiac conditions may also discover their health improving with the daily flood of lactation hormones.

In general, whatever the health of a mother, she needs to let every physician who treats her know that she is breastfeeding, so that they can select medications and procedures compatible with nursing. Keep in mind, though, that as expert as an oncologist is in cancer treatment, or a pulmonologist in asthma or cystic fibrosis, he or she may understand less about lactation. Many doctors would rather "play it safe" and ask a mother to wean rather than investigate which medications are both effective for her disease as well as safe for her baby. Some don't distinguish between those medications that appear in breast milk (most) and yet pass through the infant's gut unabsorbed (many) and therefore may be considered safe, versus those drugs absorbed by the infant gut (a few) and possibly, therefore, not safe for the baby. While little research has been done on the topic, the breastfed infant gut differs significantly from that of a bottlefed infant, and is less likely to absorb large molecules; the breastfed baby may be more resistant to ingesting foreign substances, including medications. Women being treated for a chronic or acute condition should confer with a lactation consultant in addition to their medical specialist to learn the full impact—or lack of impact—of specific drugs and procedures on breastfeeding. Medications not harmful to a nursing baby can be found for almost every illness.

Contraindications to breastfeeding do exist. Sadly, HIV infection is one, as breast milk can transmit the virus. In some developing countries, where both HIV and infectious diseases are rampant, the World Health Organization still encourages breastfeeding, as it may offer babies the best chance they have. In the United States, however, where infectious disease is not a primary cause of infant mortality, the American Academy of Pediatrics recommends that HIV-positive women not breastfeed. Some autoimmune diseases, including rheumatoid arthritis and lupus, are affected by lactation hormones, which in some cases aggravate the disease, in others coax it into remission. Some diagnostic medical procedures, including CT scans, require an injection of radioactive isotopes. These do turn up in breast milk and are not safe for babies. If a mother must undergo this sort of testing, she can express and discard her breast milk until the procedure is past and her milk tests free of the substance, then resume nursing.

A special breastfeeding challenge is the mother who has had breast surgery, for cosmetic or oncologic reasons. Plastic surgeons who reduce or augment women's breasts are sometimes oblivious to the possible future use of those breasts to feed a baby. If the surgeon's goal is to preserve the appearance, rather than the function, of the breast, he or she may make an incision around the areola and nipple, where a scar is considered less conspicuous than one from an incision across the side or bottom of the breast. If the incision is made around the areola, thereby cutting the milk ducts and nerves, the woman is five times more likely to have insufficient milk if, in time, she breastfeeds a baby.

There are surgical techniques, however, that preserve the function of the breast, keeping the ducts and nerves attached to the nipple even if it must be relocated. In breast reduction surgery, the breast tissue that is removed can be limited to nonfunctioning fat layers. In augmentation the implant can be placed under the muscle, rather than beneath the breast tissues, where the pressure and scarring it creates can interfere with lactation. If a surgeon knows that a woman may wish to breastfeed a baby in the future, he or she can employ these techniques. If surgery has already been performed, a mother who wishes to nurse should contact her surgeon to find out which techniques have been used and what their impact on lactation might be. Generally, if it is possible to express colostrum during pregnancy, the breast is probably functioning normally. (Many women who cannot express colostrum, however, do go on to nurse their babies without a problem.) If a breast has been removed altogether, the remaining breast is usually fully capable of producing sufficient milk for one baby.

WORKING MOTHERS

Working mothers sometimes assume they will have to stop breastfeeding when they go back to work. Nothing could be further from the truth; many working nursing mothers declare that continuing to nurse has made it possible for them to blend mothering and working successfully. While the working world still has a long way to go to accept and accommodate the needs of nursing mothers, and indeed parents in general, in some companies and a few fields of work progress is being made, both culturally and legally.

The invention of effective, portable breast pumps has made working and exclusive breastfeeding much easier. With a good pump and a fifteen- to twenty-minute break every four hours, most women can pump sufficient fresh milk for their babies to consume on the next day. Workplaces that provide clean and private locations in which mothers can pump and store their milk, and an atmosphere in which they are able to do so without chagrin or defensiveness, also contribute to a mother's success. (See Chapter 12 for more detail on the ins and outs of combining nursing and work.)

OLDER MOTHERS

Does the age at which a woman has her first baby make a difference in breastfeeding? Hardly ever. The standard medical viewpoint is that older mothers are apt to have more physical problems, making all aspects of child care, including breastfeeding, more of an effort. Yet, as one pediatrician with many mothers of all ages in his practice points out, the medical literature often cites population data from decades ago, when a woman of forty or more might well have been sedentary, overweight, and a smoker. Today's older mothers are far more likely not to smoke, to watch what they eat, and to exercise regularly; they present a clinical picture "that doesn't fit the literature."

In fact, breastfeeding may be a bit easier for the older mother. Life teaches us judgment, and the experienced woman may be more apt to do what seems right to her rather than to obey generalized instructions that may be inappropriate for her circumstances. Life teaches us observation skills, and she may be more likely to notice her baby's signs and signals. She may be better at taking care of herself, as well. And the experienced woman may be eager to enjoy her baby fully because she has already proven herself a capable adult in other areas.

What about fatigue? No doubt about it, motherhood is hard work. All mothers get tired. The older mother, however, may be more likely to guard against fatigue and take action to resolve it than a younger woman. She may improve her nutrition, change her schedule, or ask for help sooner than the younger mother who has not been pushed up against that particular wall in the past.

BREAST AILMENTS

A few physical problems are directly associated with breastfeeding, most a result of misinformation or interference in the process of establishing a milk supply and learning to nurse. Most can be avoided with common sense and an accurate understanding of lactation.

Engorgement occurs when the breasts become so full of stored milk that they are taut, swollen, and can be extremely painful. The areola may be stretched so flat when the breast is engorged that the baby cannot latch on and suckle. The mother may run a fever and feel sick all over. It can occur during the first week postpartum as the colostrum changes to mature milk. The mother's body is suddenly producing milk and is ready for the baby to remove it day and night. If that removal is hindered in some way—by restricted nursings, or by poor positioning or latch-on at the breast—natural postpartum fullness can swiftly become severe engorgement. Nursing long and often, with the baby in various positions and latched-on well, prevents and resolves the condition. Moist heat (warm, wet towels on the breast or warm showers) and gentle massage, as well as frequent nursing, eases it. After two or three weeks, the likelihood of engorgement decreases significantly.

Sore nipples also occur in the first week or two of nursing when a new mother may not receive enough support or accurate information on breastfeeding. Most women, especially first-time mothers, experience an initial period of nipple tenderness as the breast suddenly receives more tactile stimulation than it ever has before. This early tenderness fades at every nursing as the milk lets down, and it disappears altogether after the first couple of weeks. Sore nipples, however, are not part of the usual course of events. The baby's position at the breast—how much of the areola he holds in his mouth, how his tongue rests under the nipple, and how he draws the nipple into his mouth—can prevent or create sore nipples. Without intervention from a lactation consultant or someone else who understands lactation, a sore nipple can develop into a painful, cracked nipple. Long before that point, however, simple measures can soothe sore nipples: exposure to air and light between nursings, avoiding keeping moist fabric over the nipples, and shifting the baby's position at each nursing.

Almost every woman has experienced a yeast infection, *Candida albicans*, in her vaginal tract. The infections usually occur when a woman has been ill and taken antibiotics, or if her diet is out of balance, or she's overly fatigued or stressed. Yeast is always present in our bodies, but certain factors can cause it to have an overgrowth, which produces a noticeable irritation or pain. When the infection occurs on the nipple surface or the interior of the breast, it is called "thrush." In nursing couples, when either the mother or the baby has thrush, the other does too, and both need treatment. Clues that thrush has appeared include intense nipple pain or itchy, burning nipples, and white patches in the baby's mouth. The infection can be present without any visible symptoms, other than a baby's fussiness at the breast because his mouth is sore. If a mother suspects thrush, she should visit the pediatrician (who, with luck, will have a lactation consultant on staff), and get a prescription to clear it up, usually drops for the baby's mouth and an ointment for the mother's breast.

Mastitis, sometimes called "milk fever," is a bacterial infection within the breast, typically localized in one duct or duct system. The symptoms are fever and flulike aching, with a place on one breast that is sore to the touch. A duct blocked by secretions, swelling, or a too-tight bra is the usual genesis of mastitis. Nursing the baby in different positions, so that different ducts are drained on each feeding, can relieve a blockage; it's helpful to position the baby on alternate feedings so that her nose points to the sore place, "even if you have to stand on your head to do it," says one lactation consultant. Hot compresses, frequent nursings, and rest for the mother are often sufficient treatment; if the infection persists, antibiotics are called for.

BREASTFEEDING AND BREAST CANCER

Nursing reduces the risk of breast cancer. The longer you nurse, the lower the risk. A woman who nurses two babies for a year each reduces her risk of premenopausal breast cancer by 28 to 61 percent. Every additional year of breastfeeding lowers a woman's lifetime risk of breast cancer by 4.3 percent. (Women who carry the BRCA1 genetic mutation that places them in the highest risk category for breast cancer may reduce their risk even further through breastfeeding one year or more—by as much as 45 percent, according to one study published in 2004.) Pregnancy and birth also reduce a woman's risk of breast cancer, with a decrease of 7 percent for every child.

For years the standard medical opinion was that breastfeeding offers no particular protection against breast cancer. As is all too common, this conclusion was based on studies in which no attention was paid to duration of breastfeeding and no distinction was made between exclusive breastfeeding and token breastfeeding. If a mother ever put her baby to the breast, even if that baby received formula supplements from birth, she was included in the study data as a breastfeeding mother. Now more exact research has shown that many aspects of reproduction have a protective effect against development of breast cancer. Lactation is high on the list of protective factors, and the protection it offers is "dose related," that is, the more and longer you breastfeed, the better the protection it gives.

The likelihood of developing breast (as well as ovarian and endometrial) cancer appears to increase as the length of time increases in which a woman has high levels of estrogen in her system. During pregnancy and menopause, estrogen levels are low. Thus having children early or having an early menopause offers some protection by reducing a woman's lifetime exposure to estrogen. Lactation suppresses estrogen production, and appears to be one basis for the conspicuous protective effect of breastfeeding against the development of breast cancer in the childbearing years. Broad-scale epidemiologic studies by the U.S. Centers for Disease Control and Prevention show that premenopausal breast cancer is twice as likely to occur in women who have never lactated as in women who have regardless of their family history. A review of 47 epidemiologic studies in 30 countries suggests that if women have the average number of children, 2.5, but breastfed each child for a full year, there would be 50,000 (or 11 percent) fewer diagnoses of breast cancer each year.

While the reasons that childbirth and lactation have a

protective effect against breast and other cancers are still being investigated, the fact that they do doesn't seem surprising. When you have experienced the changes that pregnancy and lactation bring to the breast, it seems sensible to suppose that these glands were intended to function and are healthier when they do.

Human Milk

Giving milk is the characteristic that binds all mammals. From the great blue whale to shrews weighing less than an ounce; from fast-growing rabbits and slow-growing elephants; from herbivores to carnivores to insectivores, all mammals give their babies milk. All their milk is made of water, fat, special milk proteins, and milk sugars. All milk contains some of each important vitamin and mineral. If it is allowed to stand, the cream will rise. Be it the milk of a human, cow, or rabbit, it can be made into cheese or butter and will go sour in the same way. Whatever the source, milk is milk.

On closer inspection, however, milk differs remarkably from species to species. Making milk is a rather expensive process for the mother, biologically. She has to find and consume extra calories to put into the milk and to run the elegant machinery of the mammary glands. Complex molecules such as antibodies must be created for special purposes. No energy can be wasted on creating elements that her baby will not need. In consequence, each species' milk is carefully tailored to provide exactly what that sort of newborn creature needs to grow well. The milk of seals and whales is almost 50 percent fat, to enable the baby to double its size in a few weeks. Horses and cows provide milk that grows bone and muscle in a hurry, for a baby that needs to be able to run fast from the day of its birth. The milk of primates, including we humans, is specialized for, among other things, the rapid growth of the brain.

While babies can often survive on the milk of other species—dogs can nurse kittens, and goats feed lambs—substitutions are far from optimum. This is especially true if the species are very different. The problems are great when you modify the milk of hooved animals for infant human beings—if you wanted a really good match for us, you'd have to milk gorillas.

Mother's milk is for babies; cow's milk is for calves—people have been saying that for years. Feeding cow's milk to newborn babies used to involve an elaborate business of adjusting the differences between the two kinds of milk—differences that cause real problems for the immature digestive system—by adding water to dilute the protein content, adding sugar to raise the calorie content, and so on, according to various medical recipes. Mothers had to make this "formula" in their kitchens, and then sterilize the concoction by boiling it. Nowadays, corporations make up these doctored versions of cow's milk for baby food, and you can buy them ready mixed and sterilized in the drugstore and supermarket. In fact, we know so much about chemistry and nutrition that some of these synthetic foods for babies are not based on animal milk at all, but are made completely from other ingredients, such as soy beans. These ingredients supply enough calories for a baby, and the nutritional components such as protein and vitamins that we know are necessary, at least those that have been proven to date, and those that are possible to manufacture outside a woman's body.

So what's the difference between these synthetic foods and the real thing, human milk? Plenty, starting with taste and smell, the qualities that matter most in the baby's opinion. What the baby isn't aware of are the specific nutritional differences and constituents that impact infant physiology and behavior, and that protect against disease. Many of the valuable components of human milk are substances that are destroyed by heating; thus they cannot be powdered or canned or even pasteurized. In some cases, they are factors that cannot be synthesized or duplicated in a chemistry lab; they are ingredients that no artificial or modified nonhuman milk will ever contain.

THE UNIQUE PROPERTIES OF BREAST MILK

As researchers like to point out, the really wondrous quality of breast milk, the big difference between it and formula, is that human milk is alive. Like blood or skin or any other tissue, it is a living substance, full of active cells, and it is designed to stay alive for a long time. Human milk fresh from the breast contains an average of one million living cells per milliliter (roughly one-third of a teaspoon). Colostrum, the first milk after birth, contains up to seven million living cells per milliliter

The ancients believed that breast milk was "white blood," and they were not all wrong. Most of the living cells in human milk are leukocytes, or white cells, similar but not identical to those in our blood. White cells attack foreign bacteria wherever they find them. The white cells in human milk are primarily neutrophils, which take action on the surface of the baby's insides, and macrophages, which can penetrate tissues and attack bacteria there. They can kill pathogens—disease-causing organisms—by engulfing and digesting them, or by releasing toxins into or around the enemy cells and in effect stinging them to death.

These living cells in human milk are extraordinarily vigorous. In one now-famous experiment, which has been successfully duplicated several times, biologists counted the bacteria in a sample of fresh human milk, finding a fair representation of harmless skin flora (bacteria from the nipple and the breast) and a few pathogens. They then left the milk sample, uncovered, on a table in a warm room for thirty-six hours—a perfect setting for culturing prolific bacterial growth. When they retested the sample a day and a half later, the bacteria count had actually gone down. The macrophages and other protective mechanisms in the milk had been doing their work, scouring the milk for illness-causing elements and eliminating them.

The macrophages in human milk provide protection in the stomach and throughout the intestine. It's as if every swallow of mother's milk contained a tiny Pac-Man army, gobbling the germs in its path. (And if the baby happens to sputter and get some milk up her nose, these protectors do their work there, too.) While peak production of macrophages occurs right after birth, they continue to be produced in useful quantities for at least four to five months. They can survive freezing; frozen breast milk, when properly stored up to six months, continues to offer this cellular front-line disease protection when thawed. The macrophages cannot survive heating, including microwaving or pasteurization; thus they are not available in cow's milk–based products. And they cannot be created artificially; living cells come only from a mother.

ANTIBODIES AND IMMUNITIES

When *Nursing Your Baby* was first published in 1963, we could not say outright that human milk, or even colostrum, definitely provided immune factors protecting the baby against disease. That had been proven, scientifically, only for goats and cows. In fact, some medical experts argued that factors providing immunities or disease protection could not be possible in human milk; that antibodies would be excreted rather than absorbed, or that they weren't there anyway, and that humans, in any case, were not cattle.

It had been observed that breastfed babies acquired fewer infections than bottlefed babies. The method of transmission was given the credit; milk supplied directly from the breast is free of bacteria. Formula, mixed with water and placed in bottles, can become contaminated easily. Yet even infants who receive prepackaged, sterilized formula suffer from more meningitis and infection of the gut, ear, respiratory tract, and urinary tract than do breastfed babies.

Now the evidence is in, and increases with each passing year: In addition to providing optimal nutrition, breastfeeding protects against infection. Researchers have demonstrated that human milk is laced with immunity-inducing factors, including antibodies to many common infectious agents, and that these antibodies are indeed absorbed and utilized by the baby. The newest evidence shows that these and other immune factors offer protection not just in the first days or weeks of life—when the baby's immune system is immature and needs all the help it can get—but throughout lactation, from the first sip to the last swallow of human milk, and in some cases even after weaning and into adulthood.

During pregnancy the mother shares her antibodies with her fetus through the placenta, along with the nutrients she ingests. These antibodies continue to circulate in the baby's blood for several weeks after birth. The newborn immune system, however, is somewhat suppressed (perhaps as a mechanism for preventing the maternal immune system from recognizing paternal, i.e., foreign, antigens present in the fetus, and therefore rejecting the fetus). Newborns therefore have a hard time mounting an effective immune defense for the first couple of months of life; minor infections can spread quickly to become systemic.

Breast milk steps in where the placenta leaves off, providing the protection of the mother's own immune system while kick-starting the baby's ability to protect itself. The first feedings of colostrum, the creamy yellow, ultranourishing milk produced immediately after birth, are especially vital. Colostrum protects babies against many specific diseases, including polio, rotovirus, coxsackie B virus, several Staphylococci, and *Escherichia coli*, the adult intestinal bacteria that can cause particularly vicious intestinal, urinary, and other infections in newborns. Antibodies to these infective agents are present in colostrum in much higher concentrations they are in the mother's blood serum. Leonard Mata, PhD, a breastfeeding researcher working in Central America, starts off all newborns in his hospital with a "colostrum cocktail," from donor mothers if necessary. Mata reports that the reduction of illness, particularly in preterm infants, has been dramatic, even if the babies are subsequently formula fed. Of course, dairy farmers have been doing this for years; all new calves are given colostrum for their first feeding, not milk.

Pathogens, whether viral or bacterial, have specific attachment points that an antibody can recognize and plug up, so to speak, to render the pathogen harmless. A new pattern of antibody must be created for each new enemy encountered, but once the system has made that kind of antibody, it can quickly crank out more; that is why many specific diseases can be caught only once. Immunizations protect us against disease by presenting dead pathogens and tricking the system into making antibodies that fit those particular infectors—the measles virus, say, or typhoid bacteria. Then when the real thing comes along, the antibodies swarm out and shut down the initial invaders before they take hold and launch a major infection.

A nursing mother can provide her baby, through her milk, with antibodies to many organisms to which she has been exposed in the past; she can "vaccinate" her baby against them through breastfeeding. If she happens to be exposed to a new pathogen during lactation—a new variety of cold virus, say—antibody production sites in her lungs and intestines go into action. The new antibody types are packed into special white cells that actually home in on the mammary glands, where they start secreting the new antibody into the milk within two or three days of the mother's exposure. By the time the mother comes down with the cold, the baby is already getting protection from that specific virus. That is one reason for a phenomenon noticed by many nursing mothers: When everyone in the family catches a cold, the baby often has the lightest case or escapes altogether.

If a mother and baby are separated during the day, and the baby is in an environment with a different set of pathogens than the ones for which the mother has formed antibodies, breastfeeding still provides a degree of protection. If a baby exposes his mother to any new germs he has picked up at day care, her immune system creates antibodies to those infections and returns the antibodies to her baby. The system helps to protect the baby when he is with his mother, and when he is not.

SECRETORY IgA

The principal immunity-inducing compound in human milk, including colostrum, is secretory IgA (the letters stand for immunoglobulin A). Many of us have heard of gamma globulin, most of which consists of IgG, an immunity-conferring compound found in blood, which offers broad, short-term protection against many infections; it is sometimes given to people who have been exposed to, or who might become exposed to, hepatitis or other dangerous viruses. IgA is a slightly different protein, manufactured in the mammary gland and secreted into the milk by chemical pathways that were simply unknown in 1963. Secretory IgA offers protection against foreign molecules that might induce allergic reactions in the baby. Secretory IgA also provides antibodies to E. coli, Salmonellae, Shigellae, Streptococci, Staphylococci, Pneumococci, Pseudomonas aeruginosa, polio virus, coxsackie, cytomegalovirus, retrovirus, rubella virus, herpes simplex virus, mumps virus, influenza virus, respiratory viruses, rotoviruses, cholera, pertussis, and Giardia lamblia, not just in developing countries, but wherever mothers and babies may be.

Secretory IgA antibodies work not by destroying enemy cells, but by binding to them and preventing them from attaching themselves to the mucosae (the linings) of the digestive or respiratory tracts, where they could multiply and cause illness. With each feeding of colostrum or milk, secretory IgA paints the infant gut, coating the mucosal surfaces and sealing them against invading infections. Highly concentrated in colostrum, secretory IgA is found at reduced levels in mature milk. A mother produces more milk, however, as her baby grows, so that the amount of secretory IgA a baby ingests remains constant, or can even increase until solid foods are added to his diet.

Human milk is packed with other immunity-inducing elements, and more are being discovered with regularity. The function of immunoglobulins IgG, IgM, and IgD, also found in breast milk, is still being explored by researchers. Some of their benefits for the mother appear to be: Higher levels of IgD are found in the breast when a plugged duct or other reservoir of bacteria develops. Other intriguing facts are emerging about these elements. Levels of IgM in full-term newborns, for example, are 20 percent those of the adult, and take two years to attain adult levels.

Immunoglobulins supplied by breast milk supplement those levels as long as the breastfeeding continues.

Breastfeeding, in short, shelters a baby long enough for the baby's own immune system to get into gear. By the time of weaning, if nursing continues for nine months or more, the baby's body has usually encountered most of the common pathogens in its environment, and has developed a constellation of antibodies of its own. Breast milk does not stop at antibody-producing elements to protect babies from infections, and their side effects. Other factors, equally impossible to manufacture, include lysozyme, lactoferrin, the bifidus factor, lactoperoxidase, and oligosaccharides.

LYSOZYME

An important antibacterial ingredient in human milk is lysozyme, an enzyme that is also abundant in saliva and in tears. Lysozyme is harmless to human tissue; in fact, it is actually soothing and reduces inflammation and redness. When it comes in contact with certain bacteria, however, it "lyses," or dissolves their cell walls, which kills them. Lysozyme is a sort of natural disinfectant; it performs that function in our eyes, mouths, and noses, as well as inside the mammary gland, where it is produced in quantity. Human milk contains five thousand times as much lysozyme, per milliliter, as does cow's milk. Unlike some other protective elements in human milk, after an initial dip during the first month of lactation, the proportion of lysozyme per milliliter of milk actually increases, and remains thus throughout lactation, perhaps to protect babies against pathogens that may be introduced when they begin solid foods.

Lysozyme, like secretory IgA and other defense agents in human milk, is also designed to withstand the acids of the stomach, and to act throughout the baby's digestive system. Although it can be constructed artificially, lysozyme cannot be added effectively to formula, because like most enzymes it is destroyed by the heat necessary for sterilization and packaging.

THE BIFIDUS FACTOR AND OTHER NUTRITIOUS PROTECTORS

Many of the substances in human milk—fats, sugars, proteins, vitamins—that are perfectly good nutrients also do double duty as protectors. The first of these to come to scientific attention was the *bifidus* factor.

Many bacteria cannot survive in an acid medium: A favorite cure in the past for diarrhea was made from buttermilk or sour milk. The formula-fed baby develops an alkaline environment in the intestinal tract that supports the growth of many organisms, including harmful and putrefactive bacteria; consequently, the intestines are often irritated, and the stool of the formula-fed baby has the usual offensive fecal odor. Some of the sugars in breast milk, however, when digested, produce an acid environment in the intestines, in which harmful bacteria, including Shigella, Salmonella, and *E. coli*, cannot survive. As a result, the predominant intestinal bacteria of nursing babies are a harmless species called *Lactobacillus bifidus*. (Cow's milk formula–fed babies, however, have potentially pathogenic bacteria in their gut flora.) As a result, the stool of the breastfed baby has no unpleasant smell, but only a faint odor, something like yogurt. Nobel laureate Paul Gyorgy, discoverer of vitamin B_6 and a pioneering researcher in the values of human milk, discovered a growth factor for lactobacilli in human milk and found it virtually absent in cow's milk.

Waste products of bifidus metabolism make the breastfed infant's intestinal tract even more resistant to the growth of other, invading organisms. Formula manufacturers have been working to develop "humanized milks" that contain something similar to the bifidus factor, but so far no one has succeeded in manufacturing a product that can maintain L. *bifidus* in the intestines of a bottlefed baby.

Another nutritive ingredient of human milk that modifies the environment inside the baby is lactoferrin, a protein. The principal protein in cow's milk is casein; in human milk, lactoferrin makes up at least a third of the protein. Lactoferrin not only is much more digestible than casein, it also has the unusual property of being highly absorbent of iron molecules. Many pathogens, such as E. *coli* and other bacteria that cause infectious diarrhea, require free iron molecules for their metabolism. With lactoferrin mopping up the loose iron in the baby's intestines, these pathogens simply cannot grow. Lactoferrin is not present in cow's milk.

Special groups of sugars in human milk, the oligosaccharides, fight pathogens by interfering with their attachment sites. These sugars prevent Pneumococcus, an especially "adhesive" bacterium from attaching to the surface of the gastrointestinal tract. There is ten times the amount of oligosaccharides in human milk than in cow's milk.

The lipids, or fats, in human milk do much more than give babies energy to grow. One of their important functions is protective, as they disrupt and kill many kinds of viruses, including polio. There is evidence that fatty acids, produced during the digestion of lipids, protect the infant against intestinal parasites such as *Giardia lamblia* and amoebic dysentery. Spread by dogs and wildlife, *Giardia* is a common parasite throughout the United States, found in brooks, streams, and wells. On occasion, it can be passed from person to person, as can happen at day-care centers.

Recent research reveals new tidbits about the protective factors in human milk. In 2000, a new peptide was identified in breast milk that was found to inhibit the growth of bacteria and yeasts. In 2002, researchers found that human milk contains large amounts of xanthine oxidase, an enzyme that, when combined with the nitric oxide present in the infant gut, inhibits the growth of enterobacteria, E. coli, and Salmonella. As researchers piece together new clues and known facts, it becomes clear that we have just begun to understand the marvelous ways in which human milk defends the health of babies.

THE SOOTHERS: ANTI-INFLAMMATORY AGENTS

Infectious illness is usually accompanied by inflammation. The battle against infection is fought with natural toxins that kill bacteria and free oxygen atoms to burn up the invaders. Extremely effective, these toxins can irritate normal cells and cause painful inflammation. If you get a scratch on your skin, and Staphylococcus organisms move in, your body's defense system will rush to attack them. In the process, your skin around the scratch will become red and swollen. If the swelling is extreme, it may toughen the tissue permanently, leaving a scar. Sore throats, earaches, and diarrhea are all manifestations of inflammation caused by the body's attempts to battle pathogens.

The protective mechanisms in human milk, however, appear to be cunningly designed to do their work without causing unpleasant symptoms or pain. Some ingredients fight germs without causing inflammation; some negate or reduce inflammatory agents that do occur. For example, the kinds of white cells that cause inflammation and swelling while defending the body, such as basal cells that release histamines, are not the kinds found in human milk. The macrophages and neutrophils in human milk can kill bacteria without harming nearby normal cells, and without causing discomfort.

Other agents in human milk, including several vitamins, are antioxidants: They combine with loose oxygen atoms, called "free radicals," that are part of the body's disease-fighting process but that could injure healthy tissue. Many fragments of sugar and fat molecules that appear during the digestive process are also antioxidants. Like secretory IgA, lysozyme, and lactoferrin, they can persist throughout the digestive tract and protect the baby from inflammation from one end to the other.

These components of human milk, and others still to be explored, do not directly fight disease. Instead, when a pathogen does get into the baby's system, these agents deter the process of disease control from causing the baby to feel pain or sickness as a side effect. Armond Goldman, MD, of the University of Texas Medical School, was perhaps the first lactation researcher to deduce, in the early 1980s, the existence and importance of this new class of protectors in human milk. Dr. Goldman continues to explore how elements in human milk attack pathogens without causing damage or discomfort. Many elements in human milk, writes Dr. Goldman, appear to have "pluripotency," or the power to protect babies in several ways at once.

BREASTFEEDING AND ALLERGIES

Breastfed babies on the whole have far fewer skin ailments, including eczema, and other allergic reactions than do formula-fed babies. Allergies can be caused by proteins unfamiliar to the body's chemistry. Babies under two are less tolerant of alien proteins than are older children, partly because their immune systems are not yet fully mature. Newborns in particular are at risk of absorbing, and reacting to, foreign proteins because their intestines are highly permeable and can admit large molecules into the bloodstream, rather than harmlessly passing them through and out of the GI tract. This permeable condition is essential to the fetus to facilitate absorption of amniotic fluid. The adjustment to extrauterine life after birth, however, requires that the lining of the GI tract become less permeable, a process accomplished by secretory IgA, if a baby is breastfed. If the gut is not sealed, and the GI tract remains in its permeable fetal state after birth, a newborn is vulnerable to absorbing foreign proteins and other agents that can launch lifelong allergies.

Gut closure begins with the initial feedings of colostrum. It is believed that the lipids and secretory IgA in early milk coat the linings of the infant's intestines, making them impermeable to large molecules, and thus making the baby less susceptible to invasion by disease organisms. A single feeding of colostrum might reduce intestinal permeability and render the infant capable of digesting such molecules rather than absorbing them unchanged. The bottlefed infant, on the other hand, may continue to absorb whole proteins, and develop reactions or even permanent allergies to them, well into the second year of life.

Even in the fully breastfed baby, supplementation in the first four months of life may set off allergic reactions, especially when the supplement contains complex proteins such as those in eggs. The protein in cow's milk is among the worst offenders in causing allergic reactions, and this protein can be transferred from the mother's diet to the baby through breast milk. (It has also been suggested that proteins from peanuts can be transferred to a baby through breast milk and may cause, in some babies, a life-threatening allergy to peanuts.)

Several studies have shown that infants who are susceptible to cow's milk protein allergy can be sensitized by a single feeding of cow's milk–based formula, sometimes given in the hospital as a routine "extra" feeding. An infant who reacts to cow's milk in the mother's diet may well have been "triggered" by a previous feeding of formula. Thereafter, some researchers suspect, cow's milk antigens in her milk may act like booster shots, causing allergic reactions.

A baby's risk of developing allergic reactions decreases with age, and with the duration of exclusive breastfeeding. Pediatricians recommend that babies with a family history of allergies be exclusively breastfed for a full six months before any solid foods are introduced. A mother who knows that she herself is sensitive to certain foods, or that allergies to them run in her family or the baby's father's family, should avoid them during pregnancy and lactation. (There is some evidence that very susceptible babies can become sensitized to allergens, especially cow's milk protein, in the uterus.) Supplementation with cow's milk formula should be guarded against. By six months of age, when nature intended a baby to be sampling new foods, most babies have passed the danger point when allergic reactions become established.

Do fully breastfed babies, in fact, have fewer allergies? The answers vary from study to study. Not fully understood (in part because studies in this area are plagued by flawed research methods), allergies appear to have a strong genetic component. It seems that a child with a susceptibility to allergies may develop them even if he is breastfed, but that his allergies will be less severe than those of relatives who suffer from the same sensitivities, and who were not breastfed as babies. In one study that followed Finnish breastfed babies, children who were exclusively breastfed for six months without any formula or solid food in their diet had fewer cases of eczema and food allergies than children who were exclusively breastfed for three months.

The protective effect of breastfeeding against eczema is perhaps the most clearly delineated in the scientific literature. A comprehensive review of eighteen studies of breastfed babies in various countries from 1966 through 2000 found that exclusive breastfeeding during the first three months of life is associated with lower incidence of eczema in children with a mother or father who has eczema. The researchers concluded that "breastfeeding should be strongly recommended to mothers of infants with a family history of eczema."

Eczema is just one signal of an immune system rejecting a foreign protein; allergies can also take the form of vomiting, diarrhea, fussiness, runny noses, cough, asthma, and wheezing. The variety of symptoms that allergies produce confuses their diagnosis and makes pinpointing their source difficult. What is clear is that allergic diseases have increased over the last twenty years in most countries. In many cases, a sequence of allergic symptoms begins in early infancy with food sensitivity (often to cow's milk) and gastrointestinal distress, proceeding to eczema, and then to asthma, which can be severe and last a lifetime. Regardless of the piles of conflicting data on allergies, preventing the first step in the sequence, food sensitivity, through exclusive breastfeeding for the first six months seems to make sense.

NOURISHMENT

The direct protection that breast milk offers against disease is perhaps the most dramatic aspect of the benefits of breastfeeding. But the principal function of milk, after all, is to *feed* the baby.

How well does mother's milk do that? It should not be a surprise to learn that the nutritive components of human milk are tailored precisely to our babies' needs, and that these components are not easy, or even possible, to duplicate precisely.

Human milk is not designed to produce the biggest baby possible in the shortest amount of time, as we sometimes crave as evidence of overall health. It is designed to foster neural and brain development; to promote behavior and cognitive growth along with a healthy, growing body. Formula-fed infants take in more calories than breastfed infants, but they also expend a great deal more energy overall, while maintaining the same or lower activity levels. Breastfed infants gain weight more rapidly during the first three months, and then more slowly through to the sixth month; it is a different pattern of growth than that of formula-fed infants. Fortunately, in 2000, the American Academy of Pediatrics has at last updated the growth charts on which pediatricians track the weight and length of infants, so that they are no longer based solely on the growth patterns of formula-fed infants, but also reference the quite different growth of breastfed babies.

And the difference is significant. The special nutritional mix in human milk keeps babies growing at the most desirable rate for humans, while maintaining beneficial activity levels. The nutritional contents of human milk are perfectly geared to the energy needs of the human infant. Here's how:

Protein:

The protein in cow's milk is mostly casein. Casein is not very digestible and forms a large, tough curd when it is mixed with digestive juices. The infant with a stomach full of the solid curds of raw cow's milk can be in real trouble. Diluting the milk helps; heating also makes the curds smaller and softer. But they still tend to linger in the infant's stomach, so that he feels full for about four hours after a feeding (hence the traditional pediatric advice that babies be fed every four hours, an inappropriate schedule for breastfed babies). Digesting these gobs of protein accounts for the high expenditure of energy seen in formula-fed babies.

In human milk, casein forms only about a third of the protein content, and the remaining proteins, such as lactoferrin, are easier for the human baby to digest. The curd of human milk, produced from this different balance of proteins, is soft and fine, almost liquid. The stomach of the breastfed baby empties rapidly and easily, supplying a steady flow of nutrients to the baby. With a stomach roughly the size of a walnut, the breastfed newborn usually wants and needs to eat more often to fill and refill the tiny vessel with gentle breast milk: eight to ten times a day in the first two or three months of life, which in turn stimulates the mother's milk supply.

Human milk also contains a significant proportion of essential amino acids, the "building blocks" of protein, which can be absorbed and used by the infant just as they are. Colostrum is especially high in amino acids. According to Drs. Icie Macy and Harriet Kelly, authorities on infant nutrition, this bonus of nutrients probably forms a splendid basis for the rapid growth and profound changes taking place in the body of the newborn.

The human infant uses the protein in breast milk with nearly 100 percent efficiency. After the first few days of life, virtually all the protein in breast milk becomes part of the baby; little or none is excreted. The baby fed on cow's milk–based or vegetable-based formula may waste about half the protein in his diet. Some is excreted in the feces undigested. Some is digested, but cannot be utilized by the cells of the body and is excreted in the urine. To get enough usable protein, the bottlefed baby must drink a much larger volume of liquid than the breastfed baby. In taking aboard extra fluid, the formula-fed baby may also get extra carbohydrates, which may make him obese.

The mother who has had one bottlefed baby, and watched him tuck away 8 or 10 ounces or even more on occasion, may worry because her subsequent breastfed baby couldn't possibly be getting a similar volume of milk. But because he absorbs nearly every drop from the breast, the breastfed baby doesn't need to take in nearly as much. In fact, while bottlefed babies vastly increase their volume intake as they grow, the volume intake of breastfed babies levels off long before the babies begin taking other food, without affecting growth rates at all.

Water:

Eliminating unusable protein is largely the job of the kidneys. This may place quite a strain on a function that is as yet immature. For years it was widely believed that premature babies gained better on certain formulas than they did on breast milk. Finally, investigators found that the weight gain was due not to growth but to retention of fluid in the tissues. This is the result of strain on the immature kidneys, which are not yet properly equipped to eliminate unsuitable proteins and mineral salts.

Human infants get plenty of water in their mother's milk for their metabolic needs; breast milk is 90 percent water for hydration and 10 percent solids for energy and growth. Although an occasional baby seems to enjoy drinking water, during hot weather it is the mother who needs extra water, not her breastfed baby. The baby fed on cow's milk, on the other hand, needs additional water by bottle not only to regulate his own metabolism, but also to enable his kidneys to eliminate the unusable proteins and salts, especially in hot weather.

Fat:

Some of the most intensive and exciting research on lactation and infant development in recent years has been done on the subject of fat. The source of energy for the rapid growth of infants, the various fats in human milk are now understood also to be essential for optimal brain and eye development. Two prevalent fats, the long-chain polyunsaturated fatty acids docosahexaenoic acid (DHA) and arachidonic acid (AA), have been documented as so important that formula manufacturers are racing to find ways to mimic their actions by adding similar fats derived from algae and fish oil. DHA and AA, however, are not the only fats in breast milk; the brain is about 60 percent fat, and of that, 25 percent is DHA and 15 percent is AA. The role of the remaining fats is still being explored.

Besides supplying the energy for growth, human milk fat contains essential vitamins and fatty acids; nutrients that are supplied through the placenta during pregnancy and through breast milk after birth. Fat molecules enable the complete use of protein by the infant's developing body; without adequate fat, the functions of protein are less efficient.

The level and types of fat in milk vary according to the length of a nursing, the time of day, the gestational age of the baby (the milk of mothers of preemies is higher in fat than full-term milk), a mother's genes, metabolism, and diet. Women on highly restricted diets, whether low fat or low protein, may produce milk with lower levels of fat. Women in overall good health who eat a balanced diet that includes fats and proteins will produce, over the course of the day, milk with a more than adequate proportion of cream.

All breastfed infants show higher deposits of fatty acids in their neural tissues and retinas. Not surprisingly, these higher concentrations correlate directly with improved mental performance and visual acuity in the first year of life. Remarkably, according to several studies, these differences appear to last long past weaning. The differences are so well documented that formula manufacturers have begun to add synthetic fatty acids to their products. Unlike breast milk, however, these "enhanced" products have not been shown to improve brain development or vision in infancy or beyond.

Cholesterol:

Like fat, cholesterol is not a bad word when it comes to babies. Essential for nerve and cell development, cholesterol is found in breast milk in the form of lactose, the sugar in milk, and oligosaccharides, the complex sugars that fight pathogens as well as supply energy, are also found in breast milk. Human milk is relatively high in cholesterol: five to ten times higher than cow's milk, and about six times higher than what most adults consume in their daily diets.

In adults, high cholesterol levels are associated with clogged arteries and heart attacks among other health concerns. In infants, however, quite the opposite seems to be true. The plentiful cholesterol found in breast milk seems to offer some protection against developing clogged arteries in adulthood. In 2002, a team of researchers from St. George's Hospital Medical School in south London, compared more than 1,500 babies, children, adolescents, and adults who had been breastfed with those who had received formula as infants. While there were minimal differences in cholesterol levels between the two groups of children and adolescents, among the adults the results were startling. Cholesterol levels of those who had been breastfed as infants were dramatically lower than those who had been formula fed, despite the fact that breast milk is higher in cholesterol than formula. The researchers suggest that early exposure to the high cholesterol content of breast milk may improve fat metabolism in later life. Indeed, children who are breastfed are less likely to have a heart attack or stroke as adults, according to a study published in May 2004.

The levels of cholesterol in breast milk appear to be unrelated to the mother's diet. In one experiment, a group of lactating women spent four weeks on a high-cholesterol diet and four weeks on a low-cholesterol diet; their own blood levels rose and fell depending on their diet, but the levels in the milk (and in their babies' blood plasma) remained the same. It appears that some cholesterol compounds in human milk are actually manufactured in the breast, to make up any deficiency in dietary supply. In other words, the breast monitors both the amounts and kinds of cholesterol in human milk, and keeps the "good" level high, possibly facilitating brain growth, as the brain is rich in cholesterol.

Lactose, the principal sugar in human milk, includes galactose, glucose, and other compounds. Sugar-related compounds are important in the maintenance of safe intestinal flora, as we have seen, and serve numerous other functions, in addition to providing calories for energy and making human milk taste sweet, an inducement to feeding that newborn babies seem to relish.

Incidentally, lactation also seems to manage maternal blood

sugar levels, a much appreciated benefit to mothers with insulin-dependent diabetes, by drawing on the glucose for milk production. Many nursing mothers with diabetes find that they have a reduced need for regular insulin treatment as long as nursing continues.

Vitamins:

Designed to provide for babies even in times of famine, breast milk normally supplies all the vitamins babies need for the first six months, even if a mother's nutrition is compromised, and continues to be an excellent source of vitamins thereafter. While many of these essential nutrients are found in lower quantities in breast milk than in commercial formulas, they are used more efficiently by the infant's body—they have a higher bioactivity and bioavailability—and therefore meet the complete needs of newborns better even than the most enhanced formulas.

Vitamins can be divided into two groups: those that dissolve in fat, which can be stored in the body (vitamins A, E, D, and K), and those that dissolve in water and must be supplied daily by the diet. Except in very peculiar circumstances, breast milk contains plenty of the fat-soluble vitamins A and E, which are supplied from the liver and other storehouses in the mother's body, even when they are low or absent in her diet. Both of these vitamins are especially plentiful in colostrum, where they are undoubtedly valuable to the newborn, whose supplies of A and E are very low at birth. At the age of one week, the breastfed newborn has more than five times the amount of vitamin E in his system than does his bottlefed counterpart. So far, breastfeeding is the only way we know of to establish this high, virtually adult level of vitamin E, a powerful anti-inflammatory agent, in the newborn.

Vitamin D does not normally come from diet except in northern and Arctic climates, where the diet is rich in fish oils and fish liver. In the rest of the world, vitamin D is synthesized in the body through exposure to sunlight. Both breastfed babies and nursing mothers synthesize their own vitamin D in the sun. Some vitamin D is also supplied to the baby through his mother's milk and, for about eight weeks after birth, from prenatal stores.

In fact, the precursor of a hormone and not a vitamin at all, the misnamed vitamin D controls the body's ability to absorb calcium. When it is not provided by the diet, and if exposure to and absorption of sunlight is insufficient, children can develop rickets, a disease that results in brittle bones, among other complications. A highly preventable disease, rickets remains all too common among urban communities where children have little access to outdoor play areas, have dark complexions, and may not drink vitamin D–fortified milk. A vitamin D deficiency is, in short, a sunlight deficiency.

Breast milk contains insignificant vitamin D; nature did not expect babies to be kept indoors or to live in northern cities if their skin tone was designed to protect them from equatorial sun rays. The prevention of rickets and other problems stemming from vitamin D deficiency is straightforward. Just fifteen minutes of sunlight a day (for a total of less than two hours a week) is sufficient; a walk around the block in a stroller, even with a hat on, will give light-skinned babies, newborn to six months old, the sunlight their bodies need to synthesize vitamin D. Babies whose ancestors came from southern climes and have dark skin may need three to six times more exposure to sunlight than Caucasian babies to synthesize the same amount of vitamin D; a vitamin D supplement may be needed in addition to a daily walk outdoors.

The water-soluble vitamins, vitamin C and the B complex, must be supplied in the diet. Cow's milk contains almost no vitamin

C, since calves can manufacture their own. Human milk, on the other hand, contains quite a lot, regardless of the amount in the mother's diet. (Even when mothers take large supplements of vitamin C, 1,000 micrograms or more, the amount in their milk stays level, suggesting a still-to-be discovered regulatory mechanism.) Scurvy, the disease caused by a lack of vitamin C so familiar to nineteenth-century sailors, has never been seen in a breastfed baby, even where it is still found among adults, including nursing mothers.

The B-complex vitamins, a mysterious and extensive group, play a role in human and animal nutrition that is not yet entirely understood. Some are supplied by the diet. Some are synthesized in the body. In most parts of the world, at least enough B-complex vitamins for survival are supplied to breastfed babies by their mothers, whatever the diet. The notable exception is parts of Asia, where polished rice is a food staple and sometimes the only food. Polishing removes the thiamine, and whole populations may be deficient in that B vitamin, with breastfed babies perishing of beriberi, the thiamine-deficiency disease. Unpolished rice cannot be stored as long as polished rice in warm climates; it is difficult to persuade manufacturers not to polish rice when to do so is to their economic advantage.

Deficiency of other B vitamins in breastfed babies does not normally arise, even under conditions of deprivation, with the exception of vitamin B_{12} deficiency, sometimes seen in vegan and vegetarian mothers. While a vegetarian diet can be healthy for both mothers and children, the breastfeeding vegetarian must ensure that her diet has nonanimal sources for protein, calcium, and essential amino acids. If a vegetarian or vegan mother breastfeeds and does not have a sufficiently balanced diet, her baby may have symptoms of deficiencies before the mother does.

In some infant formulas, B-vitamin supplies may not be

sufficient for the needs of individual babies. Some babies have had convulsions, found to be caused by insufficient vitamin B, when they were fed sterilized products in which parts of this vitamin complex were destroyed by heating. In 2003, several Israeli babies fed the same brand of soy formula were hospitalized, and two died, of beriberi when the manufacturer left vitamin B_1 out of the recipe.

Minerals—Calcium:

Human milk contains less than a quarter as much calcium as cow's milk; this appears to be all the calcium a human baby needs, with the exception of extremely premature babies. Yet, because of the higher bioavailability of the calcium in human milk, babies absorb 67 percent of it compared with 25 percent of that in cow's milk. Babies on cow's milk–formula diets tend to grow larger and heavier skeletons than breastfed babies in the first year of life. However, they must also process and excrete all that unused calcium and phosphorus through their kidneys. At present, our understanding of babies' calcium needs is inadequate. One authority sees a need to investigate the "poor calcification" of the breastfed baby, to determine if long-term or immediate disadvantages result. Another accepts the breastfed baby as normal, and deplores the distorted growth curve based on formula-fed babies who have been "too highly mineralized" by cow's milk. We do know that babies absorb calcium from human milk much more efficiently than they do from formula. Like many other elements, calcium in breast milk is highly bioavailable; it doesn't take a lot to do the job. We also know that the calcium content of human milk remains stable even in the malnourished mother, since the mineral is drawn off the supply stored in her bones, and that in healthy mothers, this supply of calcium is completely recovered after weaning. We don't understand exactly how that recovery takes place, but epidemiologic studies of large population groups show that women who have breastfed have a decreased risk of developing osteoporosis later in life.

Minerals—Iron:

Iron is needed to make red blood cells. A baby is born with a good supply of iron and with a high concentration of red blood cells, which is presumably diluted to normal levels over the first four months. It used to be thought that human milk contains "no" iron. In fact, it does contain iron in a form much more easily absorbed by the baby. High levels of vitamins C and E in the breast milk function in making iron available to the baby's system, and lactoferrin in the mother's milk binds and recycles iron molecules that in the bottlefed baby may be usurped by bacteria. If the mother is not anemic during pregnancy, the baby's stores of iron are adequate for the first six months, until about the time that solids are added to the baby's diet. Then additional dietary iron becomes available from grains and baby cereals, some vegetables, meat, and so on.

The breastfed baby may actually absorb more iron than the bottlefed baby without receiving an iron supplement. (Formula supplements, solid foods, or even iron supplements, if given before the fifth or sixth month, may interfere with the iron absorption process.) Thus, the breastfed baby is not normally anemic.

If the mother is extremely anemic during pregnancy, her baby's prenatal stores of iron may become inadequate within two or three months, rather than five or six, and "suckling anemia" may occur. Suckling anemia is seen even in the children of healthy mothers when solid foods are withheld past the sixth or seventh month of pregnancy. In Renaissance Italy, it was customary to give babies nothing but breast milk for up to two years. The results may be detected in many paintings of the period: Representations of the Madonna and Child frequently show the Infant Christ as a pasty-white anemic older baby.

Formula-fed infants, despite the high levels of iron in their diet, have been found to be anemic as a result of "microhemorrhages," or hidden bleeding, in their intestinal tract due to chronic irritation of the mucosal lining of the intestine caused by bacteria. As formula-fed babies are more subject to anemia, an effort is usually made to have them eating iron-rich foods, including egg yolks, as soon as they begin solids. This early exposure to eggs and other high-protein foods, however, may cause allergic reactions in susceptible individuals.

Breastfed babies usually signal when they are ready for solid foods by trying to help themselves to the foods on a parent's plate. It is not surprising that just as fetal stores of nutrients begin to run low, babies begin to show an interest in new food sources. Sometimes concerns about adding iron to a baby's diet are answered by the suggestion that a little iron-fortified infant cereal be added to a baby's bottle of formula or pumped breast milk. (There is also a popular old wives' tale that doing so may help a baby sleep longer at night. It won't.) A recent study has found that adding cereal to a baby's diet before four months of age may increase some children's risk of developing juvenile diabetes. The eventual necessity of adding iron to the diet and the desirability, around the middle of the first year, of introducing the baby to new foods ("A little bagel, a piece of salami, he should know what good food tastes like," as one cookbook author puts it) should not be used as an argument to promote feeding solids to an already well-nourished breastfed baby before the fifth month.

Minerals—Trace Elements:

Trace elements are minerals—such as copper, manganese, sulfur, zinc, chromium, and many others—that occur in minute quantities and yet are necessary for healthy metabolism. Mothers deliver these minerals in their milk; for example, the breastfed baby shares the benefits when his mother drinks fluoridated water. Human milk has frequently been considered to supply insufficient levels of minerals, as the amounts found in breast milk are lower than the standard recommended daily allowances. The problem is that those official recommendations do not account for the high bioavailability of the elements of breast milk. All that is needed is supplied, and used with 100 percent efficiency. There is no waste in lactation.

Gradually, we are learning some of the roles played by these "micronutrients." Human milk is much higher in copper than is cow's milk; copper seems to be associated with iron metabolism. Zinc, the most abundant trace mineral in mother's milk, is involved in muscle tissue growth. Selenium, once considered unnecessary and in fact a poison, turns out to be important in immune-system functioning.

The diets of even well-fed mothers may or may not provide adequate supplies of all trace elements: trace element researcher Michael Hambidge, MD, states that the diet of the African Bushman mother is better supplied with zinc, for example, than the diet of an urban American woman. Suppose that a slightly inadequate zinc supply reduces a baby's rate of muscle growth by a few percentage points; the baby is still healthy and normal, and the growth reduction would be hard for a scientist to prove—but that is not optimum nutrition. Does this matter? Perhaps only to parents.

A mother can improve her trace element intake by eating a wider variety of foods. The provision of trace elements in infant formulas, however, is not in a mother's control, and is somewhat uneven from brand to brand. Where the nutritional need for a specific micronutrient has been proven, it is added to formulas as a supplement, unless it is already a part of some protein or other compound already in the mix; thus infant formulas and even some adult breakfast cereals are now fortified with zinc. Where a nutritional need is yet to be identified, formulas may not be supplied with a micronutrient. There have been some serious episodes of deficiency diseases in infants fed exclusively on one brand or another of formula, before the necessary but absent nutrient was identified and added.

Breast milk, while providing at least some of all the necessary nutrients, is also guaranteed not to contain trace elements at levels that are unnaturally or dangerously high. Formulas may contain too much of a trace element, especially when research has not yet been directed at that substance. For example, the role of manganese in human nutrition is not known, although it is present in our bodies and in breast milk in minute amounts. Manganese levels in cow's milk formulas, however, are typically ten times higher than in human milk, and in soy-based formulas up to a hundred times higher. These levels are so high that the baby's excretion system can be overtaxed. Manganese that cannot be excreted is stored in the brain. In high doses, manganese is a neurotoxin. Indeed, in several studies, children with learning disabilities have been shown to have higher than normal levels of manganese.

PEPTIDES, ENZYMES, HORMONES, AND OTHER MYSTERIES

Human milk is full of other complex substances whose functions and roles have not yet been fully determined. Some aid the infant's immature system in digestion. Amylase, for instance, is an enzyme that promotes the digestion of starches. Infants do not manufacture their own amylase until about six months of age. Cow's milk and soy formulas do not contain amylase (which in any case would be destroyed by heating), but breast milk does; as a result, breastfed babies old enough for other foods actually tolerate and digest solid foods better than bottlefed babies do. Children with the genetic disease cystic fibrosis provide a striking example; among other symptoms, the child's ability to digest food is affected by the disease. If the child is breastfed, the gastrointestinal symptoms of the disease may not manifest until the child is weaned, as even small amounts of breast milk assist in the digestion of solid foods.

Some of the compounds in human milk appear to promote the development of the baby's immune system; others, the growth and development of the intestines. Harvard Medical School research on growth factors suggests that the first few feedings of colostrum and early breast milk may contain specific growth-inducing hormones that play a major role in stimulating the maturation of the intestines of the newborn. The result is improved food absorption and protection against allergies, infections, and serious intestinal disorders. These growth factors may be of particular importance in premature babies.

Breast milk contains many of the hormones found in the mother's bloodstream. The prolactin and oxytocin of lactation presumably have the same calming, relaxing effect on the baby that they have on the mother. Another hormone, insulin, occurs in a mother's milk in higher levels than in her blood serum. Why this is true is not yet clear, but some researchers theorize it may be connected to the fact that as the frequency and duration of breastfeeding increase, the risk of a breastfed child eventually developing Type 1 diabetes decreases.

LONG-TERM BENEFITS OF BREAST MILK

Remarkably, research is accumulating that breastfeeding confers health benefits long after weaning, and even into adulthood. In addition to a decreased risk of developing Type 1 diabetes, children who have been exclusively breastfed for six months show myriad other long-term health advantages. At Oregon State University, a study of dental caries in two well-matched communities, one with fluoridated water and one without, turned up a surprise side issue. As it happened, both towns had high percentages of breastfed children, so there were many in the study. Children who had been breastfed for three months or longer had 45 percent fewer cavities than their bottlefed counterparts in the nonfluoridated community, and 59 percent fewer cavities in the fluoridated community. The three-month period of nursing seemed to be a significant factor; children who had been breastfed only two months showed lessened protection (10 percent and 20 percent fewer cavities, respectively). Never mind the toothpaste ads—if you want good checkups, start life as a nursing baby!

A well-recognized, long-term drawback of bottlefeeding as opposed to breastfeeding is the bottle-caused distortion of the infant's use of the facial muscles and the pressure on his mouth, jaws, and palate. This is considered to be a major cause of malocclusions and other facial development problems in some children, including, typically, crooked or crowded teeth that require braces and orthodontia in later childhood. One large study shows that the effect of breastfeeding on malocclusions is dose related: That is, the longer the baby is breastfed (past six months, into the second year, or more), the greater the benefit to his jaw and facial development.

One study of the relationship between infant feeding methods and obesity compared the height, weight, and skinfold thickness of 907 teenagers with their infant feeding histories. The authors concluded that breastfeeding, even if for less than two months, provided significant protection against obesity, with indications of increased protection with longer duration. Early or late introduction of solids made no difference in this study, nor did race, birth order, or socioeconomic status. A study of nearly 200,000 children, performed by the Centers for Disease Control and Prevention and published in 2004, confirmed that if a child is breastfed for at least three months, the risk of developing obesity during childhood was significantly decreased. Nursing for six months lowered the risk of being overweight at six years of age by 30 percent, and nursing for longer than twelve months versus never breastfeeding at all lowered this risk by about 50 percent. The longer breastfeeding continued, in short, the lower the risk of obesity. The study also showed that breastfeeding for any duration was also protective against becoming underweight (below the 5th percentile for weight for age and height). The results for this study were affected by race (the protective effect of breastfeeding seemed limited to non-Hispanic whites), and the researchers urge that more studies be done on the long-term impact of nutrition in early childhood.

Epidemiological studies (statistical surveys of large chunks of the population) in Sweden and the United States have shown that fully breastfed babies have less chance than bottlefed babies of developing diabetes in childhood. When the incidence of breastfeeding fell, early-onset, insulin-dependent diabetes cases rose. When breastfeeding increased, the diabetes cases fell, and the onset was delayed where the disease did occur.

A British study has demonstrated that ulcerative colitis in adults is 100 percent more common in patients whose medical history includes weaning from the breast before two weeks than in patients who were breastfed for longer periods. Similar statistical studies have shown that breastfeeding, even for short periods, reduces the likelihood of contracting several other adult diseases related to immune-system problems, including celiac disease and Crohn's disease.

Breastfeeding appears to provide a dose-related protective effect against asthma in children one to two years old. Whether breastfeeding reduces the risk or severity of asthma over the longer term is controversial, and research continues to investigate this question. It does seem clear, however, that the probability of respiratory illness occurring at any time during childhood is significantly reduced if the child is fed exclusively breast milk for at least fifteen weeks, and if no solid foods are introduced during this time.

The evidence is in that breastfeeding offers a degree of lifetime protection against heart disease and stroke. Breast milk is high in healthy cholesterol, and breastfed babies have correspondingly high levels of cholesterol throughout childhood. As adults, however, this group has significantly lower cholesterol levels than adults who were not breastfed, and therefore improved cardiovascular health. Early exposure to the high cholesterol content of breast milk seems to improve fat metabolism in adults. Adults who were full term at birth and exclusively breastfed for at least six months are more likely to have lower blood pressure than those who were not. British researchers followed nearly five thousand children born in 1991 and 1992 for seven years, and found that children who were breastfed for any length of time had slightly lower blood pressure than those who were exclusively formula fed, even after adjusting for other factors that might affect blood pressure, including birth weight and mother's education. The study also showed that the blood pressure–lowering effects of breastfeeding increased with the duration that the infant was breastfed. The authors comment, "Even a small reduction may have important population-health implications. A 1% reduction in population systolic blood pressure levels is associated with about a 1.5% reduction in all-cause mortality, equivalent to a lessening in premature death of about 8,000 to 20,000 deaths per year in the United States and the United Kingdom, respectively."

Another British study published in 2004 suggests that breastfed babies are less likely as adults to die of heart attack or stroke because breastfed babies grow more slowly in the first weeks and months of life than do formula-fed babies: "Diets that promoted more rapid growth put babies at risk many years later in terms of raising their blood pressure, raising their cholesterol, and increasing their tendency to diabetes and obesity—four main risk factors for stroke and heart attack," says Alan Lucas of the Institute of Child Health in London, and one of the authors of the study. The effects of breastfeeding on blood pressure and cholesterol later in life, the researchers emphasize, are greater than anything adults can do to control the risk factors for cardiovascular disease, other than taking medications.

At least two studies have shown that as the incidence and duration of breastfeeding goes up, the incidence of childhood leukemia and other lymphomas—white cell–related cancers—goes down. We do not yet understand the mechanism for this protection, and the evidence at present is only a statistical association, rather than the suggestion of a direct cause.

As the rush to add synthetic versions of DHA and AA to commercial formula attests, the fatty acids in breast milk appear to have a direct impact on cognitive and intellectual development. A large analysis of numerous controlled studies indicates that breastfeeding is associated with a 3.16-point-higher score for cognitive development compared with formula feeding. This difference was observed as early as six months and could be measured through fifteen years of age. The effect was dose related; the longer breastfeeding lasted, the greater differences in cognitive development. The difference was magnified in the case of preterm and low-birth-weight infants, with these babies showing a 5.18-point difference in IQ compared with weight-matched, formula-fed infants.

The discovery that breastfeeding protects health far into adult life occurred largely by accident; in the cases of the Oregon dental caries investigation and the British study of ulcerative colitis, the investigators had no idea in advance that any such correlations would show up. One wonders how many "modern" diseases, generally supposed to be by-products of pollution or of the tensions of twenty-first-century life, are physiologically related to our widespread unnatural system for feeding babies.

GRAPE JUICE AND KARMA:
ENVIRONMENTAL CONTAMINANTS IN HUMAN MILK

Whatever we eat, breathe, or touch—wood smoke, hair spray, soapy water, bubble gum, the smell of pine needles—anything that can be absorbed into the human system may be transferred and detectable in human milk. Occasionally, a mother has been startled to discover that drinking grape juice tints her milk a pale shade of violet. Volatile oils, which give most spices their characteristic odors and flavors, pass through milk unchanged. Babies don't usually care; if these were the predominant flavors of the mother's diet during pregnancy, her baby is already accustomed to them as they passed through to the amniotic fluid and were tasted by the fetus in utero. (The *Journal of Human Lactation*, however, does report one baby who refused the breast temporarily when his mother ate ten ounces of mint candies in two days.)

That's all very well for harmless food ingredients, but what about substances that might be bad for the baby? These fall into two categories: substances mothers ingest knowingly, such as medicines, tobacco, alcohol, and other drugs, and can therefore usually choose to avoid; and contaminants in our environment that we unknowingly absorb and ingest.

Alarming reports of these contaminants periodically make the headlines: REPORT OF DIOXIN IN HUMAN MILK, NURSING MOTHERS ADVISED TO TEST MILK FOR PCBS, and so on. These news reports give everyone the jitters. Are contaminants a real problem? How serious is it?

Many research projects on illness-causing agents are investigations of quantity: How much of an agent can an organism absorb before damage occurs? One answer is that, of course, anything can be bad for you in large enough quantities; people have been poisoned by ingesting too much carrot juice. Most of the substances we acquire from our environment, even those that have been shown to be dangerous in laboratories, are absorbed in tiny quantities and are probably harmless in effect.

Some environmental pollutants, however, have become public health concerns: organochlorine pesticides such as DDT, reaching us through the food chain; dioxin-related compounds, which are sometimes a product of burning and thus can be airborne; and polychlorinated biphenyls, or PCBs, oil-like substances used in industry, which may reach us in many ways.

These substances are toxic. They don't degrade into harmless substances quickly. They are fat soluble, and tend to be stored in the fat cells and accumulate in the food chain; they are found in the highest concentrations in carnivores. Female mammals that have such contaminants stored in their body fat may transfer a percentage of them into milk fats during lactation. By the time the persistence of such compounds was understood, these complicated, enduring molecules had been manufactured in enormous quantities and distributed all over the world. They can now be found almost everywhere on the planet, and in all forms of animals, including us.

Almost certainly, we have all had some lifetime exposure to these compounds, from our food, from the ground we walk on, from the air we breathe; how much and what, depends on where we live. World Health Organization surveys show that people in industrial nations have less exposure to DDT-related compounds, and more to PCBs than people in third-world countries, who in turn might show more traces of agricultural chemicals in their body fat, but no PCBs at all.

What does this mean to babies? Almost anything a mother is exposed to during pregnancy crosses the placenta and enters the bloodstream of the fetus. Prenatal exposure to environmental toxins has been linked to subtle cognitive and motor development delays in infancy and childhood, as well as to vitamin K deficiencies. If a developing fetus can be affected by pollutants through the mother's bloodstream, can a baby be affected by them through breast milk? These chemicals, sadly, can be detected in breast milk, just as they can be in the bloodstream and fat deposits of just about everyone who lives in an industrialized nation. Several long-term studies show that exposure to these compounds through breast milk, remarkably, does not cause the same adverse effects associated with prenatal exposure. One large-scale study by Dutch researchers of children in Western Europe tracked pregnant women and their babies through the age of six, measuring pollutants to which the infants were exposed both prenatally and after birth through breast milk. During pregnancy all the mothers in the study had a measurable level of pollutants in their bloodstreams, and therefore their fetuses did as well. By eighteen months of age, the effects of this exposure could be detected through neurological exams in the toddlers who had been formula fed, but not in those who had been breastfed. Despite continued exposure to PCBs and other chemicals through the small quantities unavoidably present in breast milk, the researchers found that at eighteen months, at forty-two months, and at six years, the breastfed children fared better on motor-skill cognitive-development tests than did the formula-fed group. The authors of the study concluded that "breast feeding counteracts the adverse developmental effects of PCBs and dioxins."

Of course, it is outrageous that we have contaminated the planet to any measurable extent; cleaning up our act, on individual, corporate, and governmental levels, has become a widely recognized imperative. The idea of contamination in breast milk, however, as opposed to, say, skin creams, apples, coffee beans, or our water or air supply, has grabbed a giant share of media attention for several reasons. First, it has headline-getting shock value; second, the fat in mother's milk is easy to obtain and measure, compared with human body fat or fat from carnivorous animals; in fact, mother's milk is so easy to use that it has actually become a tool for such infinitesimal quantities of chemical substances that we can identify molecular-level traces of substances, not in

parts per thousand or million, but in parts per billion or even tril-
lion. What we too often fail to do is put that information into
perspective.

When the headline reads MOTHER'S MILK CONTAMINATED
WITH . . . , the important question is not "Is this true?" but "How
much contamination are we talking about?" and "Does this level
of contamination affect a nursing infant?" It used to be that to
isolate or identify a substance you had to obtain enough of it to
weigh it. Now, using a variety of elegant new methods, tiny quantities of complex substances can be identified in an instant. For
example, in one short experiment, using mass spectrometry and a
capillary gas chromatograph, scientists identified over two hundred compounds in the *smell* of a cup of coffee. Theoretically, a
mother could probably absorb all kinds of things into her milk—
in "trace" quantities—just from walking past a coffeemaker.

Using these techniques, someone looking for, say, hexchloro-
1, 3-butadiene in a few ounces of human milk may find trace
amounts. But is this harmful? It's like coffee: Drink ten cups a day,
and the caffeine in your breast milk will without a doubt have an
impact on your baby. Walk past the coffeemaker, and one can
hardly suppose the baby will suffer, even though parts per billion of
measurable chemicals might indeed enter your bloodstream and
show up in your milk.

This hasn't stopped some people from stating that every
nursing mother should have her milk tested for contaminants.
(Test results, in any case, depend on the amount of fat in a sample and are therefore highly variable and subject to gross over-
interpretation.) Some wildly irresponsible conclusions have
been drawn in the press that babies should be fed cow's milk formulas because cows eat only grass, not meat. A poorly founded
scare tactic, this assumption ignores the fact that commercial

formulas, whether based on cow's milk or plant materials, contain contaminants as well, many of which are not screened for, and none of which are continually tested for, by the U.S. Food and Drug Administration. Cow's milk formulas, for example, can contain amounts of antibiotics, hormones high above the government's allowable levels, and contaminants, such as aflatoxins from spoiled grain, that are almost never found in human milk. The water used to mix formula powders may not be safe; the water from some farm wells can be laden with chemicals from fertilizers, and lead may be found in water from city taps. Even feeding equipment is not necessarily safe. Some rubber bottle nipples can leach a preservative, sodium nitrite, at such levels that one should really boil them in several changes of water before use. Avoiding human milk in order to avoid environmental contaminants, however, is not a well-founded strategy.

Current studies suggest that the protective elements in breast milk counteract the impact of any contaminants that may also be in breast milk. The effect of prenatal exposure to pollutants, however, remains a concern. Unfortunately, pollutants enter women's bodies many years before pregnancy occurs, and only cleaning up our environment will prevent them from doing so. While we have far to go on this front, some progress is being made. In Canada, the United States, and Europe, the levels of DDT and similar compounds in human beings were much higher in the 1970s than in the 1990s, suggesting that for these countries the peak of those contaminations is past. (In many developing countries, however, contamination levels are still severe.) An Australian study found that younger people carried smaller traces of contaminants than did older people, presumably because of the passage of effective environmental laws.

DRUGS, ALCOHOL, AND CONTAMINANTS YOU CAN AVOID

Most things a mother ingests can appear in her milk, including nicotine, caffeine, alcohol, medications, and illegal drugs. Although there are many exceptions, the rule of thumb with prescription medications is that the baby gets 1 percent of the dose the mother takes. Among the exceptions are many mood-altering chemicals, which have a long half-life in an adult body. That means they circulate in a mother's bloodstream not just once, but hour after hour. The breastfed baby, therefore, can accumulate a new dose at each feeding and, because a baby may take longer to eliminate the drugs, may build a high level quickly.

Caffeine is a particularly difficult drug for infants to eliminate. An adult will eliminate caffeine from a single dose—one cup of coffee, for example—in about five hours. A newborn baby, however, may take up to three days to get rid of a single dose, so subsequent doses rapidly add up to very high levels. While the half-life of caffeine in an adult body is five hours, in a newborn it is nearly one hundred hours (although it decreases with age until, at six months, babies can eliminate caffeine in roughly the same amount of time as an adult). One mother reported that her first-born baby was irritable from birth, and became absolutely frantic twenty-four hours a day when she brought him home. Her doctor was unable to find anything wrong, decided the baby was "allergic to breast milk," and advised weaning and feeding the baby formula in a bottle, whereupon the baby calmed right down. It took the mother years to realize that no one had asked her what *she* was doing: drinking six or eight cups of coffee a day as she tried to cope with a series of sleepless nights while caring for her increasingly miserable breastfed infant, who in all likelihood was suffering from a caffeine overdose.

If a mother smokes, there will be nicotine in her milk. One nursing mother who smoked heavily found that her baby was not gaining well. She recalled that she herself never gained weight while smoking, so she quit, and the baby began gaining at once. Smoking is strongly discouraged during pregnancy and lactation for both the health of the mother and the baby. Babies born to smokers tend to be smaller at birth than babies born to nonsmokers, and are likely to suffer respiratory ailments and other health problems. If a mother is trying to quit smoking with the help of a nicotine patch or nicotine gum, both products do deliver a level of nicotine to the bloodstream, and therefore to the breast milk. It is a far lower level than that reached by smoking, and is certainly preferable to continuing to smoke or to weaning and switching to formula. If the patch is removed at night or the gum chewed immediately after the baby has nursed (i.e., two to three hours before the next nursing), the amount of nicotine that reaches the breast milk, and therefore the baby, can be minimized.

The effects of alcohol on fetuses can be severe. To date, no safe level has been established, and pregnant women are advised to abstain completely from alcoholic drinks. Alcohol appears in breast milk at about the same level that it occurs in the maternal bloodstream. Once born, however, the nursing baby digests these molecules, rather than receiving them straight into the bloodstream via the placenta. Alcohol does enter the breast milk, in other words, but passes through the infant's gastrointestinal tract mostly unabsorbed. Unless the mother drinks alcohol to the point of drunkenness, the effect on the baby is negligible. Midwives once encouraged new mothers to drink a stout ale to bring their milk in, and it seems that the sugars from barley may stimulate prolactin production. Nonalcoholic beer has been shown to have the same effect. While the occasional glass of beer or wine is not contraindicated during breastfeeding, babies may prefer that their mothers stick to nonalcoholic beverages. In one small study, infants consumed less breast milk for four hours after their mothers drank alcohol, although they made up for it by nursing more in the subsequent eight to sixteen hours.

Marijuana stays in the system for several days, rather than several hours like alcohol. Smoking pot, like caffeine, may result in cumulative doses for the breastfed baby; it may also affect one's mothering. Drugs that affect the mental processes may also be especially bad for babies even in small quantities, since their brains and nervous systems are in a state of rapid growth. Other illegal psychedelic and mood-altering drugs that powerfully affect a mother's behavior will reach the baby through the breast milk. The baby of a mother who is a user of heroin is born an addict and will continue to receive doses through the breast milk if nursed.

Cocaine is in a class by itself. It is extremely dangerous to the fetus and to the breastfed baby. It passes through the milk with ease. Babies have died from a single dose of cocaine-laced breast milk, and from breathing cocaine smoke. Even the smallest remnant of cocaine in the mother's system can damage a nursing baby. Babies cannot handle cocaine, period.

MEDICATIONS: WHAT'S SAFE FOR THE NURSING MOTHER?

Prescription drugs, like any other ingested substance, can appear in trace quantities in a nursing mother's milk. Usually the amounts are so trivial that they make absolutely no difference to the nursing baby. Nevertheless, every time a new drug is introduced into the medical repertoire, somebody worries about what effect it will have on nursing babies. Doctors whose specialties have nothing to do with mothers and babies—surgeons, ophthalmologists, cardiologists, and so on—may prescribe drugs and forbid further breastfeeding without understanding its importance or the problems involved in stopping even temporarily. Many physicians rely on a single book, *The Physicians' Desk Reference*, for information on the safety and side effects of drugs. The *PDR*, as it is called, lists all the information provided by research done by the drug's manufacturer. Pharmaceutical companies rarely research the effect of their drugs on the babies of nursing patients, and therefore play it safe for liability reasons and simply instruct that almost every drug "is not safe for pregnant or nursing mothers." Often a drug is declared unsafe for nursing mothers and babies simply because it shows up in the breast milk, without regard to the level (usually so tiny as to be "subclinical") or how the baby metabolizes it. Medications that do reach the baby often pass unabsorbed through the gastrointestinal system and are eliminated; they have low bioavailability for the infant. A physician unfamiliar with the biology of lactation, however, is unlikely to question the *PDR*, and may forbid breastfeeding upon prescribing anything from antibiotics to aspirin. Mothers have even been advised to wean when prescribed drugs that the same physician wouldn't hesitate to prescribe in oral doses for the infant itself.

The fact is, most medications that people are normally given for transitory illnesses are safe for nursing mothers and their babies; this includes antibiotics (except for tetracycline, which can stain the baby's newly forming teeth) and anesthetics. Anesthetics given to a mother during birth may inhibit her baby's sucking reflex in the first hours of life, but anesthetics and analgesics given to a mother afterward or postoperatively will not affect her nursing baby; she should be free to nurse as soon as she wants to. Vitamins, even in megadoses, are harmless, as are single doses of most drugs.

Approximately 1 percent or less of a mother's dose of most medications is excreted in her breast milk. The mammary glands do not "store" drugs; a medication that a mother takes in the evening will be gone from her bloodstream and therefore from her milk by morning, whether she nurses the baby in the night or not. Most prescribed drugs, such as antibiotics, are gone from the system in two to four hours—that's why you have to take a new dose every four hours. In the case of many common medications, such as aspirin, the amount of drug in the mother's milk peaks ten or twenty minutes after the dose is taken, and then rapidly disappears.

When medications are prescribed for a nursing mother, the physician must consider how much of a specific medication is likely to be transferred to the mother's milk (and this depends on the molecular size of the drug, and whether those molecules will bind the fat molecules in the milk), how long the medication will stay in the mother's system before being eliminated, and the oral bioavailability of the medication to the infant (how much of a drug is absorbed through the gut before being eliminated). Drugs most likely to be transferred to the milk are those with low molecular weight, those easily dissolved in fats, those that do not bind to proteins, and those with long half-lives. Thus alcohol, with a molecular weight of 100, zips into the milk almost instantaneously, while a diabetic mother's dose of insulin, with a molecular weight of 5,000, won't appear in the milk at all. Some drugs that might seem dangerous for infants, such as the anticoagulant warfarin, bind to blood proteins and never get into the milk. Drugs that can't be absorbed in oral doses, and must be given to the mother by injection, are usually not a problem as they can't be absorbed in the baby's stomach either.

The physician must also consider the age, weight, and overall health of the infant. A full-term four-month-old baby may be unaffected by his mother's prescription drugs, while a four-month-old born prematurely may be more sensitive. Babies born with conditions affecting the function of their gastrointestinal system may be more affected by some maternal medications. Mothers of nursing newborns should not be given medications that may limit milk production, if possible, although these are less of a concern after the newborn period has passed and the milk supply is well established.

Long-term medications that may offer some risks to nursing infants include lithium and other antidepressants and sedatives, which over many months could affect the baby's developing nervous system, cyclosporins, and other immunosuppressant drugs. Radioisotopes necessary for diagnosis or treatment need not be cause for weaning. One can select the isotope with the shortest half-life, and suspend nursing for a relatively brief period (thirty-six hours or so) to allow the drug to clear the mother's system before nursing the baby again. A baby's exposure to any medication taken by his mother can be minimized by nursing the baby immediately preceding the dose, then waiting until the peak level of the drug in the mother's bloodstream has passed—usually four to five hours—before nursing again. A mother can pump her milk in advance of taking the medication to cover her baby's needs until it is safe to nurse again.

We have not included in this book a list of specific drugs and their known effects on mothers and babies. New drugs come along all the time, old drugs are taken off the danger list as we learn more about lactation, and such a list would soon be out of date. La Leche League International in Franklin Park, Illinois (www.lalecheleague.org, 847-519-0035), refers callers with medication-related questions to their Breastfeeding Information Center. Another good source is the frequently updated reference *Medications and Mothers' Milk*, by Thomas W. Hale, PhD.

VIRUSES

Several viral diseases in nursing mothers are apt to cause concern, and lead a physician to suggest weaning for the safety of the baby. As with medications, weaning is often not appropriate or necessary. Viruses, like bacteria, can be found in breast milk; like bacteria, in the milk they are generally harmless to the baby. Some antiviral components exist in the milk itself. Others, such as fatty acids that dissolve the coatings of viruses, are produced in the baby's stomach during digestion. Some kinds of viruses—respiratory infections, for instance—may appear in the stomach or intestines. In any case, a mother who has a viral infection is usually protecting her baby by producing antibodies to that very infection in her milk.

Some viruses are dangerous for a fetus, but not for a nursing baby. An example is rubella, or German measles, which may cause birth defects if passed to a fetus through the placenta in early pregnancy, but which produces only a mild illness in a baby. Another teratogenic, or birth defect–causing, virus is a common infection called cytomegalovirus, or CMV. In some parts of the United States, more than half the population has antibodies to this virus, which causes a mild, flulike illness. Full-term babies who pick up the virus from breast milk usually develop antibodies without any symptoms of illness, and thus become immune to that infection for life. In a population where this virus is widespread, girl babies especially benefit from being thus protected from possible later infection in pregnancy. We do know that CMV is dangerous to the fetus in early pregnancy, and also dangerous for preterm babies if they receive it in blood transfusions. We don't know what the effects of this virus might be from banked human milk given to preterm babies; hospital human milk banks test the milk and their donors stringently for CMV.

A serious virus for the newborn is genital herpes, so much so that babies born to women with active cases of herpes are usually delivered by cesarean section to prevent the infant from coming into contact with open lesions. Such babies may be safely breast-fed, provided the mother keeps her hands clean and follows sanitary practices.

Hepatitis B is another dangerous, infectious virus—more common than it once was because of intravenous drug use—that has been identified in mother's milk. Sometimes people are carriers of this virus even though they are not ill with it themselves. Sometimes a mother who has already nursed her new baby for two or three days is told to wean because a blood test taken from the umbilical cord at birth is hepatitis-positive. There is no clear evidence, however, that the hepatitis B virus can be transmitted via breastfeeding. In addition, a vaccine given at birth can protect babies from the infection. In one study in China of more than two hundred babies born to hepatitis B–positive mothers, and therefore given the vaccine, there was no statistical difference in the rate of infection between breastfed and formula-fed babies at one year of age, with 90.9 percent in the breastfed group and 90.3 percent in the bottle-fed group remaining free from infection. In a larger study, performed at the University of Texas Medical Center, 3 percent of the formula-fed infants and none of the breastfed infants acquired the infection after an average of five months. The authors of both studies conclude that not only does breastfeeding pose no additional risk of transmitting the hepatitis B virus, but indeed seems to offer some protection when the mother is a carrier (and treated for the disease) and the baby is vaccinated.

A virus called human T-cell lymphotropic virus, or HTLV, which can cause a type of leukemia as well as central nervous system disorders, has become endemic in some parts of Japan and Africa. As with hepatitis, some people can be carriers after they themselves have recovered from the disease. This is perhaps the first virus that has been demonstrated definitely to have the capacity to infect a baby via mother's milk, although it is not yet known whether or not the baby will develop problems in adulthood as a result. The virus is not found in most parts of the world, but presents a concern to which we have no clear answer at present.

The terrible dilemma presented by HIV/AIDS has complicated breastfeeding advocacy across the globe. The virus that causes the human immunodeficiency syndrome can be transmitted to an infant through breastfeeding, although transmission is far more likely during pregnancy. Women in developed countries who are HIV-positive are advised to formula-feed their babies to avoid any risk of transmission via breastfeeding. However, for most of the world's women who are HIV-positive, the choice of infant feeding method is not so clear. In many countries burdened by great poverty, feeding babies formula places them at higher risk of contracting non-HIV infectious diseases (with many countries suffering an infant mortality rate of 10 to

20 percent) than breastfeeding does of acquiring HIV. For these mothers, the World Health Organization (WHO) advises that antiretroviral drugs be given to the mother, and that her baby be breastfed. If antiretroviral drugs cannot be obtained (an all-too-likely scenario), the WHO encourages physicians and public health officials to give mothers nutritional supplements to strengthen their immune system, thereby reducing the risk of transmission. Treating and preventing adult HIV/AIDS and improving the overall health and conditions of their communities remains the best hope for these babies.

BREASTFED BABIES ARE HEALTHIER BABIES

The protections offered by breast milk are valuable to any child. They are, of course, particularly vital in poverty-stricken or underdeveloped areas, where rampant diseases as well as inadequate supplies and environment for formula feeding mean that a baby taken off the breast may not survive. Increasing awareness of this fact, however, has led to two popular misconceptions in the United States—especially, oddly enough, in the medical community. The first is that the main value of breastfeeding in developing nations is that it protects the baby against contaminated water and dirty bottles. That premise leads to the second misconception, that breastfeeding is not important in disease protection in developed countries because we have sanitary alternative foods for infants. A well-known and oft-cited report published in the mid-1980s by Yale University researchers purported to prove that breastfeeding didn't make a significant health difference to United States babies. (That conclusion was made possible, in part, by a failure to differentiate between briefly and fully breastfed babies.) As a result, some pediatricians began telling North American mothers that breastfeeding was "not worth the bother."

In fact, breastfeeding makes quite a difference to the health of even infants born right here in North America. A large study, published in the May 2004 issue of *Pediatrics*, the journal of the American Academy of Pediatrics, reports that American breastfed babies are 20 percent less likely to die before their first birthday than formula-fed babies; the longer a baby nurses, the lower the risk. If all babies in the United States were breastfed, the researchers state, approximately 720 infant deaths could be prevented each year.

At Mary Imogene Bassett Hospital in upstate New York, researcher Allan Cunningham, MD, noticed in his own pediatric practice that breastfed babies seemed to be healthier. Medical commentary had concluded, however, that since it was the well-educated and better-off mothers who tended to breastfeed, these babies could be expected to be healthier anyway. Cunningham decided to study the healthy, normal babies born in the hospital in a two-year period to see if there were any other significant factors.

He limited the study to the 503 babies who had made regular "well-baby" clinic visits during their first year of life, and so were seen regularly by the same pediatricians. He divided them into three groups: breastfed babies, whom he defined as those who at least were partially breastfed for longer than four and one-half months (there were 135); limited breastfed babies, meaning that lactation was maintained for at least six weeks (80 babies); and formula-fed babies, which included those who might have been breastfed in the hospital, but were weaned shortly thereafter (288). Then he tabulated in all the babies the incidence of common illnesses requiring a doctor's care, such as chest colds, ear infections, vomiting, and diarrhea.

The results were published in the *Journal of Pediatrics*. During the first four months, when all of the "breastfed" cohort were still on the breast, the formula-fed babies were four times as likely to be sick, and during the first two months, sixteen times as likely. In the course of the first year, even though some of the breastfed babies were receiving mixed feedings, and nearly two-thirds of them had been weaned by six months, the wholly formula-fed babies still had twice as many of these common illnesses.

Perhaps the breastfed babies were simply doing better because their families on average were better off. Choosing education as an indicator of socioeconomic status, Cunningham took a look only at families in which the fathers had had at least three years of college. Of the breastfed group of babies in those families, the rate of illness worked out to 62 illnesses per 100 children, compared with 91 per 100 for the limited breastfed babies and 126 per 100 for the artificially fed babies (that is, some babies had more than one illness). How about families with smokers in them? How about families with babies in day care? In each of those circumstances, the babies breastfed for at least four and one-half months had fewer illnesses than babies breastfed for six weeks, and about half as many as babies raised on formula.

As to the seriousness of the illnesses, formula-fed babies were fifteen times more likely to wind up back in Mary Imogene Bassett Hospital than were the babies still receiving some breast milk. Over the whole year, only 6 of the babies who had been breastfed for at least six weeks were hospitalized for various infections, compared to 60 of the formula-fed infants (33 for common illnesses, 14 with bronchitis or pneumonia, and the rest with major ailments ranging from meningitis to allergy attacks; there was also one loss through SIDS in this group). Other larger-scale studies in both developed and developing countries have had similar results:

- Formula-fed babies in industrialized countries are hospitalized twice as often as breastfed babies and have more severe illness from lower respiratory tract infection, primarily the respiratory syncytial virus (RSV).
- In Finland, formula-fed babies had 4.3 times the rate of otitis media, or ear infections, than breastfed babies.
- In a study performed in Connecticut, formula-fed babies were hospitalized four times more often for bacterial meningitis than were breastfed babies.
- Human milk was the best preventative for bacteremia and necrotizing enterocolitis in preemies in British neonatal units.
- Diarrhea causes the most infant mortality in developing nations, where formula-fed babies are fourteen times more likely to die from it. In the United States, they are 3.7 times more likely.
- Sudden infant death is about 20 percent less common among North American breastfed babies than among formula-fed babies.
- There is evidence for better long-term health after breastfeeding in disorders such as celiac disease, Crohn's disease, cystic fibrosis, ulcerative colitis, insulin-dependent diabetes mellitus, thyroid disease, malignant lymphoma, chronic liver disease, atopic dermatitis, and food allergies.

These studies, with more under way, confirm that breastfeeding protects babies strikingly against serious illnesses, and somewhat against all illnesses, and that the protection increases in proportion

to the extent and duration of breastfeeding. As Dr. Cunningham remarked to an audience of health professionals, "Breastfeeding is no panacea. It will not prevent all illnesses. But you
are far less likely to see a breastfed baby than a formula-fed baby
in the hospital or on the autopsy table. That is true in New
Delhi and Nairobi, and it's true in Scarsdale and in Valley
Forge."

A baby's illness, whether major or not, disrupts its parents'
life, causes anxiety and wakeful nights, and most of all is no fun
for the baby. What parents wouldn't prefer their child to have a
short case of sniffles instead of a full-blown cold, a low fever
rather than a high one, diarrhea once a year instead of five or ten
times? Parents of nursing babies can be sure that the protection
the baby is getting from his mother's milk is making their life a
little easier, too.

The human baby is remarkably adaptable. Most babies can
survive on any diet that is near adequate: Islanders in the South
Pacific have raised orphaned newborns on diets of ripe bananas,
green coconut, and water. However, while a baby can do well on
formula, there are many who, without being actually allergic, are
never entirely suited to the practice of artificial feeding. The
gradient of intolerance probably runs all the way from what is
accepted as "normal" crankiness to the obvious cases of convulsions and progressive emaciation called "marasmus." There is
the baby with rashes and eczema, and the baby with gas; the
baby who vomits sour milk after every meal, and the baby who
cries inconsolably by the hour. There is the baby who screams as
he evacuates his bowels. There is the baby who perpetually has a
runny stool and diaper rash. Some people argue that these imperfect adjustments to an imperfect diet are not in themselves
harmful—although the long-term evidence of the bottlefed

child's eventual susceptibility to colitis and other adult diseases suggests otherwise. In any case, these babies do gain weight and grow. In most cases, their maladjustments are eventually outgrown. But while the problems are occurring, they may be distinctly unpleasant for the parents, and they are undoubtedly unpleasant for the baby.

There are a few babies who can tolerate only human milk. These babies, if put on formula, do poorly from birth, and eventually are back in the hospital receiving fluids intravenously, while one brand of formula after another is tried in the hope of finding something the baby will tolerate. Sometimes the missing factor or the intolerable ingredient can be pinpointed. The baby cannot use cow's milk proteins, so a soybean-based milk is substituted; or it is the sugar, or the fat, that the baby cannot adjust to. Sometimes the fact that a particular baby is more sensitive than average does not appear at first, because he is breastfed; he thrives until a routine supplement is introduced, or until he is prematurely weaned, at six or twelve weeks perhaps, when his mother and doctor have great difficulty in finding a brand of formula that the baby can tolerate. All such babies, however, can tolerate human milk, and in some cases when no tolerable formula can be found, a source of human milk must be found, whether it is from the mother who reestablishes her lactation or from a human milk bank.

As far as infant nutrition goes, we can say with complete certainty that human milk is the only completely adequate food for human infants in the first six months, and forms a splendid addition to the diet thereafter. Even in undernourished mothers, breast milk has all the needed nutrients. Unless lactation is inhibited so that the baby does not get enough milk, he will thrive. Such individual variations that occur are easily adapted to by the baby, and the marvelous flexibility of lactation almost always ensures a good and abundant supply of milk, whatever the vicissitudes of the mother's physical environment. There are still many questions to be answered about human milk. The one question that we can answer assuredly now is whether the best food for a human baby is its mother's milk: It is.

How the Baby Functions: The Body

THE BABY'S EQUIPMENT FOR BREASTFEEDING

The newborn baby arrives in the world specially equipped for feeding at the breast. His nose is short, and tilts upward at the tip because the nostril openings are wider than in an adult. His cheeks are plumped up with two firm pads of fat that keep them from collapsing inward as he suckles. The combination of the baby's little nose and the fat pads in the cheeks form two channels on either side of the nose, quite obvious when you look for them: These channels deliver air right into the nostrils even if the baby's nose is close to the mother's breast. (In addition, if the baby's nose isn't very close to the breast or touching it, the nipple is likely to be in the front of the baby's mouth, rather than the back, which can lead to nipple soreness.)

The inside of the newborn baby's mouth is likewise designed for breastfeeding. The palate is shaped like a smooth dome, to make room for the nipple in the back of the mouth during nursing. The tongue protrudes if touched, which facilitates latching on to the breast. The protruding tongue response, however, makes it almost impossible to spoon solids into the newborn, as the tongue reflex just thrusts them out again. (This reflex probably also protects the infant against choking on objects or substances that enter the mouth accidentally.) Finally, in breastfed newborns a "sucking blister" usually forms in the center of the upper lip, and may persist for weeks. This blister is not an injury but an adaptation to the activity of nursing.

LATCHING ON

In order to breastfeed, the baby must first "latch on" to the breast. "Latching on" is the term for taking a grasp on the areola behind the nipple, with the nipple well back in the mouth, and with lips and tongue forming a seal to prevent swallowing air. In this position, the baby can milk the breast effectively.

To latch on well, the baby needs to be facing the breast directly, with the mouth wide open. Kittie Frantz, RN, a pediatric nurse practitioner and an authority on positioning and breastfeeding, advises mothers to turn the baby on his side so that the mouth is level with the nipple; the baby's face, chest, stomach, genitals, and knees are all facing the mother's body, with the area from the chest to the knees flat against her: "Chest-to-chest, chin-to-breast," advise lactation consultants. This brings the baby into the contact he was designed to maintain; and whether one is sitting up, lying down, or even walking around, the baby can be drawn close with the "baby-holding" arm by keeping one's hand on the baby's rump or the upper thigh.

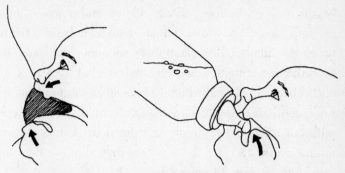

Figure 4.1 The breastfeeding baby nurses with wide-open jaws, lower lip flanged outward, and the breast tissue drawn well back in the mouth. The nipple is in the arch of the palate, out of harm's way. The tongue and gum ridges compress the milk sinuses.

SUCKLING BEHAVIOR

The mechanism by which a baby milks the breast is remarkably powerful. If you want to be impressed by a new baby's strength, just put a clean finger, pad upward, into the baby's mouth, against the roof of the mouth; you'll feel that mechanism go to work (it is an informative experience for new fathers). Suction, per se, is not, however, the main action. The baby may use the tongue and some suction to draw the nipple back into the mouth; then a combination of systems takes over. At the breast, the baby's mouth opens very wide, as if the baby were about to shout. The lips are everted, or flipped outward, against the breast, forming a seal all around the areola; thus the baby can nurse without swallowing air. The baby compresses the areola horizontally between the upper and lower jaws, forming the areola and nipple into a teat shape. The tongue comes out over the gum of the lower jaw, completing the air seal and incidentally padding the lower gum ridge, which protects the mother's areola and nipple. As the milk begins to flow, the lower jaw moves up and down, compressing the milk sinuses, or widened ducts, which are behind the nipple, under the areola (the milk sinuses are about the same distance from the nipple in all women no matter what the size of the areola). The tongue, meanwhile, in a wavelike motion from front to back, gently reaches forward, massages the ducts, and moves the milk out through the nipple and down the baby's throat. This tongue action also puts the now teat-shaped nipple deep into the baby's mouth, out of harm's way.

THE SUCKLING PATTERN

When the milk lets down, every suck is accompanied by a swallow and a breath; one can hear this as the baby nurses: "suck-hah, suck-hah, suck-hah." Episodes of letting down and rhythmic swallowing may occur several times during a single feeding, often without the mother even being aware of the ebb and flow of her milk. The baby typically nurses in a burst of four to ten or so suckling movements, followed by a short rest, and then another burst of suckling.

From time to time during feedings, the baby may engage in bouts of what is called "nonnutritive" sucking, in which the jaw moves rapidly, almost in a quiver, and no swallowing occurs. Nonnutritive sucking is most likely to occur before the milk has let down, toward the end of the feeding, and when the baby is resting. Medical staff not well versed in breastfeeding sometimes regard this as unimportant or even undesirable behavior, a sign that the baby is "not interested in the breast," is "just fooling around," or has "finished feeding." In fact, nonnutritive sucking is a normal component of breastfeeding and has several important functions: It stimulates the breast into letting down, it rests some of the baby's facial muscles while strengthening others, and it seems to soothe the baby without causing drowsiness. Most of the feeding is swallowing behavior, however; babies who swallow initially for a few minutes and then spend long periods—twenty, thirty, forty minutes—in a nonnutritive sucking can tire themselves and make the breast sore. Changing to the other side and then back again may help.

BREASTS VS. BOTTLE: EVENTS DURING FEEDING

One widespread misconception about breastfeeding is that it is somehow more difficult for the infant than bottlefeeding; that the baby has to "work" to nurse. For example, the conventional wisdom and standard medical care in neonatal intensive facilities was, until very recently, that preterm babies, once they are able to suck and swallow—and thus no longer need to be fed by stomach tube—should be given the bottle until they have mastered those actions, because the bottle is "easier" than the breast. Additional justifications were that taking babies from the incubator would chill them—the bottle can be given in the incubator but the breast cannot; and that breastfeeding takes a long time, thus tiring babies.

Paula Meier, DNSc, professor of perinatal nursing at the University of Illinois College of Nursing, found sound scientific evidence to contradict all of these assumptions. While she was still a graduate student, Dr. Meier watched mothers breastfeeding tiny preterm babies in the neonatal intensive-care unit and realized that these mothers and babies appeared to be disproving the beliefs on which standard practice was based. One baby who had been fed his maximum estimated capacity of two ounces of milk, by stomach tube, at every meal, took five ounces the first time he was put on the breast. Other babies were able to co-ordinate sucking and swallowing on the breast before reaching the gestational age when they were supposed to be able to do that, and often long before they could cope with the bottle effectively.

Meier set out to discover whether babies really get chilled while breastfeeding. It was a straightforward task, since accurate instruments exist for measuring a baby's temperature externally. Meanwhile, Meier also used an external sensor, laid harmlessly on the baby's skin, to monitor the percentage of oxygen in the baby's bloodstream. This would provide a clear indication of how hard the baby might or might not be working. Because Meier and her colleagues took measurements from the same babies, over and over, as they went back and forth between breast and bottle feeds, each baby acted as his or her own research "control," or opposite number.

On the question of chilling, the researchers found that the preterm babies actually got warmer while they were out of the in-cubator and breastfeeding. Additional research has suggested some of the reasons. First, no matter how adroitly one warms the bottle, its contents will cool during the feeding. The baby, there-fore, will receive cool liquid right into the middle of the body, which must then be warmed to blood temperature by the baby himself, a costly expenditure of calories. Breast milk, on the other hand, stays at the baby's core temperature to the end of the feeding. The baby's oxygen levels stay normal. The baby can use periods of nonnutritive sucking at the breast, without relinquish-ing the breast. Breastfeeding is easier because babies can modify it for distress-free, organized feeding; they can't modify the flow of milk out of the bottle.

CHANGES WITH AGE

By the time a baby is six months old, her physical adaptations for breastfeeding are beginning to be replaced by adaptations for eating solid foods. The sucking pads diminish, to be largely gone by the end of the first year. Incoming teeth form the "leading edge" of each jaw, although the gum ridge may persist below and in front of the lower teeth for a while. (The baby's incoming teeth do not interfere with nursing, nor do they constitute a hazard for the mother; during feedings the tongue continues to cover the lower jaw, so that the baby cannot bite and nurse at the same time.)

The action of the tongue and jaws also changes. The tongue no longer protrudes automatically, so the baby no longer shoves solid food out of her mouth in an effort to swallow it. As the baby's hands come under control enough so that she can pick up a cracker or a piece of meat, her eating equipment develops enough to make use of such items. Even though the baby loses her infantile breast-feeding specializations, she can of course continue to feed at the breast. By six months, she has considerable know-how; she does not need special equipment to nurse efficiently and comfortably. And as long as she nurses, the breasts continue to function.

BABIES WITH DIFFICULTIES:
NEUROLOGICAL IMPAIRMENT

Some babies come into the world with an immature nervous system or other developmental problem that affects their ability to suckle. A baby may suckle weakly and tire easily, or the sucking response may be less vigorous than normal. Some babies may have difficulty coordinating sucking and swallowing, at first. Many techniques now exist for improving these motor patterns and in effect teaching the baby how to suck. A lactation consultant can show you techniques and devices that will help. One can expect improvement as the central nervous system matures further, muscles get stronger, and the baby learns compensatory movements. Developing breastfeeding skills in a neurologically immature baby or one with a neurological deficit is of special benefit, as the organizing of the mouth movement patterns stimulates reorganization of the rest of the nervous system. These babies profit from patient, consistent assistance by the mother and from ongoing encouragement of the mother and her family by health-care providers.

Some neurological deficits show up as behavioral difficulties. An example is the baby who persistently arches his back and rears away from the breast after latching on. This aggravating wrenching can be forestalled if the mother holds the child under one arm "football style" to nurse, and meanwhile sits in a chair with a firm back and puts the baby's rump against the chair, with his legs vertical and at right angles to his body; in this position he can't arch his back. He is also apt to become calm because this position supports his body in the same way it was supported in the uterus.

Many babies with developmental delays and other issues, including Down syndrome, can breastfeed very well. These babies have an acute need for the closeness and the physical and cognitive development benefits that breastfeeding can give.

BREASTFEEDING THE BABY WITH A CLEFT PALATE

The baby born with a cleft lip or palate may or may not present special breastfeeding problems. Unfortunately, many craniofacial surgeons and other physicians who care for these babies rarely see fully breastfed babies. Standard medical care dictates postponing repair surgery for weeks or months after birth, by which time, if the defect has caused nursing difficulties, the mother may have long ago given up trying to breastfeed. After surgery, cup- or spoon-feeding is usually recommended for a month or more, until the repair has healed. To quote specialist R.C.A. Weatherly-White, MD, of the Children's Hospital in Denver, in the plastic surgery textbooks, bottlefeeding is universally discouraged, and breastfeeding is not mentioned at all.

Dr. Weatherly-White's work, however, suggests that there are no disadvantages and many benefits to doing the repair surgery immediately, in the first week of birth, and then breastfeeding. He and his team undertook research to test the conventional prohibition against breastfeeding after they had made the initially disconcerting discovery that some of the mothers of babies who had been operated on in the first week of life had breastfed their postoperative babies without discussing it, and without problems. Their studies demonstrated that the baby with a cleft palate or lip may breastfeed immediately after surgery without endangering the sutures. A touching photograph in one research paper shows a nursing, postoperative newborn who is clearly in some pain but also clearly avid for the comfort of the breast. The Denver researchers found that the baby will recover faster on the breast, and cry less than he would otherwise—and crying does endanger the repair.

Other researchers continue to investigate the impact of breastfeeding on the baby with a cleft palate. Breast milk not only provides babies with superior nutrition, but the act of milking the breast strengthens the muscles and influences the shape of the infant's developing hard palate and jaw bones. This is why breastfed babies rarely require braces; it is also why breastfeeding is so helpful to the baby with a cleft lip or palate repair. Nursing provides physical therapy for the oral cavity that, along with surgery, helps it to grow strong and normally. Babies with cleft palate repairs tend to have a lot of ear infections. A couple of studies have begun to show that breastfeeding these babies—even *giving* them breast milk in a bottle—significantly reduces the number of infections they suffer.

THE TONGUE-TIED BABY

A little-recognized, but by no means rare, problem is the tongue-tied baby, born with a tongue that cannot be easily extruded from the mouth. All of us have a thin strip of tissue between the underside of the tongue and the floor of the mouth, called the "frenulum." As a rule, the frenulum is attached about halfway back on the underside of the tongue. In some people, however, the frenulum is either very short or attached close to the tip of tongue, holding the tip down. This tongue-tied condition, *Ankyloglossia* in medical parlance, makes it impossible for such a person to stick his tongue out and may cause speech impediments. Since the tongue cannot protrude properly over the lower jaw, being tongue-tied also makes it hard for a baby to latch on to the breast and make a good seal. In one study, 12.8 percent of newborns examined were tongue-tied to some degree.

A tongue-tied baby has trouble staying on the breast. He may have to clamp on ferociously, just to stay in place—making the baby tired and the mother's nipples sore. Tongue-tied babies tend to be noisy nursers, gasping and grunting, and sometimes messy, with milk leaking out of the mouth throughout the feeding. They also take a long time to get a meal down, and may either nurse extremely frequently, for long periods, or give up from fatigue before they're really full, and thus gain weight poorly.

A hundred years ago, doctors and midwives routinely inspected babies' tongues at birth and clipped the frenulum with sterile scissors if it was too short or situated too far forward, and thus apt to interfere with the baby's nursing. When bottlefeeding became the norm, and being tongue-tied makes no difference in bottlefeeding, medical students were no longer taught to clip the frenulum, or even to inspect it. It is still common for pediatricians to be unaware of the problem and its straightforward treatment.

The procedure of clipping a frenulum so that a baby can nurse unhindered is easily done in a physician's office; it produces only a drop or two of blood and causes almost no pain, especially if the baby is nursed immediately afterward. Parents with a tongue-tied baby can sometimes locate a dentist or oral surgeon familiar with the problem and willing to treat it. For the mother, the instant change from fierce to gentle nurser can be nothing short of amazing. For the baby, life becomes a lot easier right away.

Tongue-tiedness is genetic in origin; it runs in families. If you or your mate, as an adult, cannot protrude the tip of your tongue beyond your lips, it is something to watch for in your babies. A giveaway occurs when the baby tries to protrude her tongue; the tongue tip will dip into a V in the middle, like the top of a valentine heart, instead of coming to a point. (You can sometimes get even a tiny baby to stick out her tongue by sticking your own out at her, since most new babies, when alert, will mimic this behavior.)

One nurse practitioner who accepts many referrals of tongue-tied babies was asked by the parents of one if she would mind also clipping the frenulum of their six-year-old son. When she did so, the boy cheered, stuck out his newly liberated tongue, and danced up and down—now he could eat an ice cream cone like everyone else. In another case, a tongue-tied father asked for the same treatment. At the instant freeing of his tongue, he also announced that he was heading for the nearest ice cream shop—and then he was going to go home and, for the first time, properly kiss his wife.

JAUNDICE

In many medical environments, one essentially normal event in newborns can create special problems for the breastfeeding family: jaundice. In the late 1960s, the pediatric community began to focus much attention on the question of neonatal hyperbilirubinemia, or newborn jaundice. Most babies, breastfed or bottlefed, become slightly jaundiced in the first week of life. Sometimes the skin and eye whites temporarily take on a yellowish, or jaundiced tinge. The jaundice usually appears on or around the third day and is gone within a week or so. The majority of these babies are perfectly healthy. They are experiencing a normal physiological process, and need no medical therapy.

Unfortunately, misunderstandings of the nature of this process and its relationship to breastfeeding have led to customs of medical intervention that can seriously compromise lactation. Parents can't know in advance if their newborn will be affected by jaundice and how much. To make sound decisions, it is wise to understand normal newborn physiology before a baby is born, and why intervention is sometimes necessary, and sometimes not.

Red blood cells are constantly being created and reabsorbed in the body. As the red cells die and deteriorate, a waste product called "bilirubin" is formed. Until birth, the mother's body clears the fetal blood of most of the bilirubin via the placenta. After birth, bilirubin is excreted through the baby's liver into the intestines, and is evacuated along with the stool. In the very early days, as the newborn's body adjusts to life outside the uterus, this excretion does not happen completely. Some bilirubin is reabsorbed from the intestines into the blood. There may, in fact, be some evolutionary advantage to this transitory reabsorption, as bilirubin has an antibacterial effect in the bloodstream.

At birth, the baby's bowel contains a black, sticky stool called "meconium," which is loaded with bilirubin, giving it that blackish color. Normally, the laxative effects of colostrum start the intestinal tract moving in the right direction, and the meconium is eliminated. Although bilirubin continues to be excreted into the lower intestines, frequent feedings during the baby's first hours and days create more feces; the color of the feces changes from black to tan or yellow, indicating that the meconium is gone, and the frequent stooling continues to empty the intestines and to reduce the reabsorption of any bilirubin that might be there.

If the meconium is not eliminated, the bilirubin within it is reabsorbed by the bloodstream, creating a temporary overload of bilirubin in the baby's system. Other contributing sources of bilirubin in the newborn include bruising during birth, which creates pockets of red blood cells that must be broken down by the liver; vacuum extraction, a birth intervention, is particularly culpable in creating this condition. Medications given to the mother during late pregnancy or labor may also contribute, by passing through the placenta and temporarily overloading the waste-processing capabilities of the newborn's liver.

Jaundice caused by this unexcreted bilirubin is called "physiologic jaundice," meaning that it is a normal process and part of the baby's maturation. The duration of this postbirth period of physiologic jaundice, and the peak levels of bilirubin in the bloodstream, depend on one thing only: how often the baby's bowel movements empty, which is in itself a result of how soon and how often the baby is fed. In a landmark study on the genesis of neonatal jaundice, researcher M. de Carvalho and his associates found that the bilirubin levels of breastfed babies could be cut in half, bringing them lower than the levels typical of bottlefed babies, by feeding the babies every two hours instead of four.

In hospitals, unfortunately, breastfed babies are apt to be more jaundiced than bottlefed babies, not because of any flaw in breast milk, but because the hospital regimen interferes with breastfeeding. The mother and baby are not always encouraged, and sometimes not even permitted, to nurse early enough and often enough in the first three days for the baby to make and pass sufficient stools to avoid physiologic jaundice. Since the visibly jaundiced babies in those hospitals are so apt to be breastfed babies, some health-care providers refer to normal physiologic jaundice, somewhat misleadingly, as "breastfeeding jaundice." Babies who are, by nature, "sippers and tasters," and like to linger over feedings, or who are sleepy in the first few days after birth, are more likely to develop normal jaundice and to be treated for it.

Common jaundice associated with breastfeeding, which is really just physiologic jaundice aggravated by hospital interventions, is visible by the third day after birth. There is, however, a real and relatively rare genetic condition called "breast milk jaundice," in which elements in the mother's milk produce a milk jaundice that appears later than the third day, peaks in the second or third week, and may last for weeks or months. It appears to be related to the fat content of the milk, and may not show up until the mature milk develops. It will usually occur in 70 percent of subsequent breastfed siblings. The researchers who identified this syndrome emphasized that it is "thoroughly benign," and no cause for weaning.

Real pathologic jaundice, in any living organism, is a symptom of liver failure and, as such, is very serious indeed. The resulting huge overload of bilirubin can damage any organ, including the brain. The most serious newborn pathological jaundice is caused by Rh or ABO blood incompatibility and is apparent at birth or soon after; other serious causes of jaundice include congenital conditions such as hypothyroidism. The bilirubin level in such cases is in general far higher than that of babies experiencing normal or benign jaundice.

The differences are important and should determine treatment options. Too often, however, and despite recommendations to the contrary from the American Academy of Pediatrics, hospital staffs consider that jaundice is jaundice, and each case receives the same treatment regardless of the cause. One common treatment of the jaundiced newborn is to put the baby under special lights, the "bili lights," that contain some of the elements of sunshine. In the 1950s, an observant nurse noted that babies placed near the windows in the hospital nursery were less jaundiced than babies near the wall, a discovery that led to the present phototherapy treatment. Of course, putting the baby under the lights usually means more separation from the mother, which is deleterious to breastfeeding. Babies can also become dehydrated under the lights and thus be especially in need of frequent nursing.

The newborn breastfed baby should get at least twelve feedings in each twenty-four hours. Frequent feeding not only causes stooling, but coats the infant gut with milk fat, which protects against the reabsorption of bilirubin: To produce both stooling and gut coating, frequency of feedings is more important than the quantity ingested.

In some hospitals, the initial feeding at the breast is customarily delayed twelve to twenty-four hours after birth: Naturally, these babies will have elevated bilirubin levels by the third day.

Much of the published research about jaundice in breastfed babies was conducted in such hospitals. Lawrence Gartner, MD, chairman of the department of pediatrics at the University of Chicago, and a leading researcher on neonatal jaundice, points out that the babies in these studies were actually coping with problems caused not by breastfeeding, but by starvation.

Other hospital practices can contribute to elevated bilirubin levels, or hyperbilirubinemia. Sometimes sugar water is given to breastfeeding babies in the nursery in the mistaken notion that it will "flush out" the bilirubin, or in the belief that sugar water, or sucrose, benefits babies by calming them. Water, however, makes the situation worse, not better. Water increases urination, but bilirubin is not eliminated via the kidneys: Water intake also does not contribute to stooling and does not coat the gut. Water eliminates thirst and makes the baby feel full for a while; both reduce the urge to nurse. The baby gets less milk, and the mother's breasts get less of the stimulation so vital to starting lactation. Researcher A. J. Nicholls, MD, and others have shown in fact that water feeds in the hospital are directly correlated with increases in bilirubin levels. Feeding water to nursing babies also contributes directly to problems of engorgement in mothers.

What constitutes a "safe" bilirubin level? The age of the baby is a factor. In very small preterm babies, bilirubin levels acceptable in a more mature baby may be a justified worry. Babies differ genetically, too, in what is "normal." Caucasian and black babies, breastfed or bottlefed, tend to have bilirubin levels that peak on the third day, at perhaps 5 to 9 milligrams per deciliter of blood, gradually subsiding to the adult norm of about 1 milligram per deciliter by the fourteenth day. Children of Asian ancestry, on the other hand (including Native Americans and South American Indians), tend to have bilirubin levels that peak later (on the fifth day or so), peak higher (at 10 to 12 milligrams per deciliter in at least 30 percent), and last longer than in black or Caucasian babies. A nurse or physician who doesn't understand this may order drastic measures for a bilirubin count that for this particular genetic group is standard.

What is considered a "safe" level of bilirubin also varies widely from hospital to hospital and doctor to doctor. When and whether a physician calls for "bili lights" may depend on how recently he graduated from medical school. Older medical literature cautions concern when levels reach 10, 12, or 15 milligrams per deciliter; some newer studies suggest 20 to 25 as the level indicating a need for intervention. The question remains controversial among researchers and physicians, with one study's authors concluding in 2001: "At present we have no tools for ensuring identification of infants with increased vulnerability to bilirubin toxicity" and urging that "relaxed guidelines" be followed "in an atmosphere of increased vigilance." As a result, some doctors have "pet" numbers; some intervene in every possible case. Very few consider disrupting lactation in the first week of life as a severe intervention.

In fact, a very common treatment for jaundice is to tell the mother to stop breastfeeding for twenty-four or forty-eight hours, and to give the baby formula feeds during that time. Blood tests will usually show that the baby's bilirubin level falls as a result (which proves little except that breastfeeding was not yet well established). Of course the effect on the mother's lactation can be devastating; one cannot just "stop nursing" for twenty-four hours in the first days or weeks of lactation, as if stopping driving, or avoiding caffeine, or engaging in some other minor inconvenience. As Jay Gordon, MD, La Leche League medical board member, points out, a rise in bilirubin indicates a family with breastfeeding problems. The most important treatment is to help that mother and baby get the nursing going smoothly.

Some physicians defend the routine use of phototherapy on the grounds that it does the infant no harm. That is not entirely true. A study by Kathi Kemper, MD, and others at Yale–New Haven Hospital, found that after phototherapy for bilirubin not only were mothers twice as likely to stop breastfeeding, but many also concluded that the baby was extremely ill. This set the family up for what has been called the "vulnerable child" syndrome, a pattern of extremely anxious parenting—many doctor's visits, for example, and an unwillingness to let the child out of sight. This syndrome may continue for years, to the child's detriment.

Caught in this medical dilemma, what can mothers do? Sometimes the "bili lights" can be brought to the mother's hospital room; having the baby near may make them both feel better. New lights have been designed for use in a special fiber-optic blanket that can be wrapped around the baby's torso so that she can nurse while being treated at home or in the hospital. Home phototherapy is an increasingly accepted option for babies with elevated but not severe bilirubin levels. Mothers who are forced to stop breastfeeding for a day or two can pump their milk, and should be taught how, lent a hospital-grade pump, and given informed support.

Kathleen Auerbach, PhD, while assistant professor of pediatrics at the University of Chicago Medical School, used a much simpler intervention in that university's large teaching hospital. When a baby was reported as jaundiced, Dr. Auerbach visited the mother during breastfeeding and provided the baby with a little additional formula though a nursing supplementer tube slipped into his mouth while he was on the breast. Often this needed to be done only two or three times to increase a baby's caloric intake while a mother's milk supply was being established, without decreasing time at the breast. The mother felt encouraged about breastfeeding, the baby was reinforced for suckling, and the mother's milk supply soon increased. Meanwhile, the supplement usually improved the rate of stooling, which brought the bilirubin down; that, Dr. Auerbach points out, had the principal effect of reassuring the medical staff, thus forestalling less amiable intervention.

DIFFERENCES BETWEEN BREASTFED AND BOTTLEFED BABIES

Lactation researchers such as Niles Newton, PhD, have pointed out that there are many obvious differences between the healthy breastfed baby and the healthy bottlefed baby; one can learn to tell them apart at a glance. The bottlefed baby is apt to be pallid and plump, with soft muscles. The breastfed baby has a glowing skin, even in winter, and good muscle tone; her body feels resilient when you pick her up. Some of these differences are no doubt due to general health; the breastfed baby is less likely to be coming down with or recovering from some germ, and less likely to look washed-out because of allergies and stomach upsets. But there are some fundamental physical differences, too.

For example, breastfed and bottlefed babies smell different. An artificially fed baby may smell sour, like curdled formula; his soiled diapers smell the way we expect diapers to smell, and if he spits up, his clothes (and his mother's) may carry a vomity odor. Breastfed babies have a distinctly sweet odor, so attractive and cuddly that it has been roughly imitated in scented talcum powder. Even the smell of their soiled diapers is not unpleasant; both their stools and spit-up smell a little like yogurt.

Breastfed babies grow and gain weight differently from babies fed formula. Breastfed babies often gain faster in the first three months and more slowly thereafter. Some babies, in fact, gain very fast at first, then slow down and grow into their weight; one nurse practitioner reports on a favorite (fully breastfed) patient, "Daniel the Porkchop," who weighed eight pounds at birth and twenty pounds at three months, but then eased up this galloping gain by six months and reached a comfortable twenty-five pounds at one year. Often by the end of the first year, breastfed babies weigh less than bottlefed babies, on the average; but typically the breastfed baby then follows a slow but steady growth curve that extends further into childhood. The bottlefed baby is often actually overweight, since he may take in more calories than he needs in an effort to get adequate nutrition. This tendency toward heaviness lasts past weaning, as four- and six-year-olds who have never been nursed are 50 percent more likely to be obese than children who were nursed for a year.

Breastfed babies tend to be more active than bottlefed babies. They tend to sit, creep, and stand a little earlier, and they have more vigor, on average, from the start. In one study, breastfed babies tested on the third or fourth day of life showed stronger arousal reactions than bottlefed babies. Another test found more physical activity in general by the sixth day of life. Several studies have shown that on the whole, breastfed babies sleep less than formula-fed babies. From the first months, the length of maximum bouts of sleep tends to be shorter (since the baby must and should waken after four or five hours to be fed). From seven months on, the total number of hours that the baby spends asleep, per twenty-four hours, dwindles. In one study, in which mothers kept daily diairies, bottlefed babies were sleeping fourteen hours out of twenty-four at thirteen months, and breastfed babies were sleeping eleven. This might sound like a disadvantage to the parents who want a little peace from a fussy baby and are glad when he goes down for a three-hour nap. But extra waking hours are valuable to the baby, giving him that much more time in the day to learn, to stretch muscles and mind, to socialize, to grow mentally as well as physically.

The exception to the normal picture of the healthy breastfed baby is the baby who is not getting enough milk, which, in the United States, can be an unfortunate result of lack of support for the mother and misinformation about lactation. The hungry baby is pale, and lacks the snap and cheeriness of the satisfied nursling. He may be fretful and cry often, or he may be lethargic, sleeping for longer and longer periods. He has less than three stools a day, and, if a newborn, may not have regained his birth weight by the tenth day. Such a baby and his mother need the help of a lactation consultant to investigate the reasons for breastfeeding problems leading to insufficiency. In almost all cases, these problems can be resolved and breastfeeding can continue to the benefit of both mother and baby.

Another difference between breastfed and formula-fed babies has become well documented. Children who were breastfed perform better on cognitive tests—IQ tests and other measurements of brain function—than children who were formula fed. The differences are most significant among preemies or babies who were of very low birth weight (known as "small for gestational age," or SGA), yet can be measured among all groups. The increase in cognitive development seems to be dose related; that is the longer a baby is breastfed, the higher his IQ score tends to be at a later age. Several studies pinpointed the type of fats found in breast milk, DHA and AA, as the elements that make this difference, and formula manufacturers duly added similar compounds to "enhanced" formulas. As research continues, however, evidence suggests that even these enhanced formulas do not equalize the long-term results between the two groups. Researchers at the Institute of Child Health in London reported in 2004 that the increase in physical growth shown in SGA babies who received the new enhanced formulas "was not matched by a neurodevelopmental advantage," and concluded "that breastfeeding may be especially beneficial for neurodevelopment in children born SGA."

GROWTH RATES

Officially, in most countries, the standard infant growth charts are based on the Caucasian, middle-class, formula-fed baby, and they present an incorrect picture for exclusively breastfed babies, babies who are not fed solids until they are four to six months of age, and babies of ethnic ancestry other than Caucasian. Several studies, including the 1992 Davis Area Research on Lactation, Infant Nutrition, and Growth (the DARLING study), have compared the growth patterns of breastfed and formula-fed babies for the first eighteen months of life.

Their current data show that, overall, breastfed babies initially gain weight more rapidly than formula-fed babies, but from the third or fourth month through the eighteenth month, they gain weight more slowly. As older children and teenagers, the breastfed group catches up; the height one reaches is dependent to some extent on genes but also on diet after weaning. People grow taller if the food supply is constant and abundant. For example, between 1920 and 1960, children of the second and third generations born to Japanese immigrants in Hawaii almost always grew much taller than their Japan-born parents and grandparents.

Still, during the nursing years, breastfed children are on the whole smaller than their bottlefed counterparts. It does not affect their health, development, or ultimate growth, and so seems to be nature's intention. Why? Researcher Margaret Neville, PhD, at the University of Colorado, asked a vital question: Is it indeed the mother's milk production that determines the breastfed baby's growth during the first year or is some other factor operating?

What Neville and her associates found, in an ingenious series of tests, is that breastfeeding mothers can almost always make more milk than their babies need (as we know). What limits the baby's growth is her own demand—her appetite. When one is giving a baby a bottle, there is always a temptation to get the baby to "finish the bottle" by jiggling the bottle until the last half-ounce goes down. But on the breast, no one sees how much went in, and only the baby can tell exactly how much she wants; when she's satisfied, she takes no more. The breastfed baby thus takes the optimum amount of milk, not the maximum possible. Contrary to our widespread assumption that bigger is better, evolution has perhaps developed human babies for whom "enough is as good as a feast." Our babies come into the world, it seems, as ecologically sound consumers.

Unfortunately, our medical definition of a healthy baby is one growing as much as she could, not one growing just as she should. Until 2001, all pediatricians relied on the same growth charts to track a baby's height and weight from birth through the age of two. These standards for infant growth, set by the National Center for Health Statistics, are based on a study published in 1976 that collected data on babies from 1929 to 1975, the vast majority of whom were bottlefed and fed solid foods within the first four months of life.

For decades, lactation consultants and breastfeeding advocates have protested the use of these growth charts as an inappropriate method of assessing the growth of the breastfed infant. Too many mothers of breastfed babies have been told, as their babies' rate of growth slows around the sixth month, that according to the chart at the pediatrician's office their babies "are not gaining sufficiently." The concern often leads to a mistaken belief that a baby is not thriving on breast milk, that formula is needed, that somehow a mother overlooked her baby's nutritional needs and did not provide optimum care. All these assumptions are false, and all are caused by outdated, inaccurate, unquestioned statistical charts. Change is on the way, however, as new charts that reflect the normal healthy growth of the fully breastfed baby have been researched and have been made available to pediatricians as of 2001.

How the Baby Functions: Behavior

INNATE BEHAVIOR IN BABIES

Many of us were once taught that human beings, unlike animals, are not governed by instinct, but we learn most of our traits and behavior though external events—as if we came into this world as blank chalkboards, waiting to be written on. We once believed that newborns are little more than bundles of primitive reflexes. We now understand, however, thanks to the work of Marshall Klaus, T. Berry Brazelton, and other developmental researchers, that from the moment of birth, babies are individuals able to respond, interact, and learn. They are provided not only with suitable physical equipment, but also with a wonderful assortment of innate, or inborn, behavioral skills, including a surprising amount of built-in social behavior, to help them survive and thrive in their new world.

There are several varieties of innate behavior. Simple motor patterns triggered by external stimuli—coughing and sneezing, for example—are called reflexes. The grasp of an infant's hand, which will close automatically on anything that touches the palm, is a reflex. A more complex level of innate behavior consists of motor patterns produced in response to internal or external stimuli. Facial expressions and some vocalizations, for example, are expressed automatically in response to feelings, and in turn are recognized as social signals by others. Much innate behavior consists of combinations of reflexes and motor patterns into which learned behavior is quickly interwoven.

Some innate behavior shows up at birth; other innate patterns, such as those related to sexual activity, surface when they are needed later in life. An example is the following response. Once a baby has learned to walk well, he is likely to follow anyone moving suddenly away from him; he is compelled by an innate urge. If you move quickly away from a creeping baby, he will quietly watch you go. Move quickly away from the same child, now a run-about two-year-old, and he will make haste to follow you and, if he cannot keep up, will burst into roars of protest. You need not be a parent to elicit this automatic response; one can sometimes see a toddler, frustrated by the sight of older children running past him in play, screaming furiously until someone picks him up. The utility of this response is obvious. The toddler, old enough to stray but not old enough to keep up with adults on foot, is thus protected from being overlooked and abandoned if his elders suddenly decide to go somewhere else.

Biologists have found that behavior crucial to survival for individuals or for a species, such as an infant's ability to attract attention or adult reproductive behavior, is particularly likely to be innate. In mammals that includes infant suckling. A newborn colt, for example (or any baby hooved animal), is programmed to get to its feet as soon after birth as possible. Innate mechanisms then dictate that it will move toward the nearest large object and make shoving motions with its nose. The nearest large object is likely to be its mother. Shoving along the mother's flank, the baby will shortly be blocked by a leg; if that is a front leg, the mother eventually will respond to the shoving by moving, and the baby will have to start over. If it is a hind leg, the shoving will bring the baby's lips in contact with the udder. Presto! Breakfast. It doesn't take the colt long to *learn* to go straight to the udder, and to the right mother, as well. But the first motions that get it on the path to survival are dictated by its genes just as surely as are the color of its coat and the number of ears and legs it comes with.

Primate babies have a number of innately urged actions to help them find food. When a baby chimpanzee is born, it immediately grasps whatever it can with its hand and starts to crawl. Since it usually grasps the hair on its mother's abdomen, its crawling takes the baby chimp up her body, with or without her help, to her breasts. A newborn human baby shares with other primates the habit of clenching his fists, especially when hungry, and of shoving his feet in a "neonate crawl." If left quietly on his mother's abdomen after birth, a baby just minutes old will crawl up to her breast, pushing his legs into her abdomen to propel himself. While moving up, he may turn his head from side to side. Drawn by the scent of amniotic fluid on the nipple, he opens his mouth widely and, after several attempts, grasps the areola of the nipple. (Pain medications given to a mother during birth may keep her baby too sleepy after birth to exhibit this behavior.) Like the baby chimp, he grasps tightly in his fists any part of his mother's clothes or anatomy he may come in contact with. This further ensures that he will not lose contact with the breast. (Many a newborn baby seem to nurse more steadily and happily if they are holding something—their mother's finger or a lock of hair—in their fist.)

INNATE RESPONSES IN BREASTFEEDING

To locate the right place to suckle, the human baby, like other young mammals, has a "grope" reflex. In the newborn human, it consists of turning his head and "reaching" with his mouth in the direction of any touch on his cheek. If his mother picks him up, his head is apt to fall into the crook of his mother's arm, bringing the breast near his cheek. When the nipple touches his cheek, he swivels his head toward the touch. If the whole breast bumps his cheek, providing generalized stimulation, he may shake his head back and forth very fast as if to home in on the stimulus.

Once the baby has located the breast, another reflex comes into play; a touch on the center of his lower lip makes the baby gape his jaw. Thus, even an accidental touch of the nipple in the center of the lip, as the baby gropes for the breast, produces exactly the right wide-open mouth for optimal latching on. The mother helping her newborn get started at the breast can lift her breast with her free hand and move the nipple to trigger the opening of the mouth on purpose.

Some lactation specialists teach new mothers to touch the nipple to the baby's lower lip so that the baby opens wide, and then to quickly pull the baby in close, plopping that wide-open mouth right onto the breast; this helps forestall the baby's learning to latch on to the breast with his mouth half open, or to grasp the nipple first and then "walk up" the breast with his jaws, both of which increase the likelihood of nipple soreness.

In our culture, women don't always have a chance to see other mothers nursing, and thus to learn from observation how to hold a baby in an optimal nursing position. An inexperienced mother may let the baby lie horizontally in her arms, as we do when we bottlefeed a baby; that is the feeding position she has seen most often, after all. At the breast, though, a baby lying flat on his back has to turn his head to nurse; the result is a baby that is valiantly trying to nurse while looking over his shoulder and inevitably tugging on the nipple itself, causing abrasion. Or the mother may hold the baby too low, so that his head is tilted back instead of facing the breast squarely. This is a highly awkward position in which to swallow—try it yourself—and again puts uneven and abrasive pressure on the areola and nipple.

Proper positioning at the breast, beginning with observing and understanding the innate reflexes already in place to help the baby get started, prevents a host of tiny problems that may interfere with establishing breastfeeding.

THRESHOLDS

The strength of responses such as groping and latching on, and the ease with which they are produced, can vary. A hungry baby will respond to a touch on the cheek or mouth far more vigorously than a full one; psychologists say that his "threshold" to the stimulus of touch has been lowered. A really hungry and vigorous baby may suck anything that touches his lips, such as his father's arm. There are also individual differences in the strength of the suckling responses, which are subject to the same variations as are all the other hereditary features of living creatures. One baby never gropes or gapes very strongly, and the mother must patiently teach him to latch on. Another baby turns toward the slightest touch, and the brush of his baby blanket on his cheek may make him turn and grope frantically.

An accidental light touch on the cheek may continue to induce a groping response in such a child for years. The 1960s version of a reality television show, *Candid Camera*, once showed a pretty woman "accidentally" annoying a man sitting next to her by letting the long feathers on her boa hat brush his face. The man was trying to be polite, to ignore the tickling feathers, and make conversation; but every time a feather brushed his cheek, he unconsciously opened his mouth and turned his head toward the touch. It was the grope reflex, still operative in the grown man.

External circumstances can also alter a baby's response threshold temporarily. Pain medications given to a mother during labor may dull or confuse her baby's reflexes for the first few days of life. A baby who has been allowed to wake and cry until she is really ravenous may have such a low threshold that she can't organize herself sufficiently for an innate reflex to operate. These babies tend to do better if nursed at the first peep of wakefulness or at early signs of hunger, such as rooting around and thrusting the tongue out, before prolonged crying disorganizes the baby completely.

LEARNING IN THE NEWBORN

Babies arrive with a little advance information; they have done some learning in the womb. For example, researchers have shown that newborns can identify and recognize their own mother's—although not their father's—voice, from birth. They have learned, already, something abut the cadences of their own language; newborns whose mothers read a particular story aloud, repeatedly, from birth, appear to perk up and listen carefully to the tale being read after birth by another voice, showing that they recognize its familiar sounds. (They even show a preference for familiar stories by sucking more while hearing it than when listening to a new story.) Babies in the uterus have also gotten used to other noises in their environment. Pregnant women who live near airports are apt to give birth to babies who are not wakened by the sound of jet planes landing and taking off. They are even introduced to the popular culture of their birth place. A British researcher found that newborns whose mothers regularly watched a popular soap opera during pregnancy stopped crying when they heard the show's theme song, while babies whose mothers were not fans of the show did not respond to the song at all. The surprisingly keen hearing of newborns, and preference for familiar sounds, assists them in locating and focusing on the sound of their mother's voice right from the beginning.

Babies learn as much before birth through their sense of smell as they do by listening, and rely on it far more after birth. In utero they are bathed in amniotic fluid that has a scent created by their mother's diet, environment, and genetics. Able to use their sense of smell from the twenty-eighth week of pregnancy on, they know their mother's unique scent as well as her voice, and after birth are drawn to it. A newborn baby will turn his head toward a pad soaked in his mother's breast milk, and away from a pad that carries the scent of a stranger's breast milk. While turning his head toward the source of dinner is clearly a useful skill, a baby also finds simple comfort in the all-over scent of his mother, whether he is breathing in the odor from her breasts, neck, underarms, or a recently worn garment.

Much else that newborns do is innate and spontaneously manifested, without any additional learning through experience being necessary. Crying, startling, yawning, and squinting at bright lights are all responses that are programmed into the genes, or, in the scientists' usage, are "hard-wired." A lot more behavior in human babies is partly innate and partly learned, and is capable of being modified or "soft-wired." The suckling pattern is a good example. Some elements of it are innate—groping, moving the tongue appropriately, and swallowing. Others—how wide to open the mouth, how the lips behave—must be learned, and for good reason. Mothers and breasts come in many sizes and shapes, and babies must be flexible enough to adapt their nursing behavior to their own mother's body. For the breastfed baby, this very first experience of life involves learning and discovering. This kind of active learning—finding out how to attain your own goals by your own efforts, how to make the world work for you, instead of just passively enduring events—contributes mightily to launching and guiding a baby's cognitive development. Current research on the question of why fully breastfed babies perform better on cognitive performance tests than formula-fed babies focuses on the composition of breast milk, and on nutritional elements that may enhance brain development. Future research may look into the action of breastfeeding itself, and how babies' involved, multilayered experience of breastfeeding contributes to their ultimate intellect. At the very least, it is clear that the happily breastfed baby starts life with a huge experience of his own capacity for attaining life's joys.

NIPPLE CONFUSION

Lactation consultants and other breastfeeding-savvy professionals have long been concerned about causing "nipple confusion" if a newborn is given a few meals with a rubber-nippled bottle as well as at his mother's breast. Feeding from a rubber nipple requires a completely different movement of the baby's tongue, lips, and jaw than does nursing at a breast. To keep air out and milk in, the baby must purse his lips as if he were whistling, rather than open his mouth wide, as if about to shout. If the milk flows

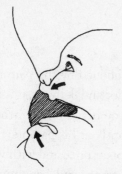
Figure 5.1 The baby's mouth, tongue, and jaw positions during breastfeeding.

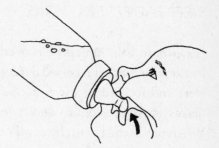
Figure 5.2 The baby's mouth, tongue, and jaw positions during bottlefeeding.

continuously and fast, the baby must stop sucking in order to breathe. Many babies quickly learn to pull the tongue back into the mouth and plug up the nipple, to stop the constant flow. As nursing is a learned action, spurred by innate urges, will simultaneously learning to feed on a rubber nipple confuse the beginning nurser? If a baby refuses the breast but accepts a bottle, many lactation consultants believe, it may be because the mouth shape and movements learned first on a bottle don't work for breastfeeding. Controlled studies have yet to identify "nipple confusion" as the cause of a baby refusing to nurse, but have shown that babies fed with bottles or given pacifiers in the first week of life are more likely to be weaned before they are a month old. Even without absolute proof of the existence of nipple confusion, lactation consultants and the World Health Organization are sufficiently concerned about its likelihood to recommend that if supplementary feedings are needed in the first week of life, they be given to the baby by cup or spoon, and that pacifiers be avoided altogether.

SLEEP AND REST PATTERNS

A newborn baby, unless he is overly subdued by the pain medications his mother received during labor and delivery, is usually
alert and focused in the first couple of hours after birth. He
makes active eye contact and stares raptly at his parents' faces.
When put to the breast, he may latch on at once and with vigor,
or he may lick and play, showing interest and beginning to
learn. The skin-to-skin contact they share as the baby nestles to
his mother's breast and nurses for the first time, enveloped in
each other's scent and presence, is unlike any other experience
in life.

This initial, early meeting is a powerful one. And yet, if a
mother and baby cannot spend the first couple of hours after
birth caught in each other's rapture, they'll catch up later.
Maternal-infant attachment among primates is not an "imprinting" process, the way it is among birds and other animals. No
studies have shown that mothers and babies who do not experience this initial birth-propelled period of bonding become any
less attached to each other than those who do. We take a long
time to develop our rich relationships. Studies have shown, however, that if a mother and baby are able to take full advantage of
this natural period of alertness, their first days together in the
hospital tend to run more smoothly. The baby is more likely to
begin nursing easily, and his mother is more likely to feel comfortable caring for him.

This early wakeful period is followed by a sleepy period,
in which both mother and baby can rest from the birth experience. This may last two to twenty hours. The newborn
may then begin to nurse every two hours or so. Research shows

that parents can also expect one or more episodes of "cluster" feeding, in which six or seven feedings take place within a three-hour period. The baby may nurse twenty minutes, rest twenty to forty minutes, and then nurse again. Following home births, one or more episodes of cluster feeding tend to occur soon after birth. In hospital births, perhaps due to the pervasive use of various medications during labor, cluster feedings will occur somewhat later.

Cluster feedings tend to occur at night. After a bout of cluster feeding, the baby will go into a deep sleep, often for several hours. To the parents, it may seem that the baby "was up all night and wanted to nurse constantly," as the cluster feeding took place from midnight to 3:00 a.m. The baby's subsequent several hours of deep sleep may then coincide with the hours when the parents must be waking up to tend to other children or get ready for their day.

Frequent nocturnal feedings may serve in the early weeks to establish breastfeeding and plentiful milk production. Prolactin, one of the milk-making hormones, peaks in its levels during the night. Cluster feedings at night ensure that the breasts are sufficiently stimulated to bring a mother's milk in as soon after birth as possible.

These nocturnal tendencies may be attributed to the fact that the newborn comes into the world with a well-established temporal pattern of activity and rest periods, based on maternal activity before birth. During the daylight hours, when a mother is walking about, her movements gently lull the baby to sleep. At night, when the mother is still, the baby wakes up and moves around; nighttime kicking bouts are a familiar complaint of pregnancy. When the baby is born, for the first few days or weeks, it may stay on "uterine time," to the dismay of the rest of the family. As the early weeks pass, most babies begin to pick up on the cues of light and dark that govern the rest of us, as long as they are roused often for feeding during the day.

STATES OF ALERTNESS

It seems obvious that one can tell at a glance whether a baby is awake or asleep. Researchers, however, have found that newborns actually exhibit many states of awareness. Marshall Klaus, MD, has named these states "quiet alert," "active alert," drowsy, crying, light sleep, and deep sleep. Parents soon learn the difference between light sleep and deep sleep, because if you put down a dozing baby too soon, she will cry. The alert states are less obvious. During the quietly alert phase, babies are content to look and listen, absorbing the universe; the actively alert stage is good for socializing and play. Family members who are inattentive to these stages may attempt to play too vigorously when the baby is drowsy, or leave her to cry when she is in a quietly alert state and would be calmed not by food or sleep, but by a chance to see what's going on around her.

Remarkably, babies seem to be able to control their levels of alertness and receptiveness, in the interest of self-preservation. While some babies relish all kinds of stimulation right from birth, others seem to be swamped by receiving too many intense sensations at once. These are the babies who may nurse better in a darkened room, who may cry out at loud noises, or who just don't enjoy being jostled or passed around. Such babies may simply "shut down" if the world becomes too eventful; they may appear to be asleep when in fact they have withdrawn temporarily from sensory overload.

INDIVIDUALITY

The behavioral doctrine that personality and social behavior are created by life experience has put an unfair burden on parents through the years. Now, partly from studies of identical twins raised separately, scientists agree that babies are individuals from birth, and that genetics has at least as much influence over what we do and who we become as does environment. Our temperaments are inborn, although the way in which they are revealed is very much affected by life experience.

Mothers, of course, have known this all along. Every baby manifests its own individual style from birth. Some are frustrated easily and express their discomforts; others are consistently calm. Some meet new experiences head on, and others seem to pull back and think things over from a distance. Some seem to love lights and noise and activity, while others get rattled and cry out, or shut down, if the world is too stimulating.

Nowhere are these newborn differences more apparent than in the breastfeeding interaction. Some babies are very businesslike; others—mothers call them the "gourmets"—taste and play between small bouts of more focused activity at the breast. Some are impatient and can't wait for even an instant to start nursing, while others dawdle. Each baby will interact with his mother differently, and personality clashes are possible. A patient mother and an impatient baby make a workable combination, for example, but an impatient mother with a leisurely baby may have some learning of her own to do.

EXPRESSING EMOTION

The newborn baby communicates in many ways besides crying. Facial expressions, for example, are present from birth. It was once believed that human facial expressions are learned rather than innate. If that were true, a newborn's facial expressions could not possibly "mean" anything. Ethologists, who study the evolution of human behavior in its natural setting, have demonstrated that facial expressions are genetically governed signals, conveying our feelings and emotional states; the great majority of these facial "gestures" are common to all humanity. Cultural fashions and learned behavior may be an added overlay, of course. For example, among the New Zealand Maoris, sticking your tongue out is a warrior's threat; in parts of China, that same gesture indicates surprise; and in the United States, a tongue thrust out expresses derision. But in any country and in all human tribes, most facial expressions are the same. An angry man scowls, a frightened child widens the eyes, people who are joking raise their eyebrows, and so on.

Still, when regarding a small baby in our arms, we try not to credit what our eyes and instincts tell us. Seeing a tiny smile crease a newborn's lips, a mother may say, "Look! She's smiling!" and then quickly correct herself—"I know, it's just gas . . ." It may not be fair to babies, however, to maintain that these fleeting expressions "don't mean anything." The newborn smile is not yet an intentional social smile, but it is triggered by pleasure—a smile of satiety and comfort. Similarly, the expressions of perplexity, wonder, curiosity, misery, and bliss that flit across the newborn face are innate responses to the baby's feelings of the instant, and convey the same meanings that they would in any person. Babies may not be aware of their emotions until six or seven months, but they certainly have emotions right from the beginning. Mothers and fathers can see the baby's tiny expressions and respond to them; when the baby's face suggests emotions of interest and friendliness, it's "only natural"—an innate tendency—for parents to feel interest and friendliness right back. Researchers Marshall and Phyllis Klaus write, "The facial expressions of newborns are strikingly similar across all cultures. It seems that when expressing the common emotions of fear, sadness, joy, disgust, and anger, the human face speaks a universal language."

THE SENSES: WHAT BABIES SEE

While babies are able to hear and taste quite well at birth, their sense of sight is less well developed. The visual world for newborns is a blurry place. Their only point of clarity rests about eight inches from their eyes; the rest of the room disappears into a fuzzy haze. As it happens, eight inches is the distance between a nursing baby's face and his mother's face; all he needs to see right now are his mother's eyes, and other nearby faces.

Indeed, faces are a baby's favorite sight in these early weeks. They are more interested in patterns (two dots and a line) that resemble a human face. They will look longer at a smiling pattern than at a frowning pattern. They are most intrigued by real faces, and can make steady eye contact from birth.

Babies can not only see their caregivers' faces, but can respond to their facial expressions. They are wonderful mimics, in fact. If, in talking to a small baby (less than a month old), you open your mouth wide, after a short pause the baby will open her mouth wide, too. Raised eyebrows, a smile, a squinched-up nose—all these will produce tiny but strenuous efforts in the same direction. Perhaps the easiest facial mimicry to demonstrate is sticking out the tongue; do this to a very young baby and, if the baby is watching and in the mood (i.e., the quiet alert state), the baby will stick out her tongue, too. She may become still and transfixed with fascination, or she may wriggle all over in her effort to create what she is seeing. It may take her several visible false tries. You are observing an innate response—that is, looking at facial expressions and the urge to imitate them—combined with learning: Yes, I see what you're doing, but *how* do I get my face to do that?

Gradually, experience connects the visual wires in a baby's brain; building the astonishing ability to see close up and far away; to see every shade of color; to perceive shape, texture, depth, and motion; to identify even never-before-seen objects; and to coordinate what the hand does with what the eyes see. By six months, most babies fully enjoy the richness of visual detail in the world around them.

WHAT BABIES HEAR

Babies begin hearing sound long before they are actually born; just ask anyone who has been to a rock concert when they were more than six months pregnant—some babies kick so hard at the amplified sound that the mother has to leave. Of course, the primary sound in the baby's amniotic pool is her mother's heartbeat. It has been found that a low tone, broadcast at a rate of about eighty beats per minute, is soothing to babies in hospital nurseries. The tone simulates the maternal heartbeat, which has dominated each infant's experience for nine months, and which would still be present were she lying next to or near her mother.

Low-pitched sounds cross the placental barrier to the baby before birth better than high-pitched sounds. The exception is the baby's mother's voice, which may be higher than other sounds in his world—his father's voice, for example—but comes from within his mother's body. It is no surprise, then, that after birth the sound of his mother's voice catches and keeps his attention better than any other.

After birth, high-pitched sounds are easier for babies to hear than low sounds. That may be one reason why we tend to talk to babies in high-pitched voices. Slow-motion filming has shown that babies do more than listen to our voices. They dance. One can easily observe a wide-awake, comfortable baby wriggling and waving his arms when his mother talks to him. What only the camera can show is that these movements are made in rhythm with his mother's speech, and follow the tempo of her stresses and pauses as if the singsong chat in which mothers indulge were music. To a baby's ears, it probably is the most beautiful music in the world.

SMELL AND TASTE

The amniotic fluid in which a baby bathes before birth is uniquely scented and flavored by the mother's diet, genetics, and environment. From the end of the first trimester, when fetal taste buds mature, to the end of pregnancy, developing babies suck, swallow, and taste amniotic fluid. From the twenty-eighth week of pregnancy on, odors from their mother's environment can be detected in the uterine bath.

Research has shown that the familiar taste and scent of the mother's amniotic fluid help a newborn recognize his mother after birth. Immediately after birth, a baby prefers to nurse on a breast moistened with amniotic fluid, and is calmed simply by the scent of it. One study suggests that unwashed babies are better organized—more able to bring their hands to their mouths and self-soothe—than babies who have been washed clean of amniotic fluid.

Just as her amniotic fluid has been flavored and scented by the dominant flavors in her diet—whether garlic, soy, or paprika—so has a mother's milk. When a baby nurses for the first time, he revisits a familiar buffet of spices and oils. Her breast milk's odor is as unique, recognizable, and comforting to her baby as its taste. Within a few days of birth, a baby recognizes and turns toward the unique scent of his mother's milk, and will turn away from the scent of a stranger's breast milk.

Recent research provides evidence that mothers are also uncannily skilled at recognizing their babies' scent. In one study, mothers of one-day-old babies were presented with three T-shirts recently worn by three newborns, and could correctly and quickly identify the little shirt worn by their own babies. It is known that during pregnancy, a woman's odor changes, becoming a blend of her own and that of her fetus, as odor is a result of genetics as much as diet. Mothers, apparently, have some familiarity with the scent of their own babies long before birth.

THE SENSE OF TOUCH

The experience of being touched and held is essential to infant growth and development for all mammalian babies. Without it, mammals lose their ability to become social animals. Rats that receive no handling from infancy become savage, while the rats that are handled daily are placid and tame, even when the daily handling is followed by an electric shock. In the classic experiment by researcher Harry Harlow at the University of Wisconsin, baby rhesus monkeys raised in the company of a "mother" made of bare chicken wire with a baby bottle of milk attached would go to "her" for food, but spent the rest of their time cowering in a corner, and screamed with fear at any change in their environment. The monkeys raised with "mothers" made of padded chicken wire that didn't supply food nevertheless clung to the soft padding, like baby monkeys do to real monkey mothers, investigated new objects with normal monkey curiosity, and showed fairly normal development. The ability to touch their mothers, rather than to derive nourishment from her, allowed the second group of monkeys to survive mentally intact.

The skin of a new human baby is far more sensitive than that of an adult. It flushes and mottles at every sensation. The whole skin is a sense organ, especially aware of contact with someone else's body. A fretful newborn can often be soothed if one merely holds him, naked, against one's own bare skin. For many months after birth, a baby's mouth also functions as a primary organ for sensing by touch, as if it were an extra hand. Any new object to be investigated is not only held and looked at, but mouthed. The infant's mouth has been described as the center of his neurological functioning; as the oral patterns of behavior come into synchrony, the rest of the nervous system follows.

The sense of touch also tells the baby about his position relative to gravity, whether he is still or moving, and whether he is being held tightly or loosely: this is called the "kinesthetic sense." It is through the baby's kinesthetic awareness, through being touched and moved and handled, that a baby first locates himself and makes contact with reality. It may be that the need for physical contact is especially acute during the critical period of the first hours and days after birth, when we so often isolate babies. To replace the warmth of body contact and the snugness of uterine existence, babies in hospital nurseries are often swaddled, or wrapped tightly in blankets, so that their arm and leg movements are restrained. Indeed, swaddled babies cry less than unwrapped babies. Babies carried in front packs or slings, rather than strollers or carriages, fuss less as they are enveloped in the touch, scent, and motion of their mothers' bodies.

Breastfeeding, of course, necessitates a great deal of simple physical contact between mother and child. Breastfed babies are likely to be carried about more by their mothers and everyone else in the family (who model their care of the baby on what Mother does). Carrying the baby, or as some mothers say, "wearing the baby," in a pack or sling not only calms him, but offers the additional benefit that he is able to see and learn about the world from an adult's height and viewpoint, where all the interesting action takes place, rather than from the knee-level viewpoint of a stroller. Breastfeeding mothers are more likely to buck the cultural influences to teach babies to be "independent," an idea that leads to leaving babies in cribs and playpens, feeding them with plastic bottles, picking them up as little as possible, and pushing them in chairs at arm's length.

Prolonged and frequent body contact with adults may contribute to self-regulation of the baby's physical functions. We have seen that body heat is affected by close contact; the infant's heart rate and breathing may also be stimulated and regulated by close contact with others. Breastfed babies, for example, are much less likely to show periods of apnea (pauses in breathing) during deep sleep than formula-fed babies, which may account for their reduced risk of dying from sudden infant death syndrome (SIDS).

As the Harlow research indicates, an infant's physical contact with his mother—touching—guides behavioral development as much as social interaction—smiling and talking—does. Advances in the care of premature infants include "Kangaroo Care," an age-old practice, now standard practice in leading U.S. hospitals. In 1983, in a hospital serving the poor in Bogotá, Colombia, neonatologists Edgar Rey, MD, and Hector Martinez, MD, lacked incubators for the preemies in their care, or even reliable power to run the equipment they did have. They resorted to placing preemies upright and skin-to-skin on their mothers' chest, with their heads turned to the side to place their ears next to their mothers' hearts. The babies were carried night and day. Like marsupials, their mothers' bodies became their incubators. The mortality rate among their patients fell from 70 percent to 30 percent. Catching the attention of researchers, Kangaroo Care began to be studied, its benefits becoming clear with each new investigation. Both preemie and full-term babies kept in physical contact with their mothers in the generous quantities provided by Kangaroo Care sleep more than infants in traditional care, and transition through sleep and waking cycles without crying. Their heart rates, respiratory rates, and body temperatures are more stable. They are eight times more likely to breastfeed spontaneously, and their mothers more likely to let down their milk without delay. Preemies in Kangaroo Care gain weight more rapidly and stay in the hospital half the time of babies who are not carried. At six months, babies who received Kangaroo Care as newborns score significantly better on both cognitive and motor development scales. Babies seem to need the touch of their mothers' bodies in quantities guaranteed by breastfeeding as much as the milk itself.

Is it possible that the anxiety and social ills that mark our culture are in part due to the custom of depriving our infants of copious quantities of body contact? The American culture prizes independence, and so we strive to teach it to our children as early as possible, leaving them in firm-surfaced cribs, feeding them with cool, rigid rubber nipples and plastic bottles, picking them up as little as possible, and pushing them about in plastic or metal chairs rather than carrying them against a parent's body. Perhaps, rather than teaching them to thrive in our culture, we are creating a culture in which it is difficult to thrive.

THE STANDARD-CARE BABY: A CULTURAL COMPROMISE

Some physicians and other medical-care providers differentiate between "unrestricted" breastfed babies, who are breastfed in a biologically appropriate manner, and "standard-care" babies who may be breastfed, but who remain subject to many cultural restrictions on their care. Pioneering breastfeeding researcher Dr. Niles Newton identified unrestricted, biologically normal breastfeeding as the technique "practiced by traditional and preliterate cultures and, in the United States, by . . . members of La Leche League." In recent years, many mothers and families have adopted biologically appropriate ways of caring for their babies, including unrestricted breastfeeding, in a spreading practice called "Attachment Parenting."

Unrestricted breastfed babies are put to the breast whenever they want, for as long as they want. They are given no bottles. They are never left alone to cry. They are carried about, and held in laps and arms, whether awake or asleep, for most of the day. They sleep with or near the parents at night, which facilitates night feedings, for at least the first year. They receive solid foods only after six months; breastfeeding continues well into or through the second year.

Standard-care babies may be breastfed, but often on a schedule. Instead of averaging ten to twelve nursings a day in the first month, they may be limited to eight, to accommodate a three-hour schedule, or just six, if on a four-hour schedule. Feedings are terminated as soon as the baby is deemed "finished"; nonnutritive sucking, playing at the breast, and falling asleep on the breast are discouraged. Nursing purely for comfort is not considered desirable. The mother's breast, as a result, receives far less stimulation, and milk production decreases.

Standard-care babies sleep alone, often in their own room, from birth. They may be allowed to cry for long periods. They tend to be put down in a crib or some other baby-holding device whenever they are not being fed, dressed, or bathed. Bottle feedings are introduced regularly, from the first weeks, and strained baby foods by four months or so. Nursing is routinely delayed or curtailed for reasons such as, "She just ate—she can't possibly be hungry again," "I'll wait until he's really ready," "It's not time yet," "She's just using me as a pacifier," and "He's just fooling around now." The baby, in general, is thus not allowed to make the decision to nurse or not. Breastfeeding may cease entirely by six or eight months if not earlier.

Although still sufficiently unusual to be called standard care, it is not unheard of for babies to be breast milk–fed, but not breastfed. A mother may begin pumping her milk in the hospital or soon after, perhaps in preparation for returning to work. She may decide that her baby prefers feeding from the bottle to feeding from the breast, but knows that breast milk is superior nutritionally to formula. Within weeks, the baby is fully bottlefed with pumped breast milk.

Standard-care babies, while receiving the nutritional and immunological advantages of breastfeeding, at least in the early weeks, are somewhat deprived (or in the case of the breast milk-in-a-bottle baby, fully deprived) of the comforting and developmental aspects of the nursing relationship. One study compared sixteen mother-baby pairs practicing unrestricted nursing with sixteen fully breastfed standard-care pairs. While weight gains and general health were similar in the two sets of babies, the standard-care babies, at two months, cried 35 percent more than the unrestricted-nursing babies. Statistical analysis demonstrated what would seem to be common sense: The infants who were fed and held more frequently cried less, and infants who were fed and held less frequently cried more.

THE OLDER BREASTFED BABY

Behavior at the breast changes as the baby grows. A newborn may take half an hour or longer to reach satiety; the older baby is finished in a few minutes. The newborn concentrates entirely on suckling during nursings; by four months, the baby can nurse and be aware of the rest of the world at the same time; in fact, he may turn his head or interrupt himself at any interesting new noise or voice.

From three months on, the baby smiles and plays at the breast, letting his mother know how much he enjoys nursing and being near her. By four or five months, the baby often wants to play with his mother's face while nursing, and may like to feel her teeth and mouth with his free hand. For many babies, nursing continues to be an important source of nutrition, with four or more nursings during the day, including one night or early morning feeding, through the first year. And long after nursing ceases to be a major source of calories, it continues to be a comfort—at bedtime, when a child is ill or frightened, and whenever a little love and cuddling seem to be in order.

How long do babies "naturally" breastfeed? Is there a biologically normal time for weaning? The matter appears to be highly variable; individual babies differ, and adult expectations vary from culture to culture. The general food supply is a factor, as well; weaning can be a calamitous event in a community with scanty alternate foods for infants and toddlers.

In the few societies still unchanged by the industrialized world—rare communities found here and there in the Amazon, on the Kalahari, and other isolated spots—babies are breastfed for two years or more. Babies are spaced by several years as unrestricted breastfeeding performs its role as a natural birth control. Presently in the United States, babies are weaned most commonly by six months. Lactation consultants and others favoring unrestricted breastfeeding recommend "baby-led" weaning, in which babies are allowed to outgrow nursing at their own pace, which, like all developmental milestones, is a little different for each baby. These babies tend to wean themselves gradually anywhere from early in the second year of life to late in the third year. Often the weaning process is so gradual that a mother one day realizes that her baby hasn't nursed lately and must, therefore, be weaned.

Although the earliest age at which babies spontaneously wean themselves—refusing the breast and preferring other food—seems to be about nine months, this early self-weaning may in fact be induced by breastfeeding practices that cause the milk supply to dwindle until it is no longer of interest. Some mothers find that their first baby weans himself well before his first birthday, but subsequent babies wean themselves much later. Only one preliterate culture, in New Guinea, is on record as weaning all babies from the breast at nine months; it is reportedly a very restrictive and unpleasant culture in other ways as well.

Mothers sometimes get tired of nursing before babies do. The mother's feelings, a subsequent pregnancy, or social pressures may all contribute to the weaning process and the time weaning takes place. The American Academy of Pediatrics' newly issued recommendation that babies nurse a full year and beyond as long as mother and baby desire may help to reduce some of those social pressures. To date, little research has been published on the effects of long-duration breastfeeding on children. Subjectively, a mother is likely to feel that the closeness she shares with her baby while breastfeeding is even more enjoyable and complete as the baby grows old enough to be a sociable companion as well as a nursling. Perhaps a nursing mother's love, lap, and milk provide our exploring, experimenting toddlers with a home base, a firm foundation of security, that makes them all the more confident as the time for independence approaches.

A Parent Is Born: The Innate Behavior of Caretaking

INSTINCT AND THE NEW INSECURITY

In 1850, a new mother learning to take care of her first baby might have felt nervous, but she was bolstered by the firm conviction that whatever she did was right. Only a mother knew what to do for her infant, and she—by the grace of God, having become a mother—would be able to feed and care for her infant, thanks to her "mother instinct." Today, however, parents feel a distinct insecurity about child rearing in general, as shown by the proliferation of parenting advice columns, books, magazines, talk shows, and famous experts. Indeed, motherhood itself is widely questioned, and the question is not "how?" but "why?" Parenting magazines and other popular authorities seem to take parental anxiety and doubt for granted. What ever happened to mother instinct?

We are coming to understand that instinct is not a blind, inflexible force but a series of nudges, of small reflexive responses to internal or external stimuli that, added together, tend to produce certain patterns of behavior. There is room for lots of variation, however. Innate behavior does not operate mechanically in every animal, every time; even ants have been found to display individuality in their behavior. It is only by a long and careful observation of many individuals that the patterns of innate behavior can be seen.

We now know that unrestricted breastfeeding elicits and promotes appropriate mothering behavior. So it is perplexing to read the current medical research literature in which breastfeeding is seen as an *outcome* of a mother's nurturing feelings when it is in fact a cause. The psychological literature is even more astonishing. Whole schools of thought and research on parent-child "attachment" have arisen in which breastfeeding is completely ignored. A monograph titled "Growing Points in Attachment Theory and Research," supposedly a review of all significant new research on parent-child attachment, includes not one reference to breastfeeding. It's as if one were to study the marriage bond without considering sex.

LEARNING AND INNATE MOTHERING

It seems puzzling that humans, with all their advantages of brainpower, face the care of an infant with minimal instructions from Mother Nature, while any cat or cow or rabbit has the genetic programming to raise babies, knowing exactly what to do from start to finish. But is that really true? Do animals have a real advantage over us? The truth is that with animals as with people, experience is a factor in successful mothering.

Every person who has raised horses or dogs or any other animal knows that mammal mothers do not do a perfect job the first time. Some horses are so nervous with their first foal that they must be restrained by force before they will let it nurse. Laboratory rats may lose some or all of their first litter through inexperience—letting the babies get chilled, go hungry too long, or stray from the nest.

Many dogs are quite incompetent with their first litter. When puppies are born, they, like other animal babies, move toward the nearest large object; when their noses make contact with fur, they grope around until they eventually find the nipples. An inexperienced female may get up and down a lot at first, giving her babies no chance to start suckling. As one kennel owner put it, "It looks as though the bitch is puzzled. There they are, ten babies, and she thinks she ought to do something about them, but she isn't sure what. Finally she gives up, and lies down to rest—and it happens!"

Experimenters have found that animals have a chance to practice some aspects of baby care before the babies arrive. If a female rat is made to wear a collar throughout life, so that she cannot reach her body and never has a chance to lick herself, she does not know how to lick her babies as they are born. Then they have a hard time functioning normally and making contact with her; generally, they do not survive. If a rat is deprived of the experience of carrying things in her mouth, she will not know how to build a proper nest or how to retrieve her babies if they stray. Some house cats arrive at maturity without good carrying experience. A new mother cat, for all her aplomb, may not know how to pick up a kitten. She may spend half an hour taking it by a paw, by the nose, by the tail, before she discovers the scruff-of-the-neck hold. The cat that has had a chance to hunt, kill, and carry mice will pick up a kitten properly on the first try.

Observation can be important, too. A chimpanzee that was reared in the London Zoo and had never seen a baby of her own species was so horrified at the sudden appearance of her first baby in her hitherto private cage that she leaped backward with a shriek of terror, and could never thereafter be persuaded to have anything to do with it. Her second, born a year later, she accepted only after her friend the keeper demonstrated its harmlessness and showed her how to hold it. Gorillas are even more susceptible to problems of inexperience. For many years, gorillas born in captivity had to be taken from their mothers and hand-raised if they were to survive. Zoos have now learned that captive gorillas should be kept in compatible groups instead of alone or in pairs. In these colonies, when a young and inexperienced female gives birth, older females not only watch her and the baby, but tend to coach or reprimand her if she does something hazardous, such as holding the baby by one limb or upside down. One zoo had success in breeding a solitary female gorilla when a keeper persuaded a woman friend to bring her nursing baby to the zoo after hours and breastfeed in the aisle of the gorilla house, so the pregnant female could see how it was done. The gorilla watched with every evidence of interest, and was indeed able to feed and raise her own baby when it arrived.

IS THERE A BONDING PERIOD?

Scientists have long recognized that many animals have strict mother-infant bonding periods. In 1935, ethologist Konrad Lorenz, MD, demonstrated in geese a phenomenon known as "imprinting," in which the newly hatched bird recognizes as its parent whatever it sees and hears on first hatching, whether that is an adult goose or a professor making gooselike honks. The subtle detail was that imprinting can occur only in a brief, critical period after hatching; subsequently, the gosling can never learn to recognize or follow a parent or parent substitute. Helen Blauvelt, PhD, demonstrated the existence of a similar critical period in goats. Ordinarily, right after the birth of a kid, the mother smells and licks it, lets it nurse, and from then on recognizes this infant as her own, and will accept no other. The instant formation of attachment is called "bonding." If the mother is separated from her offspring immediately after birth for as short a period as one hour, she may never accept it; the critical period has passed and they never become the inseparable couple necessary to the baby's survival.

Does such a period exist in primates, including humans? No, we are in general more flexible than other species; our adaptability is one of the secrets of our success. We bond to our adopted babies just as we do to our birth babies. We are often separated from our babies at birth for an hour or more, and still become deeply attached parents. Humans, whether mother and baby or adult couples, become attached to each other over time, developing and deepening their relationships through a long series of interactions.

In the 1970s, however, researchers began to study maternal-infant behavior immediately after birth, and discerned a sensitive period following birth, in which mother and baby are primed in many ways to greet each other and launch their lifelong attachment. This period does not make or break bonding, but it does seem to nudge the process.

Following a normal delivery, depending on the medications given the mother during labor, a baby is highly aroused for about two hours. The hormones, including adrenaline, that flood the baby under the stress of labor stimulate his nervous system to make him more alert than he will be for the next several days. They dilate his pupils, luring his parents to return his steady gaze. His sense of smell is more developed than sight and hearing at birth, and he employs it immediately toward his mother. Her scent is somewhat familiar, as it is created by the same genetic and environmental factors that made the scent and taste of her amniotic fluid unique. As they cuddle and he is brought to the breast for the first time, the baby is enveloped in his mother's scent, learning it well and finding it deeply comforting. Within days after birth, a newborn can recognize the scent of his mother, either on a piece of clothing or from breast milk on a pad, and will turn toward it and away from the scent of a stranger.

A baby's sense of touch is also highly developed at birth. "Kangaroo Care" (see pages 164–65), the simple yet potent practice of placing preemies skin-to-skin on their mothers' chests for prolonged periods, demonstrates the importance of early touch to long-term, overall health and emotional well-being. New studies are being performed to evaluate the impact of early contact on full-term infants, as well as on preemies. In one such study, published in *Pediatrics* in 2004, researchers looked at the effects of skin-to-skin contact initiated ten to fifteen minutes after birth. The Kangaroo Care infants stayed with their mothers, in the skin-to-skin, chest-to-chest position, for an hour or more, while the standard-care babies were briefly held by their mothers and then taken back to the nursery. Four hours after birth, the researchers observed all the infants for an hour and found that those who received Kangaroo Care slept longer, were mostly in a quiet sleep state, startled less, and indicated less stress overall. The researchers urged that future studies examine the impact of extended, early touch on mother-infant interaction, infant temperament, and attention-related skills in the early weeks of life and beyond. If these studies, as the evidence suggests, reveal a pervasive and enduring effect of skin-to-skin contact, then the quantity of maternal-infant touching built into the act of breastfeeding becomes very significant indeed.

Hospitals are beginning to attend to the importance of early touch, allowing mothers and babies to be together undisturbed after birth. With the evidence from numerous studies that a mother will breastfeed more successfully and for longer periods when she is permitted to have early contact with her baby, the opportunity to nurse her baby within the first hour of birth, and rooming-in with her baby twenty-four hours a day, the World Health Organization (WHO) and UNICEF developed the Baby-Friendly Hospital Initiative in 1991 to promote successful breast-feeding in every country. Currently forty-two U.S. hospitals and birth centers have received the "Baby-Friendly" designation by following its ten steps (see Resources), including allowing mothers and babies to be together undisturbed for the first hour or more of life. Many more hospitals now routinely give mothers—and fathers, too—a quiet hour immediately after birth in which to play with and get to know their babies, and encourage nursing and skin-to-skin contact during that hour. Hospitals are more willing than they once were to delay giving a baby the still legally required silver nitrate eye drops (which sting) or ophthalmic antibiotics until after the first hour, so that a baby can keep his eyes open and see his parents' smitten faces. Hospitals in which a relatively high percentage of mothers leave their newborns behind have seen dramatic drops in abandonings after instituting WHO Baby-Friendly policies. A hospital in Thailand reported a drop in abandonment from 33 per 10,000 to 1 per 10,000; another in St. Petersburg, Russia, saw their rate cut in half; and hospitals in the Philippines and Costa Rica have had similar experiences.

INNATE TENDENCIES IN NEW MOTHERS

Like their babies, parents are usually alert and focused after a normal birth. With emotions heightened by the birth experience, they begin a series of interactions with their wide-awake baby, urged to do so with innate tendencies common to all parents.

In 1960, researcher I. Salk, knowing that babies are soothed by sounds simulating the maternal heartbeat, made the startling observation that the great majority of mothers, regardless of past experience or right- or left-handedness, held their babies on the left side, over the heart. This observation has proved to be so sound that medical staff can use it diagnostically. The mother who does not hold her new baby on the left (like the mother who does not look at her baby while talking about it) may be at risk, suggest studies, for parenting disorders, including neglect and abuse.

Almost every new mother experiences an irresistible urge to unwrap her new baby and look at it all over when he is first brought to her from the nursery. If the nurses discourage this, the mother may do it secretively and try to wrap up the baby again exactly as it was. But do it she will, with the inevitability with which a little girl of two or three will strip the clothes off a new doll.

Many of the ways we touch our babies have innate components. If a newborn is lying on his back, mothers tend to put a hand flat on the baby's chest, middle finger aimed at the baby's chin, and rock it slightly, in a gentle, rousing gesture. Holding the baby vertically against one's shoulder and patting it between his shoulder blades is also a mildly stimulating behavior. Both stir the baby to social interaction. A new mother tends to orient herself so that the baby is looking straight at her, and their heads are angled the same way, or face-to-face; researchers call this position *en face*. Mothers of preterm babies in incubators may bend over to put themselves *en face* to the baby lying on its side. It's common for a new mother to place the baby in her lap, facing up, and spend long periods—many minutes, even hours—face-to-face, looking into the baby's eyes, talking to and touching the baby. One lactation consultant who works with many teenage mothers teaches them to breastfeed in the so-called football hold, with the baby under one arm, looking up, so that the baby's eyes look straight into the mother's eyes. This position tends to make the mother laugh, talk, and play with her baby, bolstering her confidence and attachment to her baby, a fundamental step in preventing parenting disorders.

FATHERS AND INNATE BEHAVIOR

Fathers exhibit innate behavior in many of the same ways mothers do. Fathers, like mothers, respond to infant vocalizing by vocalizing themselves. Both tend to begin contact with a new baby by touching the arms and legs, then by touching the body with the fingertips, then with the whole hand (men tend to stroke the baby with the back of the fingers, which women do not). Men also tend to regard the baby *en face* and will twist themselves around to do so, if the baby is lying down, and they make regular and continuing eye contact.

Men are also susceptible to instant bonding to an infant at birth (although, like women, they are also quite capable of developing equally strong bonds through later exposure). In the last twenty years, fathers have assumed the role of their partners' labor coaches and companions; their presence at birth has strengthened families by all measures. The hour of birth can be an emotionally intense period for fathers. Yale University psychiatrist Kyle Pruett, MD, in his book *The Nurturing Father,* quotes a man who had been present for this daughter's birth: "'She opened her eyes and looked at me—*right at me*. Perfect! Just perfect. The doc cut the cord and put her on my wife's belly, and I touched her. I was sort of afraid because she was so small and soft, but she opened her eyes again when I touched her—like she liked it. A shiver went up my back.'" Dr. Pruett comments, "What a lucky little girl and mother. There appears to be no turning back from such experiences. This father seems hooked for good." Men are designed to be nurturers, just as are women.

Irinaus Eibl-Eibesfeldt, in his landmark book *Human Ethology*, looks at human behavior as it occurs in the natural setting in preliterate cultures. His studies show that even in the most warlike tribes it is not considered unmanly for a warrior to play with an infant; men as well as women spend a lot of time with babies and toddlers. Fathers share food with babies and toddlers, cuddle, fondle, and kiss them, respond to them in sensible and competent ways, and feel and display affection from the first days on. A father has his own way of comforting a baby and rocking it to sleep, tending to snuggle the baby's head in the spot on his chest just under his collarbones, with his chin lightly resting across the baby's head. William Sears, MD, calls this position "father nursing." Studies have been made of American fathers who take a strongly nurturing role with their babies and small children. Interestingly, both sons and daughters of these nurturing fathers tend to exhibit high levels of nurturing behavior (toward pets and younger children) themselves.

There are differences, however, between the ways in which men and women interact with babies that are consistent across cultures, whether the parents are Eipos in New Guinea or suburbanites in North America. Fathers play with babies more often than mothers, but clean them far less. Mothers feeding toddlers, for example, are far more likely than fathers to wipe the baby's face and hands during the process. If a baby chokes, coughs, sneezes, or starts crying, the father is apt to draw back and wait for order to restore itself, while the mother is more apt to intervene. And fathers interact with babies more actively than mothers. Fathers are much more likely than mothers to hold babies high in the air, to bounce them, and as they grow older, engage in tickling and physical play. Babies learn to expect this; as early as eight weeks, an awake and alert baby will respond to the father's approach with hunched shoulders and evident excitement. The world over, mommies are a comfort, but daddies are *fun!*

BABY TALK

One phenomenon in parents that is hard to explain without reference to innate behavior is baby talk. Every mother and father in the world—every grandparent too—speaks two languages: their own language, be it English, German, Russian, Tagalog, or Yanomami, and baby talk or, as researchers have dubbed it, "infant-directed speech" or "parentese." Baby talk has absolutely universal characteristics: It is high-pitched, repetitive, and often ends sentences with a rising tone, "Are you a pretty baby? Hmm? Pretty baby?"

Like all innate behaviors, baby talk has purpose and value. Babies are attracted to high-pitched sounds; so both men and women raise their voices just about an octave when they talk to babies. Repetitions and questioning may help babies to focus on the sounds more easily than they can on sounds in many-worded sentences. Baby talk is a prelude to the way we talk to toddlers: "See the dog? Look, there's a dog! Can you say 'dog'?" It is the first step on the path to learning language. Perhaps most important, baby talk signals to the baby that this voice is directed at *him*. Out of the sea of voices around him, even a small baby knows, from the tone and tempo, when he is being personally addressed, and he responds with pleasure. Baby talk is a powerful behavior for looping even very small babies into the social circle.

While infants may be preverbal, they are not preemotional. Several recent studies indicate that even very young babies are quite skilled at reading the emotions of their caretakers. Some fascinating new research suggests that baby talk not only teaches infants the rhythms and sounds of their native language, but also communicates the emotions of their caretakers. When adult-directed speech is full of emotion, observed the scientists, it matches infant-directed speech in pitch and tempo. The scientists concluded that baby talk is not actually unique. What makes it distinct from adult speech, however, is "the widespread expression of emotion to infants in comparison with the more inhibited expression of emotion in typical adult interactions."

In the 1930s and '40s, with the advent of "scientific" child rearing, baby talk was denigrated, even forbidden. It was "silly"; thought to set the baby a bad example: Mothers were told, "Don't talk like that; the baby will never learn to talk properly!" The prejudice continues: in 1990, a syndicated newspaper cartoonist devoted several strips to the amusement afforded by father and grandfather secretly giving way to forbidden baby talk whenever they were alone with the baby. In fact, the almost irresistible strength of the urge to coax response from a baby in this "undignified" manner is evidence for the innate nature of the behavior.

Baby talk surfaces again in adult life during courtship and in affectionate exchanges between lovers. Similar infantile exchanges are common in many species of birds and animals during courtship. In house sparrows, for instance, when a pair is being formed, the female chirps and flutters her wings like a begging chick, and the male offers food. While lovers might be embarrassed to have their pet names and baby talk broadcast in public, this undignified behavior is by no means trivial; the use of baby talk, signaling intimacy and willingness to be open emotionally, is quite appropriate to courtship and pair bonding.

ADULT RESPONSES TO BABY SIGNALS

Regardless of the presence or absence of early bonding experiences, we grow attached to babies. To facilitate this hold on adult emotions, babies have a large armory of attributes that function as social signals for eliciting attachment. All animals give and receive social signals with facial expression, posture, and vocalizations, and deliver a complex range of essential messages: "Get off my hunting ground!" "Don't hurt me, I'm a harmless subordinate." "Look out! Danger!" "Hey, I found something to eat!" "Shall we dance?" Konrad Lorenz called these kinds of signals "social releaser," a stimulus automatically supplied by one animal that triggers or releases a specific mood or emotion, often leading to action, on the part of other animals in the same species.

A social releaser can be a sound, such as the wailing cry given by a chicken when a hawk passes overhead, making every chicken within earshot run for cover. It can be a scent—the odor of the urine of a female fox, mink, or dog in heat that arouses mating behavior in the male. It can be a gesture—the way a puppy rolls on its back, exposing its vulnerable throat and belly, to plead for mercy. It can be a pattern, such as black or white markings on the tails of many birds, or the phosphorescent array of lights on the sides of some deep-sea fishes, conveying the message to others of the species, "Come with me, we are the same kind."

Human babies automatically present many social-releasing stimuli, to which all other humans are programmed to respond. Lorenz pointed out that the whole appearance of a human baby is a social releaser. For basic anatomical reasons, babies are born with disproportionately large heads, bulging foreheads, and large eyes, compared with adults. The very features that adapt the baby for breastfeeding—the fat pads that round the cheeks, the short nose and chin, the small mouth with elevated upper lip—also contribute to a characteristic look that makes us say, "Oh, how cute!" whether we are male or female, old or young, and whether the possessor of these attributes is a baby human, calf, raccoon, or squirrel.

Soft cuddly contours and very short limbs complete the picture that seems to us innately adorable; this combination of characteristics may be seen in dolls, stuffed animals, and many cartoon characters. Think of Mickey Mouse, or Alvin the Chipmunk, or Bambi, variously possessing big head, big eyes, button nose, no chin, tubby tummy—all baby signs. Many a career in commercial art has been built on painting pictures of children and adults that are appealing solely because the eyes are about five times the normal size, triggering the "cute" response.

Interestingly, human babies are not born with this full display of "cuteness," but develop it from about eight weeks on; people unfamiliar with newborns are sometimes taken aback by their appearance. They may describe a new baby as looking like "a little old man," a decidedly uncute comparison. The newborn apparently has enough other qualities in its favor to ensure its appeal to the crucial people, its parents. Only as the baby grows older does it need to be able to promote affection and forestall aggression from all the other people in its social world, no matter their age, sex, or familial relationship.

Social-releaser stimuli often consist of behavior. The baby's grasp reflex, besides helping him hang on to the mother, serves as a social releaser. At the Yerkes Laboratory in Florida, where chimpanzees have been carefully raised and studied for years, it has been noted that a female that has just given birth is apparently very impressed when her baby reaches out with its little hands and takes hold of her. It is this touch of hands that tells her the baby is one of her own kind. In humans, touching of hands conveys friendship in a simple, universal—and therefore instinctive—way. The firm, responsive way a newborn baby grasps one's finger is a moving experience for both parents. It triggers affectionate behavior.

One easily observed social stimulus presented by all young animals is the infant distress call. This is the cheep, cheep, cheep of a hungry chick, the earsplitting ki-yi-yi of a puppy caught in a fence, the bawling of a strayed calf, the wail of a newborn child. The infant distress call is usually loud, rhythmic, and distinctive. It is not easily ignored. All animals, including humans, react to the distress call of their own species by exhibiting anxiety and distress of their own. As Benjamin Spock, MD, has said, "The cry of a young baby is like no other sound. It makes parents want to come to the rescue—*fast!*" It does indeed. It also makes unrelated people highly irritated, adding social pressure to a parent's desire to stop the noise. That is what a distress call is meant to do: get on your nerves, make you feel distracted and upset until you find a way to put a stop to it. Cry researchers, therefore, believe inconsolable crying—when a young baby cries for an hour or more even though the baby has been fed, burped, changed, and rocked—may serve the purpose of inducing interaction as a parent tries and *tries* to discover what will comfort the baby. Crying helps parents become tuned into their new baby.

An interesting social releaser in very small babies is sounds other than crying. From the first weeks of life, breastfed babies murmur as they nurse. Little coos and hums that seem to express pleasure and relaxation can be heard throughout the feeding. A toddler may make the same little singing sounds when he is happily playing by himself, and one can hear the same class of sound—little sighs, and murmurs of comfort—from an adult who is enjoying, for example, a good back rub. Richard Applebaum, MD, points out that bottlefed babies do not vocalize during feedings, or, if they do, that the sound is apt to be sputtering and grunting rather than cooing, melodious murmuring. The artificial configuration of mouth and throat during bottlefeeding may hamper the baby's ability to vocalize and eat at the same time. It is possible that the baby does not feel the same sublime enjoyment at the bottle as at the breast, and so has no emotions of comfort and pleasure to be expressed in pleasant sighs and murmurs. Certainly the nursing baby's little song is received by the mother as a message of comfort, contentment, and love, and thus serves to strengthen the nursing bond.

Smiling is a potent social releaser. A newborn baby, when his stomach is full, often smiles—a fleeting grin—as he falls asleep. While the baby is still very small, four to eight weeks old, this smile of satiety becomes a true social smile. Premature infants begin social smiling at about six weeks after the date when they should have been born, as opposed to their actual birthday. Babies who are born blind also begin smiling in their second month. Smiling seems to be an essential human developmental milestone, as basic a function as walking and grasping. At first, the releasing stimulus for this smile is a pair of human eyes. When the baby sees you looking at him, he smiles. Smiling as he catches your eye is a very valuable instinctive response, and it in turn acts as a releaser for social behavior from the parent, or indeed from almost any human, even another child or a grouchy old man; in fact, siblings and grandparents often first feel deep, abiding affection for the baby in the family when she begins to smile at them.

PHEROMONES

One special class of social releasers is scent. Scents used as social signals in lower animals are called "pheromones." In insects, these scents are single compounds giving single messages; in mammals, both the compounds and the messages are more complex, but the phenomenon of scent-triggered behavior is very widespread. Dogs, for instance, use scents to mark their territories and advertise their own presence, and recognize instantly the odor of a female in season. We humans are less aware of our pheromone-like messages. In fact, we do all we can to erase them, with cosmetics, bathing, deodorants, and laundering. Still, you may have noticed "good" scent markers—the enjoyable scent of the room or the clothes of a much-loved person—and the "bad" scent markers, such as the sharp, sour smell of a shirt you may have worn during a stress-filled situation.

Scent signals are particularly profuse in the crucial area of reproductive behavior, even when we are not conscious of them. Researchers have discovered that when women of reproductive age live together as housemates, after a few months their menstrual cycles fall into synchrony. There may be some evolutionary advantage to this; if all the women in a traveling tribe menstruated simultaneously, the whole group could stop and rest once a month for three or four days. Scent signals appear to be the mechanism for this phenomenon. Women who live in close association with a man tend to reach menopause later than single women, not, the researchers say, because of sexual relations but of exposure to male body scent. In both sexes, pubic hair and underarm hair are scent traps, concentrating these reproduction-related messages; we recognize that a woman clasping her hands behind her head is in a provocative pose, but we don't usually stop to think that she is also sending a scent message.

The fact that the nursing baby smells good is probably more important than we think; it is not just that smelling nice reinforces close contact with adults. Scientists are trying to learn more about our capacity for smell. Each new discovery suggests that the olfactory ability of mammals is closely related to the emotional and language learning centers of the brain. Infants presented with a familiar odor during a mildly painful medical procedure (a blood draw) cry less than infants presented with an unfamiliar odor or no odor. Newborns move their arms and legs in a more organized manner in the presence of their mothers' scent. While studies have not been done on human infants, other mammalian newborns have a heightened period of odor sensitivity for a few days after birth, so that they learn to recognize their mother by scent alone; if prevented from smelling their mother, infant rats do not form an attachment to her. In humans, infants recognize the scent of their mother's amniotic fluid immediately after birth, and her body and milk soon after. Most human mothers can recognize their newborns by scent alone within the first few days of birth. Mothers of older babies who pump their milk during their working day find that their letdown reflex can be triggered by smelling a nightie worn by their baby. Nursing babies transition to sleep in a crib more easily if they are put down on a piece of clothing their mother has recently worn. Scent appears to be crucial at every state of the reproductive cycle; lactation and caregiving behavior are certainly among them.

BREASTFEEDING—THE GREAT TEACHER

Both on the inborn and the learned levels, breastfeeding teaches new mothers how to be mothers. The innate needs and urges of the mother are met by breastfeeding. The frequent close body contact reassures mother as well as child—we all need hugs and cuddling, and babies can give this comfort as well as get it. Breastfeeding requires and creates attentiveness to and interest in the baby's moods and signals. A nursing baby is easy for his mother to understand; the comfortable interaction in a well-established lactation builds up a mutual communication, not dependent on words, that lasts long beyond weaning. As Niles Newton, the social biologist and lactation researcher, has said, "Breastfeeding nudges other aspects of maternal behavior."

The hormones of lactation have a powerful effect on behavior. If prolactin is injected into male rats, they will retrieve baby rats and lick them. In humans, males as well as females have prolactin in their systems; researchers have found that prolactin levels increase in men who are nurturing small children. Prolactin levels are high during pregnancy, and in a breastfeeding mother will continue to be high for as long as a year.

The hormone that triggers mothering behavior most powerfully, however, is oxytocin. Dr. Niles Newton and her husband, Michael Newton, MD, were the pioneering research couple who first demonstrated that humans have a letdown response triggered by oxytocin, and that the release of oxytocin and the letting down of milk could be inhibited by emotional disturbance. (They demonstrated this in a famous experiment, by tying a string to Niles's big toe as she nursed one of their four babies. If Michael, in the next room, unpredictably jerked the string during feedings— an annoying though not painful event—weighings showed that the baby got less milk.)

Oxytocin production can be reduced by emotional disturbance, but the reverse is also true, and very important for the nursing mother. Oxytocin release in itself triggers emotional tranquillity and strong nurturing feelings—and unlike prolactin, which has a long-term, slow effect, oxytocin works its magic instantaneously. Laboratory animals that have never had litters will exhibit mothering behavior within one minute of receiving a dose of oxytocin directly into the nervous system. No matter what her species, every time a mother's milk lets down, she is being primed on a very fundamental evolutionary level to cuddle and nurture. (Oxytocin is also the hormone of lovemaking, released during sexual climax in both men and women.)

Many mothers are conscious of the soothing, almost euphoric side effects of oxytocin release during breastfeeding. It can be the high point of a working mother's day, as all the stresses of a day at the office evaporate when she sits down to nurse her baby; "Better than a martini," declares one. A nursing mother is sometimes quite overwhelmed by how much she adores her particular baby, as the baby nestles up to her breast. We now know that the flood of oxytocin, as her milk lets down, is the physical mechanism for that emotion.

Niles Newton points out that the survival of the human race depends on reproduction, and that the continuance of reproductive behavior depends on the "voluntary satisfaction" to be gained from those largely self-initiated behaviors, coitus and breastfeeding. "Sexual intercourse," Newton has said, "is well-known to foster bonding and care-giving behavior, especially if repeated frequently with the same individual." The same, of course, is true of breastfeeding.

Various studies have found that women who practice unrestricted breastfeeding become physically different from bottle-feeding mothers, not only in hormonal levels, but in galvanic skin response (they are calmer), heart rate (which alters, as the baby cries or is soothed, strikingly more than the heart rate of bottlefeeding mothers), and thermal skin responses as the mother's breast heats and cools in response to the baby.

If lactation is suppressed, prolactin levels fall abruptly after delivery, and breastfeeding's multiple daily flushes of oxytocin don't occur at all. This hormonal "crash" may be a major factor (in addition to separation from the infant and lack of social support) in the "baby blues" and even more severe postpartum depression, which is far more common among mothers who are not breastfeeding. Not only are all innate urges being frustrated, but the sustaining, love-and-tenderness-inducing hormones are rapidly draining from the system.

The mother who breastfeeds feels this hormonal deprivation much later—on weaning—and much more slowly; as the baby gradually nurses less and less often, the mother's body is weaned from lactation, too. Even so, many women feel some sadness on weaning, especially those who do not plan to have another child. This is not just hormonal; as Niles Newton says, it's only natural: "We *like* to breastfeed."

Helpers and Hinderers: How Breastfeeding Was Saved, and Why the Job Is Not Yet Done

Through most of human existence, mothers have breastfed their babies; it is among evolution's most elegant and effective inventions to encourage survival. Regardless of the perfection of the system provided by nature for infant nutrition, however, human society has invented reasons from time to time that suggest to mothers that they are better off not breastfeeding their babies.

The most enduring social myth regarding breastfeeding is that doing so is a sign of poverty, and not breastfeeding is a sign of privilege. In previous centuries, the rich could afford to hire wet nurses, women who made their living by feeding another woman's baby, as well as (or instead of) their own. To abstain from breastfeeding, therefore, was a luxury, and evidence of a noblewoman's delicacy. Witness this grandmother, observed by Aulus Gellius in Rome in A.D. 600:

"When he had asked how long the labor had been, and how severe, and had learned that the young woman, overcome with fatigue, was sleeping, he . . . said, 'I have no doubt that she will suckle her son herself.' But the young woman's mother said to him that she must spare her daughter and provide nurses for the child in order that to the other pains which she had suffered in child birth might not be added the wearisome and difficult task of nursing."

The belief that a well-born woman was too delicate to nurse was surely supported by two other ideas unrelated to the health of babies and mothers. The first was the widespread belief among pre–nineteenth-century physicians that if a woman was sexually active during lactation, her breast milk would curdle. Clearly every devoted couple would be in the market for a wet nurse, if they could possibly afford one, and they trusted the word of their physician. The other was the desire of aristocratic families to have many children to wed to other highly placed families, thereby increasing a family's wealth and influence. Lactational amenorrhea, or temporary infertility caused by breastfeeding, spaced pregnancies too far apart for maximum lifetime childbearing.

Whether task or pleasure, performed by mother or mother-substitute, until this century, breastfeeding was the only safe way to feed babies. Artificial or substitute foods often spoiled or were contaminated with bacteria, especially in hot weather; the resulting diarrhea—the dreaded "summer flux"—killed babies who were not breastfed.

When relatively safe artificial feeding of babies was first developed in the United States, like the services of a wet nurse, it quickly became a status symbol. The baby bottle seemed the tangible evidence of the modern woman's liberation from drudgery and ignorance. Feeding a baby by clock and scale was "scientific" and therefore superior to old-fashioned methods. Those who could afford the paraphernalia and the expensive doctors' advice took up bottlefeeding first. As hospitalization for childbirth became customary throughout the nation, the accompanying systematized care of the newborn made breastfeeding physically less feasible. The medical profession began to assume a position of authority in all matters of infant care and feeding. Soon bottle-feeding was not only fashionable and medically approved, but seemed to be the only method possible for most women. The people who continued to breastfeed were those too poor to buy bottles and the ingredients for formula—rural women or recent immigrants who "didn't know any better." Formula feeding became the norm, and breastfeeding the rare exception.

It was not until the cultural reformation of the 1960s and '70s that a reevalution of breastfeeding began. Individuals and organizations began promoting and developing programs to improve the experience of childbirth, which along with infant feeding had become highly medicalized. Women began to ask for natural labors in which they could be conscious participants, they requested that their babies "room-in" with them rather than staying in the hospital nursery, and that infant care become altogether less invasive. This more harmonious approach to childbirth was accompanied by a new focus on breastfeeding.

Once again, the parents who were quick to espouse these new movements tended to be the well educated and affluent. This trend has continued into the twenty-first century, as the woman who is most likely to breastfeed in North American is white, educated, and middle class or wealthy. Disadvantaged mothers may still regard the baby bottle as a status symbol, visible evidence of money to spend. Even more likely, these mothers are easy targets for formula manufacturers' marketing campaigns, as well as their contributions of vast quantities of free formula to social service agencies.

PREJUDICE AGAINST BREASTFEEDING

The mother today who chooses to breastfeed expects her decision not only to be accepted, but applauded. So it's apt to be
a shock to her the first time she discovers herself being criticized,
subtly or openly, for nursing her baby. Antibreastfeeding prejudice may be expressed as old wives' tales, pessimistic predictions,
pointed jokes, or open hostility. Criticism may come from such
unexpected sources as one's family, medical-care providers, employers and co-workers, or even close friends. Perhaps a woman's
trusted obstetrician, whom she had assumed would heartily endorse her intentions, offers harmful misinformation (such as
scrubbing her nipples with a towel to prepare them for nursing)
or skepticism that undermines her confidence even before
breastfeeding begins: "Well, if it doesn't work out, you can always use formula." Or a nurse in the hospital, who comes osten-
sibly to help her at feeding time, may accomplish the same by
leading her to expect breastfeeding to be difficult, or by com-
menting that her baby doesn't seem to want to nurse but sucked
down a bottle in the nursery. Or perhaps her own mother constantly questions whether the baby is "getting enough" or insists
that all nursing take place behind a closed door in complete privacy, or a woman friend reveals that she finds the idea of breastfeeding repugnant. Or her husband doesn't want her to nurse the
baby if it's a boy.

Nobody ever gets used to being a target for prejudice. The experience can deflate even an experienced nursing mother. How
does this unreasoning attitude arise? Like all prejudices, it is
based on fear and ignorance. The fear of loss of social status is especially enduring. One mother, herself a childbirth instructor,
was astonished to find that her army officer father firmly held the

view that nursing a baby is a sign of ignorance and poverty, and he felt ashamed that she was breastfeeding.

In some social groups, on the other hand, a curious reversal of prejudice has arisen. While bottlefeeding mothers are assumed simply to be misguided—more pitied than censured—breastfeeding mothers who treat nursing casually rather than passionately may feel they are somehow not up to snuff. A mother returning to her job after a few weeks of maternity leave may find a previously friendly neighbor openly disapproving, because the working mother won't be available to nurse her baby during the day. Breastfeeding itself can become competitive; the mother who nursed for two years may feel superior to the woman who nursed for six months. In some circles, nursing a child for four or five years is a badge of honor. This fashion for passionate breastfeeding, often branded by others as fanaticism, has caused a prejudicial backlash of its own. Fear of being labeled a fanatic or an "earth mother" may be enough to lead a woman to wean early or not to breastfeed at all.

The main cause of prejudice against breastfeeding, however, has to do with sex. We have come to regard the female breast almost exclusively as a sexual object; breastfeeding can be perceived as prurient or obscene. This sexual association has many repercussions. A husband can feel ambivalent, if he had thought of his wife's breasts as his private treasure and now they are so visibly promised to the baby. Women may feel shy about nursing, especially in front of male relatives, and men may find the whole idea embarrassing. Physicians are not immune; one mother who had just given birth reported that her obstetrician—who, after all, probably knew more about her private parts than she did— blushed when he happened to come into her hospital room while she was breastfeeding.

If the breast is comparable to the genitals, then the substance that comes out of it must be the equivalent of semen or urine; so breastfeeding becomes an unclean act, and spots from leaking milk are embarrassing. Again, medical personnel are not immune. In one intensive-care nursery, when a baby developed a rash, the attending physician instructed the head nurse to treat the rash by putting a little fresh mother's milk on it; she recoiled, saying that she didn't like the idea of putting her hands in "that stuff." Nursing mothers who have returned to their jobs encounter this attitude whenever someone suggests that the appropriate place for them to pump their milk is a bathroom stall.

The sexualizing of the breast has far-reaching effects. It is taboo to expose sexual organs in public; therefore, nursing where people can see you is shocking. A New York writer reported that he and his family were asked to leave a restaurant because his wife was "exposing herself in public" by nursing their baby. Many nursing mothers have been asked to leave shopping malls by security guards attempting to protect the public from indecency. Breastfeeding mothers have been forced to serve on juries for extended trials. Mothers have been fired from their jobs for pumping their milk on the premises. Defending the rights of nursing mothers in court has become a small but active forensic specialty; problems range from charges of lewd conduct and public nudity to judges who cannot understand why the divorced father of a breastfeeding infant cannot have custody for the weekends.

State by state, and even at the congressional level, lawyers and other advocates are working to protect the right of a woman to feed her baby wherever she goes. State-by-state laws have been enacted spelling out the fact that breastfeeding a baby is "an important and basic act of nurturing that must be protected in the interests of maternal and child health and family values," and that "a mother has a right to breastfeed the mother's child in any location, public or private, where the mother and child are otherwise authorized to be present, irrespective of whether or not the mother's breast is covered during or incidental to the breastfeeding" (Montana Code § 50-19-501, 1999). Thirty-four states have laws that protect a mother's right to breastfeed to varying degrees (in Maryland, she is required to do so "with discretion"). While sixteen states have no laws regarding breastfeeding at all, even states that do rarely protect a woman's right to work in a way that accommodates breastfeeding her infant. This patchwork of state laws is being addressed at the national level by Carolyn Maloney, U.S. congresswoman from New York. Representative Maloney has drafted legislation to protect and promote breastfeeding in every state, for every woman. In 2001, her Right to Breastfeed language was inserted into the federal budget, ensuring a woman's right to breastfeed her child on any portion of federal property where the woman and her child are otherwise authorized to be. In 2003, she introduced the Breastfeeding Promotion Act, amending the Civil Rights Act of 1964 to protect breastfeeding by new mothers, provide for a performance standard for breast pumps, and tax incentives to encourage breastfeeding. Her bill also clarifies the Pregnancy Discrimination Act to protect breastfeeding under federal civil rights law, ensuring that women cannot be fired or discriminated against in the workplace for expressing milk or breastfeeding during breaks or lunch hours. That the simple, most beneficial, utterly harmless act of nursing a baby requires legal protection to this degree is testament to its place among all the other qualities of humanity, from race to gender to sexual preference, that have long been targets of blind prejudice.

And like other targets of discrimination, when not a victim of outright prejudice, breastfeeding is often treated as though it simply doesn't exist. There are pediatric textbooks with entire chapters on infant feeding in which breastfeeding is not mentioned. A booklet on sexual development and reproduction, printed by the New York State Department of Health for use in high schools, described and illustrated such details as the growth of pubic hair, and the development of a human embryo, but never mentioned the female breast, as if even the New York State Department of Health did not know what breasts are for. Plastic surgeons may reduce or enlarge a woman's breasts without asking if she ever plans to have a baby and, if so, would she like to preserve their breastfeeding function. A nursing mother may run into this blind spot about breastfeeding even in her own home. Relatives, seeing her holding the baby closely, may repeatedly try to look at the baby's face, or even to take it from her arms, without seeming to realize the baby is nursing.

Europeans, who are far more relaxed about the function and appearance of the female breast, sometimes think that we in the United States have very unusual ideas about milk in general. Many other cultures make use of animal milk in cooking or as a source of butter and cheese. But Americans are virtually alone in considering that animal milk is indispensable for growing children or that it is even a suitable food for adults. Certainly no other species of mammal includes milk in adult diet; from a biological standpoint, the idea is quite impractical. Could it be that our reverence for cow's milk is a confused expression of our breast taboos in North America?

The impact of the embedded prejudice against breastfeeding and lack of consistently effective support for new mothers in North American is in the numbers. Despite all we know about the benefits of breastfeeding and what needs to be done to help mothers succeed, and although breastfeeding rates have increased slightly since 1990, women who choose to breastfeed their babies for more than a few weeks are still a minority. At the time of this writing, 71 percent of women in the United States breastfeed either exclusively or in combination with formula while in the hospital; only 35 percent of mothers are still nursing at six months, and most supplement with formula.

MEDICAL ATTITUDES

In the last thirty years or so, the medical community has experienced a sea change in its attitude toward breastfeeding. Where once few physicians received any training in breastfeeding, now the American Academy of Pediatrics and the American Academy of Family Physicians have become staunch advocates of breastfeeding, promoting it to patients, educating both practicing physicians and medical students about its benefits and how to teach and manage it, and advocating for it in public health policy.

This relatively newfound enthusiasm and understanding began to be acquired through shrewd observation over years of practice, seeing women whose milk supply seemed to be dwindling who redeveloped their lactation, women who breastfed twins, or weathered illnesses without giving up breastfeeding, or women who held down demanding jobs and fully breastfed their babies, too. These object lessons enabled doctors to encourage other mothers in the same circumstances, rather than just prescribe formula at any sign of difficulty. In the last decade or so, the medical community has drawn on rising mountains of irrefutable scientific data to solidify its stand in support of breastfeeding.

Now even the smallest towns usually have at least one physician with breastfeeding expertise, or with a certified lactation consultant on staff. (Some physicians have even studied and passed the lactation consultant certifying exam themselves.) And as parents in general have become more sophisticated about breastfeeding, physicians who solve problems by telling the mother to switch to the bottle may find her switching to another doctor instead.

Potholes in the road remain, however. One example of an enduring institutional bias against breastfeeding is pediatric growth charts. Every well-baby checkup at a pediatrician's office includes an insertion into a baby's individual growth chart of her progress. Parents and pediatricians track a baby's growth along these charts, each little dot indicating whether a baby is in the 5th, 10th, 25th, 50th, 75th, or 95th percentile of weight or length or head circumference of all babies her age. If a healthy baby is born at the 25th percentile, she'll probably continue to grow at the same rate, and when she is in third grade or a freshman at college, is likely to be still be in the 25th percentile of children (or coeds) her size and weight. That is the size person her genes intended her to be. If she drops several percentiles on the charts in a short space of time, however, her growth chart serves as a warning signal to her pediatrician that there may be an underlying problem, illness or perhaps malnutrition.

Most commonly used pediatric growth charts, however, are based on information collected by the Fels Research Institute from 867 infants born between 1929 and 1975, a group of babies of which 75 percent were formula-fed and just 17 percent were exclusively breastfed, and few for more than three months. In addition, the infant formulas used at that time were higher in total proteins, total fats, and saturated fatty acids than are current formulas (which have evolved to match more closely the proportions of nutrients in human milk). These infants also were far more likely to have been given solid foods before the age of four months than babies are today. The growth charts most widely in use, in short, are an entirely inappropriate method of measuring the growth of the exclusively breastfed infant.

For breastfed babies do grow differently than bottlefed babies. While they reach developmental milestones at the same or earlier ages as bottlefed babies, are just as active (or more so), and experience illness less often, breastfed babies gain less weight in their first year than babies fed formula. In fact, it is quite normal for a breastfed baby to decrease its rate of growth between four and six months. A pediatrician who is unaware of this difference may mistakenly diagnose a sudden failure to thrive simply by the change in the arc on the growth chart, rather than by observing a perfectly healthy breastfed baby. Many a mother has been told that her breast milk is not providing sufficient calories, and supplementation is necessary. The opposite, however, may be the case. The high bioavailability of nutrients in breast milk enables babies to get all the energy and vitamins they need with less volume; the breastfed baby's growth is appropriate and normal, while the formula-fed baby grows heavier and faster than is ideal.

The good news is that as exclusively breastfed babies become more common, the pediatric community has begun to recognize the problems caused by inaccurate growth charts. The World Health Organization is at this writing developing revised charts for international use. In 2000, the U.S. Centers for Disease Control and Prevention published a new set of infant growth charts. These charts, however, still do not differentiate between the growth pattern of breastfed and bottlefed babies, and therefore remain inherently inaccurate.

Growth charts are just one example of many tripwires still in place for mothers who wish to breastfeed. In its 1997 Policy Statement on Breastfeeding, the American Academy of Pediatrics lists many other obstacles, including: a lack of commitment from many physicians to support and inform their patients (created perhaps by a lack of training in medical school about breastfeeding); insufficient breastfeeding education for obstetric patients;

hospital policies that continue to disrupt and separate mothers and babies; inappropriate instructions to wean; early hospital discharge in some populations and lack of timely routine postpartum home visits; maternal employment in the absence of workplace facilities and support for breastfeeding, portrayal of bottlefeeding on TV and in movies as the norm (and a bizarre paucity of images of breastfeeding mothers); and the astonishingly successful marketing campaigns of the formula companies.

THE WORLD'S MOST SUCCESSFUL MARKETING CAMPAIGN

Imagine you are a student at a business school. Your professor assigns a project: Invent a product that will compete with another product already in worldwide use, a product that is perfectly designed, impossible to replicate, adjusts to the needs of its recipients, is convenient and pleasurable to use and—get this—is entirely free. Not only should your invention compete with this established product (and cost a lot), but your new product should push the established, perfect, free product out of the market, making it obsolete and even ridiculed.

That is, of course, precisely the challenge taken on by the makers of infant formulas, one with which they have achieved astonishing success. The lure of the market was too much; every new human being on the planet, after all, is a potential new customer. How did they manage it?

Infant formula was first manufactured in the 1920s for use in emergencies only, to feed foundlings or babies whose mothers had died in childbirth. By the 1940s, as more women began to support the war effort by working outside the home and as hospital childbirth became more common, infant formula took on the sheen of modern science. In a time when the world was looking forward to a sleeker, safer future, anything produced by a laboratory was assumed to be superior to things made in a home, and certainly preferable to something that came out of a body.

At the same time, the mechanization of large dairy farms in the twentieth century resulted in huge surpluses of whey from cheese manufacturing, as well as vast quantities of inexpensive milk. A market for all the waste and surplus products of this burgeoning industry was needed. Various "milk modifier" products, including "humanized milk" were invented and hawked to mothers as a modern source of infant nutrition. They were sold not only as food for babies, but as the keys to freedom and convenience for mothers, along with washing machines and electric toasters.

Marketing campaigns not only presented infant formula as the modern, scientific alternative, but re-created the image of breastfeeding as a dicey enterprise: "When breastfeeding fails, try Lactogen." Suddenly not only was breastfeeding old-fashioned, but possibly ill advised as well. The generous populating of doctors' offices with posters, pens, and other freebies covered with the logos of formula makers also provided a visual connection between formula brands and trusted pediatricians, suggesting with their mere presence to every visiting mother that her doctor approved of formula. Breastfeeding had no logo with which to compete, no marketing budget to spend on promotional paraphernalia.

By 1966, just 18 percent of babies were breastfed when they left the hospital, and fewer for more than a few weeks after that. Breastfeeding in North America was nearly eradicated.

And that is not the worst of it. A worldwide market, after all, was waiting to be tapped. By the mid-1950s, several multinational corporations undertook aggressive marketing of bottle-feeding and formulas in underdeveloped countries. Milk company advertisements plastered buildings and decorated roadsides from Guam to Guatemala, picturing enormous healthy babies—who owed their health to the use of this or that canned or powdered substance. From this ubiquitous propaganda, mothers in these developing countries, just as women in the States did, gained the impression that breast milk is not good enough. In fact, some companies dressed their village sales representatives in nurses' white uniforms to underscore the presumed health benefits of their products.

The immediate results of artificial feeding in a destitute area without running water, or in village without a monetary economy, are disastrous. A mother cannot make up a sterile baby bottle in a sewage-strewn slum without clean water or even a pot to boil it in. A single contaminated feeding is sometimes enough to send a baby on the downward spiral of infections, diarrhea, and dehydration that soon ends in death. Families making seventy-five cents a day can hardly spend ten dollars a week on infant formula. A mother in these circumstances may use a spoonful of precious powdered baby milk in each bottle rather than the specified cupful, diluting it so thinly that the baby soon starves.

From South Africa to Singapore, hospitals and clinics began to build rehydration centers, designed to treat the ever-growing overflow of infants dangerously dehydrated by diarrhea, brought on by artificial feeding. They were the victims, not of poverty and infectious disease (as the breastfed baby is well protected against both hunger and infection), but of a highly successful marketing plan. By 1960, D. B. Jelliffe, MD, and his wife, Patrice Jelliffe, United Nations trailblazers in the area of maternal and child health, were pointing out in World Health Organization (WHO) meetings and publications that this disastrous scenario was occurring all over the world, and with ever-increasing frequency.

By 1970, the health consequences of corporate promotion of infant formula were becoming obvious in many underdeveloped countries. Public opposition to these practices grew and became manifest in class action lawsuits for irresponsible marketing, public protests, and organized boycotts. In the United States, opposition to Nestlé, one of the largest and most aggressive marketers of formula in developing countries, led in 1977 to an organized boycott of all the company's many products that gradually spread to ten countries and lasted seven years.

In 1981, the U.N.'s World Health Organization adopted an International Code of Marketing of Breast-Milk Substitutes, limiting or prohibiting such practices as inaccurate advertising, gifts to health-care providers, and the giving of free samples of products to new mothers. Although the international corporations lobbied vigorously against it, the resolution, now generally known as the WHO Code, was ratified by all of the participating nations in the early 1980s (with the exception of the United States, which did not agree to it until 1994). Since then, some nations have passed even stricter codes of their own in an effort to reinstate breastfeeding as the standard, thereby reducing infant mortality, public health costs, and contributing to population control.

The Nestlé boycott was called to an end in 1984, after Nestlé agreed to abide by the WHO Code. The company also signed an agreement with the International Nestlé Boycott Committee in which they promised to keep their marketing practices within the intent of the Code. Four years later, after the Boycott Committee found that Nestlé had continued to violate the Code by promoting bottlefeeding and other products that interfere with breastfeeding in developing countries, the boycott was reinstated and remains in effect at this writing. It was also expanded to include products made by American Home Products, the second largest manufacturer of infant formula in the world.

With the increase of breastfeeding in North America, formula manufacturers have seen what must be an alarming decrease in their U.S. sales. Their marketing efforts to American mothers must therefore be retooled. Less likely to believe that formula is superior to breast milk than they once were, American mothers are being pitched a variety of new messages. The angle today is that, of course, breastfeeding is best for babies, but "no formula is closer to breast milk than Brand X." The fact that no formula comes close at all to the composition of breast milk is not mentioned.

Recent research showing that breastfed babies have higher IQs than formula-fed babies—about eight points higher even years after weaning—has received a fair amount of coverage in the popular press. The data were clear and convincing: breast milk improves cognitive development during lactation and long after weaning. Researchers isolated several fatty acids present in breast milk—docosahexaenoic acid (DHA) and arachidonic acid (AA)—that are now understood to be essential for optimal brain and eye development. Formula makers are rushing to include versions of these acids, made from algae and fungi, in "superbaby" (and super-expensive) formulas. They are being widely marketed as a way to enhance a baby's IQ and eyesight. "DHA and ARA," declares one advertisement, "are important brain and eye building nutrients. That's why only Enfamil has Lipil, a unique blend of DHA and ARA, important nutrients also found in breast milk that promote brain and eye development." Another brand's advertisements call the acids "important building blocks." Free samples of the new formulas are being sent to hospitals and directly to mothers in gift packages after their babies are born (along with entry blanks for college scholarship sweepstakes, "Helping you nourish your baby's potential now . . . and in the future").

In breast milk these particular fatty acids do seem to support brain and vision development. As for the fungi/algae-based versions found in formula, however, current research suggests that they do not contribute to brain and eye development in the slightest. Indeed, the American Academy of Pediatrics has declined to endorse these new "super-baby" formulas because of their "unknown adverse effects." In a study from the Institute of Child Health in London, researchers compared the cognitive development of three groups of healthy yet small-for-gestational-age newborns who were fed standard formula, formula "enriched" with DHA-ARA oil additives, or were breastfed. By eighteen months of age, the group fed formula with additives showed no neurodevelopmental advantages over the standard-formula group. In fact, the baby girls in this group, for an as-yet-undiscovered reason, showed a significant disadvantage. The breastfed group scored higher on neurodevelopment scales at nine and eighteen months than both groups of formula-fed babies. The researchers conclude, "Use of enriched formula for [full-]term small-for-gestational-age children should not be promoted. It seems that breastfeeding may be especially beneficial for neurodevelopment in children born small-for-gestational-age." Meanwhile, the company that supplies the fungi/algae-based DHA-ARA oils used all "enriched" formulas—there is just one—enjoyed predicted global sales of $100 million in 2004.

BREASTFEEDING REBORN

In spite of the best efforts of formula manufacturers and other entities, breastfeeding has survived. Since the first edition of this book was published in 1963, the medical world has taken enormous strides to understand breastfeeding and to help mothers succeed at it. Where once the American Academy of Pediatrics (APP) offered its members little education about helping mothers breastfeed and accepted enormous grants from the formula makers, the association now adamantly urges that *all* babies (with rare exceptions) be exclusively breastfed for the first six months, and that breastfeeding continue at least through the first year, and beyond as long as both mother and baby desire. (While any effort is to be applauded, the federal government, via the U.S. Department of Health and Human Services' initiative, Healthy People 2010, sets a goal of 75 percent of mothers breastfeeding their babies in the hospital, and just 50 percent continuing breastfeeding until their babies are five to six months old, targets that fall far short of the AAP's recommendations.)

It quite possible that none of the progress toward reestablishing breastfeeding would have happened if a couple of nursing mothers had not attended a picnic one day in 1956 in Franklin Park, a suburb of Chicago.

LA LECHE LEAGUE: THE BEGINNINGS

They were ordinary young mothers, the kind you might meet in church or pass in any supermarket. They were unusual in those days, however, because they were both breastfeeding. As often happens when someone nurses her baby in public, the other mothers at the picnic began to talk about their own attempts and failures to breastfeed. The two nursing mothers were very sympathetic. Like many nursing mothers in that era, each had had real difficulty in nursing their first babies, and had not been truly successful until subsequent babies came along. They agreed that they might have been successful from the beginning if they had known another experienced nursing mother to consult for encouragement and advice.

From that picnic conversation came the idea for an organization to enable nursing mothers to get together and help each other. Its name, La Leche League, was taken from a poetic Spanish title for the Madonna: *Nuestra Señora de la Leche y Buen Parto* (Our Lady of Bountiful Milk and Easy Delivery). Seven nursing mothers were the founders of La Leche League. They started by reading all they could find about lactation, and by discussing breastfeeding with interested doctors. Then, armed with facts and the experience of nursing their own babies, they held a series of four meetings for those friends of theirs who were expecting babies. Discussions were led by nursing mothers on various topics: the advantages of breastfeeding, the art of breastfeeding and overcoming difficulties, childbirth, the family and the breastfed baby, nutrition, and weaning.

By the time the third series of meetings was under way and La Leche League was a year old, there were three groups. One physician, Caroline Rawlins, MD, filled her car with expectant patients and drove sixty miles to the monthly meetings. The young organization began receiving national publicity. Hundreds of phone calls and letters from nursing mothers came in every month. La Leche League published the first edition of its manual on breastfeeding, *The Womanly Art of Breastfeeding*, in 1958. An article about La Leche League, excerpted from the first edition of this book, was published in *Reader's Digest*. Membership grew by the thousands.

A growing group of physicians became champions of La Leche League over the next few years. The league began to hold conferences for professionals on lactation research and support for mothers, as well as on lactation and parenting issues for families. In 1974, the American Medical Association accredited the league as a provider of continuing medical education credits for physicians. In 2002, the league presented its 30th Annual Seminar for Physicians on Breastfeeding. More than 3,000 physicians have attended the seminar through the years. The league estimates that each attending physician extends his breastfeeding education to assist 6,000 nursing mothers, for the benefit of a total of 18,000,000 nursing couples.

Now called La Leche League International, the organization has more than seven thousand leaders in fifty states and forty-six foreign countries, and accredits another thousand leaders yearly. Almost 41,000 have been accredited over the past forty-five years. League leaders counsel, by mail, e-mail, phone, and in person, almost 100,000 nursing mothers a month—over a million a year. Their telephone hotline, 1-800-LA LECHE, is contacted more than ten thousand times a month, and their Web site, www.lalecheleague.org, received more than two million visitors in 2002. The remarkable growth and influence of La Leche League is testament to the commitment of nursing mothers to their babies and to one another.

LACTATION CONSULTANTS

With much credit due to the work of La Leche League, a new kind of breastfeeding adviser has evolved to become an indispensable health-care profession. By the 1980s, many women, in and out of La Leche League, had spent decades studying lactation, identifying and assessing breastfeeding problems, counseling nursing mothers, and teaching practicing physicians the fundamentals of breastfeeding support. Women began to feel the need for an organization that would serve those whose skills and knowledge had reached the professional level. Furthermore, as breastfeeding became more popular, RNs, midwives, and other women of varied backgrounds were beginning to call themselves lactation consultants and to charge fees for advice. Some form of licensing or testing seemed to be needed to ensure that everyone who was offering paid consultation would be providing accurate information to mothers.

So La Leche League funded the formation of a certification organization, the International Board of Lactation Consultant Examiners (IBLCE), to devise an exam by which one could become a certified lactation consultant. The International Lactation Consultants Association, or ILCA (pronounced "ilk-a"), was formed for consultants and others who passed the rigorous exam and are entitled to use the initials I.B.C.L.C.—International Board Certified Lactation Consultant—after their names. Its membership includes onetime La Leche League leaders, MDs, nurses, physical therapists, midwives, mental health professionals, and others who have invested years in working with nursing mothers. Known as "LCs," they are employed by hospitals, pediatric and obstetric practices, birthing centers, and in private practice. They can be found almost everywhere, from urban centers to farming communities. The association holds annual conferences and scientific meetings for medical professionals interested in lactation, and promotes breastfeeding worldwide.

A NETWORK OF SUPPORT FOR NURSING MOTHERS

What has evolved through the efforts of individual breastfeeding advocates, La Leche League, ILCA, and a host of community-based organizations is an interactive network of support for the nursing mother, in which each level of assistance bolsters the others. The La Leche League leader provides friendship, accurate information, and practical guidance. When a problem arises that is out of her range of expertise, she can refer the mother to a lactation consultant who provides trained expertise, specifically in breastfeeding. If the LC spots a medical problem—which may be anything from a neurological issue in the baby to a mother with walking pneumonia—she can refer the mother to a breastfeeding-oriented physician. The physician can then work with the mother and baby to address the medical issue in a way that preserves their breastfeeding relationship.

The system interacts, also, in reverse: Busy practitioners who may not have the time or the training to sort out a nursing mother's problems can refer her to a well-prepared and experienced certified LC. If an LC feels that a mother would benefit from peer support, spending time with other mothers who are more experienced in breastfeeding than she may be, the LC can put her in touch with her local La Leche League chapter.

RESEARCH AND RESEARCHERS

Helping mothers breastfeed—and teaching medical-care providers to help them, too—has played the critical role in saving breastfeeding in the last forty years. Just as fundamental, however, have been the advances in our scientific understanding of the process and relationship—to demonstrate why and how breastfeeding works, so that it cannot be treated as another parenting fad. This is the province of basic research.

Whenever a new field of research opens up, in any branch of science, there are those who deride it as insignificant. Human lactation has long suffered under this judgment, and been dismissed as an unsuitable area for serious researchers. A small but growing cadre of physicians and researchers in basic science, however, are contributing to the growing knowledge of the astonishing composition of breast milk and the lifelong benefits of breastfeeding. One writer has dubbed them "lactophiles," and they are plunging down investigative trails in all directions. Human lactation research is occurring not just in medicine but also in fields such as biochemistry, immunology, psychology, pharmacology, and public health. A computer search of current research in lactation will turn up dozens upon dozens of recently published studies. Even the popular press peppers its reports with regular announcements of a newly discovered benefit of breastfeeding. While we don't yet understand every aspect of lactation, the facts are pouring in that it is undeniably among biology's more extraordinary phenomena. Unlike twenty or thirty years ago, advocates for breastfeeding now stand side by side with the scientists to restore it in the lives of mothers and babies.

Part Two

The Art of Breastfeeding

Before the Baby Comes: Preparing to Breastfeed

The months when you are nursing your baby can be among the most pleasant of your life. However, it's up to you to make them so. Hospital care and community life in North America are not always set up to accommodate the needs of the nursing mother. It takes a little advance planning if you are to avoid some circumstances, common in our society, that make giving birth and breastfeeding less pleasant and less successful than they should be. Experienced nursing mothers, who have successfully breastfed several babies, generally make the kind of arrangements that are suggested here, so that they themselves are free to relax and enjoy the new nursing baby without unnecessary obstacles to their physical well-being or their peace of mind.

CHOOSING A HOSPITAL

It is possible to find competent medical care, even in a town where you are a stranger, by selecting an accredited hospital or health maintenance organization and going to the doctors on its staff; or you can ask your previous health-care provider to recommend someone in good standing at your new location.

But how can you find the kind of care that not only is medically competent, but will give you the emotional support and practical help you want, both in giving birth and in nursing your baby?

One place to start is with the hospitals. Medical attitudes and policies toward nursing couples have come a long way. Natural childbirth techniques are widely accepted, if sometimes more in theory than in practice. Comfortable birthing rooms, complete with rocking chairs, wallpaper, and draperies, can be found at many hospitals. If arrangements are made in advance, a midwife may attend you throughout your labor and birth. Your partner, too, will be able to stay with you throughout your labor and birth, even if you have a cesarean section.

Many hospitals have not only learned to accommodate breastfeeding mothers and babies, but have restructured their entire maternity services to give mothers and babies the best possible start to breastfeeding. Winchester Hospital in Massachusetts is one. Offering prenatal breastfeeding classes with a certified lactation consultant to teach breastfeeding to mothers in their last trimester of pregnancy, the hospital also provides every mother who chooses to nurse with individualized LC support after birth. Nursing immediately after birth and rooming-in until discharge are encouraged. The hospital holds weekly group sessions in which nursing mothers gather for months after birth to socialize, share tips, and ask questions. Their Outpatient Lactation Center also provides ongoing breastfeeding education and assistance for women and their families. Winchester has even opened a "Lactation Boutique," which rents and sells breast pumps, along with pillows, stools, bras, and other nursing aids sometimes of use to nursing mothers. Hospitals such as this one have learned that helping mothers succeed in breastfeeding not only keeps their youngest patients healthier, but creates a deep loyalty toward them among the women (who make most of the health-care decisions for their families) in their communities.

However, there are differences among hospitals. In some regions of the country, comprehensive lactation support and baby-friendly maternity care are available at most hospitals. In other areas, you may need to search for this sort of care, and sift through a hospital's marketing information to discover if it is giving real service or lip service to mothers who wish to nurse their babies. A search on the Internet is a good way to start. Hospital Web sites tend to either advertise lactation-friendly policies or emphasize their technological expertise—level II special-care nurseries and sophisticated fetal monitoring equipment—over their supportive-care services for mothers and babies. Many teaching hospitals expert in treating sick newborns and other special cases nevertheless give their well newborns and new mothers equal emphasis. If so, their Web site will cover both types of care with equal detail and pride.

As you search for your hospital, beginning on the Web, followed by tours of the premises and interviews with the staff, ask a few searching questions:

- What obstetric pain management techniques are offered at the hospital?
- Are options such as an "epidural lite" or nonmedicate pain relief encouraged? (All too often, obstetric medication sedates a newborn for hours after birth, delaying a successful first nursing.)
- Will the hospital allow you to nurse your baby immediately?
- Will the hospital allow you to stay together undisturbed for the first hour or more after delivery—even if you have had a cesarean section?

- Will your baby spend any time in a central nursery, or does the hospital encourage mothers and babies to "room-in," to stay together day and night until discharge?
- Will your partner be encouraged to spend the night, and are sleeper chairs provided on the maternity floor for this purpose?
- Are breastfed babies routinely, if ever, given sugar water or other supplements in the nursery (a practice detrimental to successful breastfeeding)?
- Are breastfed babies ever given pacifiers in the nursery (also detrimental to breastfeeding)?
- Are there certified lactation consultants on staff? How many? If you request a consultation with one, will she come to your room within the next hour or two?
- Do they give breastfeeding classes or just show videotapes? Does the hospital offer "individualized" or "one-on-one" breastfeeding support? Is that support provided by nurses who are well informed on breastfeeding initiation?
- Does the nursing staff consist of mother/baby specialists who will care for you as couple, rather than nurses who look after the babies and other nurses who see to the mothers?
- What sort of postdischarge support and resources does the hospital offer nursing mothers?
- Finally, does the hospital carry the WHO/UNICEF Baby-Friendly designation, certifying that it provides an optimal environment for the promotion, protection, and support of breastfeeding?

Many hospitals have come a long way from the old days when mothers and babies were routinely separated and breastfeeding widely mismanaged—but not all. Too often newly invented "family-centered" policies have been thought up by the hospital's marketing department, rather than by lactation consultants and others who understand the real needs of a new mother and her baby. If a hospital touts its wallpapered birthing rooms and gift baskets for new parents, yet doesn't say a word about support for nursing couples, keep looking.

CHOOSING A DOCTOR

Through pregnancy, labor and delivery, and the postpartum months, a woman and her baby will be cared for by many different medical professionals, from nurse practitioners to obstetricians, anesthesiologists, pediatricians, family physicians, and lactation consultants. Each has the ability to affect the breastfeeding relationship. Prenatal nurse practitioners may be your first source of breastfeeding information. An obstetric anesthesiologist may select pain medications and doses that will help keep your baby alert and ready to nurse immediately after birth. An obstetrician may arrange with a hospital that all her patients are allowed an undisturbed hour with their newborns after birth. A pediatrician may be informed on breastfeeding and support it fully, or may be focused on rapid weight gain in early infancy, and quick to suggest supplementation. A lactation consultant may visit a mother once in the hospital, or make a series of house calls over the first six weeks to ensure that a mother and baby are nursing well and happily. Family-practice physicians specialize in taking care of mothers and babies as single units, an especially fitting mission for the breastfeeding couple. Such care is not only very convenient if you both happen to become sick, but can circumvent breastfeeding problems that may arise if only one of the nursing couple is treated. In one informal survey, mothers reported that family-practice physicians were actually more experienced and more helpful about breastfeeding than specialists in pediatrics or obstetrics. If you are planning to use specialists, however, here are some guidelines. (While you may be restricted in your choice of doctors by the kind of health insurance you carry, you can expect that at least some of the doctors on the approved list will be the kind you are looking for):

The Obstetrician:

Your obstetrician's job is to keep you healthy during pregnancy and to help you give birth to your baby. Your obstetrician will not supervise your lactation, and indeed may not know much about how to nurse a baby. (It is the pediatrician, or the lactation consultant on staff in the pediatric practice, who handles most questions on breastfeeding.) However, your obstetrician may be responsible for any physical problems involving the breasts—infections, say—that may arise after the baby is born. Also, you will still be in your obstetrician's care while you are in the hospital, so her attitude can make a great difference to you in the first days of breastfeeding. She may help you put the baby to your breast as soon as ten minutes after birth, if you like. She can make sure you do not receive any drugs to suppress lactation and will prescribe mild pain relievers or anything else you may need to help you relax and be comfortable enough for your milk to flow easily. She should be capable of helping you if problems such as engorgement or nipple soreness arise.

The obstetrician who is not interested in breastfeeding and is not convinced of its importance will not be able to give you this kind of help, and is much more skillful at suppressing lactation than at keeping it going. The male obstetrician whose wife did not breastfeed or worse, whose wife "failed" or weaned early, may actually be obstructive. Although you can probably lactate with perfect success without any help from your obstetrician, it will be at least a convenience for you if he is supportive, and it may save you a few arguments in the postpartum days when you will want to be peacefully getting to know your baby without having to argue with your caregivers.

To find the kind of obstetrician you want, you may have to shop around a little. The most "brilliant" doctor, or the doctor all your friends go to, may not be the one for you. Look first for a doctor who has breastfed her own children or whose wife has happily done so, and who has a majority of patients who breastfeed. Find a doctor who believes in the principles of natural childbirth. While both you and the doctor may shy away from the term "natural childbirth" as smacking of faddism, nowadays every doctor with a real understanding of and consideration for maternity patients uses a great many natural childbirth techniques and gives the patient a vote in how the birth should be managed. Such an obstetrician is more likely to be helpful and experienced about breastfeeding.

When you have a list of possibilities, make an appointment with each one for a consultation. If you later decide that this is not the doctor for you, the consultation will have cost you less than a full examination. (In addition, once a doctor has done a full pelvic exam on you, you may feel committed to asking that person to be your obstetrician.) Sometimes you can easily spot the obstetrician who is especially skilled with natural births; her outstanding characteristics are apt to be gentleness and endless patience. She seems interested in you as a person, not just as a pelvis; she listens to everything you ask, with no hint of intolerance. She is not in a hurry, no matter how full the waiting room is. She is gentle, never brisk or rough. She explains everything she does, at great length, without condescension. This care and patience may make the office visits longer, but may make the birth easier and will foster the development of mutual trust and respect between patient and physician.

Occasionally, a physician will be very annoyed to find that you are "shopping" for medical care. This is not the obstetrician for you. The doctor who has had experience with normal childbirth and who has seen many happy nursing mothers will understand very well why you are being careful to select a physician who appreciates these matters.

The Pediatrician:

It is a good idea to pay at least one visit to your pediatrician before the baby comes. Your obstetrician will be glad to recommend one or two pediatricians and may be able to suggest someone who is especially interested in breastfed babies. The hospital nurses or your childbirth educator may be able to tell you which pediatricians in your area are the greatest champions of mother's milk for babies.

Pediatricians are more accustomed than obstetricians to mothers who shop for a doctor. They aren't apt to resent being questioned. However, don't start out by asking bluntly, "Are you in favor of breastfeeding?" You're putting the pediatrician on the spot; he doesn't know whether you want him to say yes or no, and he may feel defensive. You can tell him that you plan to breastfeed, and would like to have rooming-in (if it is available), and see what he says. If he tries to talk you out of both, you probably have the wrong doctor.

Ask him how many of his mothers breastfeed, and for how

long. If he doesn't know how many, or gives a number lower than 50 percent, or starts explaining why so many mothers quit early these days, then you can suspect that he is not helpful to the breastfeeding mothers in his practice. If 60 percent or more of his mothers breastfeed, and if he seems proud of them, you can be fairly sure he gives them help and encouragement. Finally, you can ask if he has children himself, and if they were breastfed. If they were not, the doctor may regard the question as impertinent. If they were, he will enjoy telling you so; if his own children were breastfed a year or more, you will know that this doctor is personally acquainted with the normal course of lactation.

Suppose you already have a pediatrician you are satisfied with, but who does not encourage breastfeeding or is in favor of it but does not really understand how it works? His lack of interest in the management of lactation has nothing to do with his skill at preventing complications with measles or clearing up middle-ear infections. You need not feel obliged to change to another doctor just because you two don't see eye to eye on breastfeeding. Don't let him shake your confidence. You can ignore misguided interference. You can nurse your baby satisfactorily on your own or with the help of a La Leche League leader or certified lactation consultant. He may even learn from your experience and be more helpful to his next nursing mother, especially if you are open with him.

YOUR EMPLOYER

It is just as important to talk with your employer before your baby is born as it is to confer with your obstetrician and pediatrician. The ease of nursing and returning to full- or part-time work after your baby is born can depend on your employer's attitude and the arrangements you have made in advance. Learning to combine motherhood and work is as intensive a task as the initial transition to motherhood itself. Breastfeeding while working is relatively straightforward (and discussed in detail in Chapter 12), but the stresses of blending your old identity on the job and your new identity as a mother can be tumultuous. Consider the demands and flexibility of your job now. Can you arrange an extended maternity leave of at least four months? If not, can you transition back into work on a part-time schedule or arrange to work at home a couple of days a week for the first six months? Check with your company's personnel department; they may already have policies or programs in place to assist new mothers with the transition. If not, research what their competitors are doing (check out *Working Mother* magazine's annual list of 100 Best Companies on the Internet for descriptions of successful programs for new mothers), and tell your company how those competitors manage to keep their valued employees (who happen to be nursing mothers) on staff. Once you're a nursing working mother, you'll need to pump your milk every three to four hours for fifteen to twenty minutes. You'll need a clean, private place to do that (not a bathroom stall) with an outlet for your electric pump, and a refrigerator in which to store your milk. If your employer does not support your needs and rights as a nursing mother, write your boss or personnel department a memo explaining all the benefits to the company of helping you to continue breastfeeding (a sample letter is included in Resources). Then check out the laws in your state. A few, California for example, require employers of all sizes to meet the needs of nursing mothers.

YOUR DAY-CARE PROVIDER

You will also want to meet and settle on your day-care provider before your baby is born, if at all possible. Knowing your provider, whether she comes to your home or is or at a family day-care center, during your maternity leave will ease your mind and allow you to relax and focus on your baby. If your child-care arrangements are set, you and your baby can stop by the day-care provider every once in a while before you return to work, and you can begin to build a comfortable relationship with each other. If your provider is new to breastfeeding, you can share information with her on the importance of breast milk, and how she should handle it and feed your baby once you return to work. (More detailed information on the handling and storage of breast milk can be found in Chapter 12.)

"CONTRAINDICATIONS"

You may nurse your baby if you have a cold or the flu or some other mild, contagious disease. Breastfed babies show remarkable immunity to such ailments and often escape getting sick even when the whole family comes down with a "bug." However, a mother with whooping cough or active tuberculosis (not just a positive skin test) should have no contact with her baby at all, since these very contagious diseases are dangerous for her newborn; in such cases she, or course, cannot breastfeed. In developed countries, mothers who are HIV-positive are advised not to breastfeed.

It used to be thought that a mother with Rh factor incompatibility could not breastfeed. That is not true. Rh antibodies may exist in the milk of an Rh-negative mother, but they have no ef-fect on the baby. Genital herpes, however, can be a serious threat to the newborn; nevertheless, even mothers with active herpes infections can usually breastfeed safely provided they take proper precautions (see Chapter 9, pages 252–53). Hepatitis B is a viral disease that poses serious dangers to the newborn, but there is no sound evidence that it can be transmitted through breastfeeding. Other chronic infections should be handled on a case-by-case ba-sis in consultation with one's doctor.

The diabetic mother can breastfeed successfully, with careful management. Breastfeeding, in fact, is less likely to cause prob-lems than is pregnancy; some mothers find that their blood sugar is more stable and their need for insulin actually decreases during lactation (see Chapter 2, page 55). Furthermore, there is signifi-cant evidence that breastfed children are themselves less suscep-tible to developing diabetes than are formula-fed children (see Chapter 3, page 117 Since diabetes has some genetic elements, the mother who is diabetic may be especially interested in this protective aspect of breastfeeding her babies.

Mothers receiving chemotherapy or radiation treatments may be asked not to breastfeed. However, in some cases, an alternate drug can be prescribed that does not endanger the nursing baby. When planning a diagnostic radiation procedure for a nursing mother, the physician and technicians may consider using a min-imal radiopharmaceutical dose and longer imaging time to pro-tect her baby and their nursing relationship. Epileptic mothers sometimes have a medical conflict if they wish to breastfeed; some drugs prescribed for epilepsy adversely affect the nursing baby. If you or your doctor are in any doubt about the safety of the medication you must take, send for La Leche League's publi-cation on medications and breast milk, which is supervised by the league's medical board and is frequently updated to reflect current research, or refer to the American Academy of Pediatrics' most recent report (2000 or later) on drugs and breast milk.

You should not be taking any illicit or "recreational" drugs during pregnancy, but if you are, now is the time to stop. All such drugs—including nicotine, caffeine, alcohol, and marijuana—pass through the milk and can affect the baby. Cocaine is especially dangerous to small infants; it passes through the milk, and it can be fatal even in a single dose.

If the mother is desperately ill from some chronic disease, her doctor may justifiably forbid her to breastfeed. However, the mother who is temporarily incapacitated after a difficult or surgical delivery is better off breastfeeding than not. Lactation gives her an excuse to get more rest during convalescence, and saves her from the multiple chores of bottlefeeding. The hormones of lactation relax her and ease tensions, which will aid in her overall convalescence. Lactation can be of the same benefit to the mother with a heart condition or with another chronic illness than can be managed and monitored.

THE PHYSICALLY DISADVANTAGED MOTHER

The disabled mother deserves more than ever to breastfeed her baby. A mother who relies on a wheelchair or who is blind will find breastfeeding infinitely easier than trying to cope with bottles and mixing formula. It is no more difficult for her than for any other new mother to learn to nurse, and she gains a sense of joy in her self-sufficiency that goes far to combat any feelings she might have that she cannot give her child as much as other mothers do. Kathy Beaudette, a blind La Leche League group leader, says that breastfeeding is "the only way to go" for a blind mother and her child, and that it offered for her, even after weaning, "the miraculous closeness to my son that only touch could bring." La Leche League International offers a variety of loan material about breastfeeding and child care, including its book, *The Womanly Art of Breastfeeding,* on tape and in Braille.

CLOTHING

Wearing a well-fitting brassiere during pregnancy will help prevent loss of breast shape. In late pregnancy and during lactation, you can expect to be about one full cup size larger than you used to be, with variations upward depending on the amount of milk present. If you started out as a skimpy A, you will probably be no larger than an ample B, and will get adequate support from any well-fitting bra. If you started out as a B or C, you will probably need the sturdy maternity bras. By six months after weaning, your breasts will be back to their previous size and shape. Many mothers find their figures have actually improved.

Before you go to the hospital, pack two or more nursing bras in your suitcase. These are made with a flap that lowers so you can feed the baby without losing support. Bras do get wet from milk, at first, so you will need at least one to wear and one to wash. Nursing bras may be bought at lingerie shops, maternity shops, department stores, or through mail-order catalogs. The plain cotton drop-cup type is generally affordable and comfortable. If you don't want such institutional-looking underwear, you can find very pretty nursing bras, costing slightly more, at some better stores or online.

When you are nursing, you need clothing that gives easy and discreet access to the breasts. One mother was given as a "welcome home" present a new dress that buttoned up the back! Not only did it have to be removed entirely to nurse the baby, but it took two people or a contortionist to get it off and on. Invest in nighties that open in the front and sweaters or shirts you can unbutton or lift from the waist.

BREAST CARE

No breast care is necessary in the first six months of pregnancy. In the last three months, it is probably wise to stop using any soap on the breasts. The skin secretes protective oils that help to make the nipple and areola strong and supple. By scrubbing with soap, you remove this natural protection. The protective skin secretions are mildly antibacterial; it seems likely that nature is already on the job, guarding your breasts and preparing them for the job of nursing.

The nipples are highly sensitive right after you give birth, for good reason: to respond better to the stimulation of the baby's suckling, which triggers the hormones that make and release the milk. Proper positioning in the first days of nursing can help prevent sore nipples from developing. Despite common belief, fair-skinned women are not more likely to develop cracked nipples than others, but mothers who have had trouble with sore nipples with previous babies may have trouble again. One theory is that our clothing overprotects our nipples so that they become sensitive. To desensitize the overprotected nipples, doctors sometimes recommend scrubbing with a rough towel or (horrors!) a brush; a Connecticut clinic has found that it is simpler and less uncomfortable to trim a circle of material from the cups of your brassieres so that the breast is supported but the nipple exposed, allowing some gentle chafing against clothing. (You may wish to stitch around the openings to prevent unraveling.) Better yet, if at all possible, simply expose your bare breasts to air and sunshine occasionally.

Some women have nipples that are flat or retracted. The hormones of pregnancy tend to improve the shape of the nipples, without any other help. Truly inverted nipples will retract when pressed between thumb and forefinger; these are uncommon. The standard advice is to pull the nipple out daily with the fingers; however, research indicates that this does not improve the shape, and most women dislike doing it. Wearing bras that are open at the tips will help, as the edges of the cut-away circles push gently on the margins of the areolas, which makes the nipples more prominent. Once lactation begins, the nursing of the baby will soon draw the nipple out normally in any case; however, retraction will recur when the baby is weaned.

The mother whose nipples are so inverted that she fears she will never be able to nurse can achieve normalcy with breast shields or shells worn regularly during the last weeks of pregnancy. Once fitted, the shield will provide a constant pressure that causes the inverted nipple to press out. The Medela Breast Shell Kit and Breast Shields are inexpensive; and are available through La Leche League and lactation consultants, and on some online sites (see Resources). Be selective when purchasing a breast shield; some brands can be uncomfortable. Models with multiple air holes are preferable to models with one or just a few. (Please note: Breast shields are useful only to correct inverted nipples and can be damaging if used otherwise.) One experienced lactation consultant, a nurse working for a group of obstetricians, feels that retracted nipples are seldom seen in women whose love life involves a lot of breast play. Some couples tend to avoid the breasts; others make much of them. It is of course a matter of personal preference. However, it seems at least possible that the tender attentions of a lover to this highly erogenous area are part of nature's way of preparing a woman's body for the task of nursing a baby.

If your nipples are pierced, it would be wise to remove the nipple rings before your baby is born to allow your breasts to prepare for lactation without potential complications caused by a foreign object in the nipple. The minimal scar tissue caused by most piercings is unlikely to cause any difficulty during breastfeeding.

Research indicates that it is unwise to put alcohol or other "hardening" agents on your nipples. These irritants, although sometimes recommended by health-care personnel, are worse than useless because hard, dry skin cracks more easily than soft, supple skin. Anointing the nipples with oils and creams is apparently harmless, if the preparations are water soluble and rinse off easily, but they don't do much good, either. After the baby is born, anything you put on your nipples is likely to enter the baby's body, so read the labels and package inserts; if a product is "not for internal use," don't use it on your nipples.

HELP AT HOME

If you want to enjoy the first weeks of nursing your baby, instead of struggling through them exhausted, you will need a support system. New mothers through time have been surrounded by a covey of female relatives and neighbors who help out and assist her in learning to care for her new baby. Twenty-first-century mothers in the United States have no fewer needs than those mothers of a hundred or a thousand years ago. The support system can consist of a partner, relatives, neighbors, friends, or a professional "doula" (the age-old term for a woman who helps a new mother through delivery and during the newborn period), but do put one in place before your baby is born.

It is tempting to believe that we can manage any challenge, any transition on our own. Single mothers are sometimes especially

determined to accomplish the early postpartum weeks without relying on others for assistance. But you must protect your returning strength in these first weeks, or you may become too stressed
and exhausted for the letdown reflex to work well, and for it to
deliver sufficiently high-fat milk for your new baby. Partners may
also be feeling the strain of new child-care responsibilities. Some
are not accustomed to doing more than minimal housework, and
their spouses may become impatient seeing how long it takes
them to clean up the kitchen or prepare dinner. Partners may unconsciously take their emotional cues from the new mother, and
add to her exhaustion and stress rather than being a calming and
helpful influence. (New research suggests that very young babies
also pick up on the emotions of their caregivers, and respond
with similar expressions of tension or calm.) All too soon, a new
mother will find herself helping out, and getting overtired, which
is bad for morale and for her milk supply.

The answer of course, as it has been through time, is a doula.
Anthropologist Dana Raphael promoted the term "doula" for the
woman who traditionally helps a new mother in preliterate societies. While the mother recovers from childbirth and gets to
know her new baby, the doula sees to the cooking and other
household chores and looks after the mother. She is the woman
(and the occasional man) who "mothers the mother," in the
words of researcher John Kennell. Often the doula is the new
mother's own mother, but she might also be a sister, neighbor, or
friend. Most cultures take it for granted that new mothers need
this kind of support. Our culture seems to take it for granted that
new mothers can sink or swim on their own, even if they have
been sent home from the hospital with a newborn just hours after
giving birth. Whether your doula is a relative, a friend, or a professional, find one and make a place for her in your life during the
first few weeks after your baby is born.

If your mother, mother-in-law, or some other relative offers to help out for the first few weeks, and is a truly helpful, nondisruptive presence, accept the offer gladly. However, if she must stay with you, you may feel called on to act as a hostess. And if spending time with her is ever a strain for you, consider making other arrangements. One grandmother customarily spends a week taking care of each new mother in the family—but she stays, not with the parents, but at a nearby motel. "Most of the work that needs to be done is daytime work," she points out, "and the parents need their privacy in the evening—and I need mine!"

Grandmothers who live far away often feel better about the separation from you and your children if they can be of help right after the birth. If personal help is not practical, probably one of the nicest baby presents a grandparent can give is the money for a few weeks of paid household help. However, do look out for yourself and line up a doula one way or another. In some cases, the baby's father can take paternity leave for two weeks or so, to help out. One new mother had her own mother visit and help out the first week and her husband's mother the second week. A single mother enlisted the services of her best friend's seventeen-year-old brother, who turned out to be a superlative errand runner and launderer, and a pretty good cook.

If you go to a health maintenance organization (HMO) for your health care, find out if they offer a home-care service for new parents. Several do, and it is becoming more common. (The incentive for the HMO and insurance companies is that offering postpartum support to new mothers allows them to curtail her hospital stay to forty-eight hours or less.) If the service is arranged before your baby is born, a mother's helper can come to your house for several days after you return home to help out in any way necessary, whether straightening the house, making a few meals, or doing the shopping. (Some insurance companies restrict postpartum care to breastfeeding support, which is a little nonsensical, as mother support equals breastfeeding support.) You may need help for longer than three days, however, and often this service is provided only if you leave the hospital within forty-eight hours of giving birth.

Independent services may exist in your area that provide the same kind of help for as long as you need it. Fees charged by private services vary from reasonable to extravagant. Although the cost may not be covered by your medical insurance, a crucial week or two of help may be well worth it. Look in the Yellow Pages under "Home Services." Some states provide state-funded "homemaker" services. Some retired La Leche League leaders have gone into business as doulas, and will provide you with not only tender loving care, but good breastfeeding advice as well; they may advertise in a local parents' newspaper or on the Web.

Sometimes a neighborhood in which there are a lot of young families can organize to make things easier for a new mother. For instance, a neighbor can take the toddler or older children for the afternoon, so that the new mother can nap (it is wise to institute this as a routine before the baby is born). One Chicago neighborhood full of young families has organized a round robin in which each family takes a turn doing the housework and providing a cooked dinner for the household where there is a new baby. Since there are some twenty families in on the arrangement, the mother who comes home with a new baby receives twenty days of having her housework done and her family's dinner prepared for her.

The one kind of help you don't need is a baby nurse. You may find yourself cleaning house and cooking meals for the nurse while she takes care of your baby. However, almost every city has a visiting nurse association, and you should certainly consider taking advantage of this service. It may even be free in your area. See if your medical insurance covers the cost, then ask your doctor to arrange it, or ask the nurses at the hospital before you are discharged; sometimes the visiting nurse is part of the service normally provided for each new mother. The visiting nurse can tell at a glance how the baby is doing, can help you with baths and other new tasks, and will also keep a weather eye on your own state of health. She is a good source of advice about diaper services and other methods of saving your energy. In almost any city or suburb, you can search the Web for "Nurses" or "Sitting Services" in your area, or look in the Yellow Pages, for trained, experienced mother's helpers.

Couples in which both parents must work long hours sometimes rely on live-in help. Organizations exist in large cities that train and place European-style "nannies" or "au pairs" who care for children twelve or more hours a day. If you elect to go this route, be aware that a nanny poses a risk for the nursing mother if she is not supportive of breastfeeding. One New York City mother warns from experience: "Some nannies hired through an agency actually charge more for taking care of a breastfed than a bottlefed baby. Others will not be openly critical but will say things like, 'The baby's not interested in nursing anymore,' when it's obvious to the mother that isn't true." Ask during the interview if the person nursed her own children, and for how long; some older women believe two to three months is quite long enough, and after that will offer little support and possibly the reverse.

MATERNITY LEAVE

If you plan on returning to your job after the baby is born, arrange in advance for as much time at home on maternity leave as possible. Many women have returned to full- and part-time work as soon as six weeks after the birth and continued to nurse their babies successfully right into toddlerhood. Nevertheless, the longer you can manage to stay at home full time, the more relaxed you'll be, and the more secure you'll probably feel about your nursing relationship. Eight weeks of maternity leave are now protected by the federal Family and Medical Leave Act of 1993. While considered a huge victory for working mothers, the act in reality offers a bare minimum of support and protection, requiring employers with fifty or more employees to allow eight-week unpaid leaves for employees to care for family members, including newborn babies. Smaller businesses do not need to offer any leave at all, and no employer is required to provide a paid leave.

Therefore, it is essentially up to your employer how to define your maternity leave. A majority of companies, except for very small businesses, offer eight weeks of paid maternity leave, and often an employer will agree to another four or more unpaid weeks. Save your vacation time, if possible, and add it on to your weeks of maternity leave. If you can possibly manage it financially, a leave of six months or more has numerous benefits for both you and your baby, allowing you time to learn about each other and transition comfortably into this new stage of your life.

If you cannot manage to take additional leave, don't despair. It is quite possible to return to work full time and continue nursing your baby, without formula supplements, for as long as you wish. You will find, in fact, that continuing to breastfeed will be a wonderful source of support and confidence during the early months of combining mothering and working outside your home. (See Chapter 12, "The Working Mother: How Breastfeeding Can Help.")

SHORTCUTS

After you have arranged for help in the house for two weeks, and perhaps have set up a way for any older children to be away from home for a couple of hours a day, try to organize as many shortcuts as you can to lighten your workload in the first month you are home. Here are some suggestions from experienced mothers:

- If you plan on using cloth diapers, arrange for a diaper service for the first few weeks at least. This saves a tremendous amount of work. If you live in the country and cannot get diaper service, buy a few dozen disposable diapers for the first several days at home. (While many mothers continue to use disposables until their child is toilet-trained, other mothers use cloth diapers exclusively because they are more comfortable for the baby and less damaging to the environment.)
- If you can possibly afford it, now is the time to purchase major appliances you may not have. A washer and a dryer are more important than living room furniture. A dishwasher or a microwave oven will be worth more to you than wall-to-wall carpet. There will be time for interior decorating again in years to come, but while your children are very small, the most important purchases are those that reduce drudgery and give you more time and energy for your family, particularly if you plan on returning to work.
- If you have a toddler already, a high school girl or boy can be a great help by coming in for an hour or two after school to supervise bath and supper and to play games.

- Stock the cupboards with quick, nourishing foods, with the emphasis on proteins. If you are alone with the baby most of the day, you may not feel like going to the kitchen and cooking, but you need plenty of nourishing food, especially at the start of lactation, or you will feel tired and depressed. You're less likely to skimp, or to fill up on coffee and doughnuts, if something that is better for you is easily available. Stock up on high-protein foods such as quick-cooking oatmeal, cheese, canned tuna, sardines, salmon, baked or refried beans, and tofu. A blender can produce instant high-protein milk shakes if you don't feel like cooking.

- A microwave oven can be a godsend to a family with a newborn. Frozen dinners can be made piping hot in five minutes. These days, a huge variety of prepared foods for the microwave can be found. Look also for dinners in a pouch that can be heated quickly in boiling water. However, commercial TV dinners, whether for the microwave, oven, or stove, usually don't have enough nutrition in them to satisfy a nursing mother's appetite. You can probably make less expensive and tastier dinners yourself before the baby is born and freeze them. The servings should be generous and should include your favorite meals and desserts; make the first days at home a time for treats. You can freeze meals for your other children, too. Then, even if your partner is not comfortable in the kitchen, either of you can produce a hot meal quickly.

- You and your partner may well find that you simply don't have time to market during the first weeks. Even in these days of supermarkets, you might be able to find a neighborhood store that will take an order by phone and either deliver it or hold it until it is picked up. Some urban areas have entrepreneurial chefs who have created home delivery services of your choice of one, two, or three hot meals a day. Or ask a neighbor to shop for you from a list you have prepared.

- Address your birth announcements ahead of time.
- Even if you have a washer and dryer, you may wish to cut down their use to a minimum for a few weeks by sending your sheets and towels out. Some laundries have a linen delivery service, which, just like a diaper service, will supply you with clean sheets and towels, pick them up weekly, and substitute new ones. That means you can have clean sheets and towels every day, if you wish, without doing any laundry or buying any extra sheets. These services are listed in the Yellow Pages under "Linen Supply Services." If a nearby dry cleaner or Laundromat offers wash-and-fold services, consider taking just the baby's things to be done. If the charge is by the pound, it will cost very little to do an entire layette of tiny shirts and sleepers. (Check to make sure they do not use fabric softener, which can irritate the skin of some babies, and which reduces absorbency of the clothing.) Whatever means you choose to reduce the laundering task, get the system in place and try it out before the baby comes.

DIET AND REST

Now, in late pregnancy, is a good time to learn to nap. Any book on natural childbirth, such as *Childbirth Without Fear*, by Grantly Dick-Read, one of the originators of the modern concept of natural childbirth, will teach you relaxation techniques that will help you fall asleep in the daytime. A nursing baby is usually less trouble at night than a bottlefed baby. But he will be hungry, and only you can feed him, so you are bound to lose a little sleep. To keep your spirits up and your milk supply bountiful in the first weeks of lactation, it will help if you have practiced and learned the knack of napping—really sleeping—once or even two or three times during the day. Ideally, in the first few weeks, you'll be able to sleep whenever the baby sleeps.

Pregnancy is also a good time to improve your own eating habits. You may not feel like going to the trouble of changing your ways once you are preoccupied with the new baby. You don't need to change your diet radically, or eat things you hate, to eat right. Just concentrate on good nutrition, on getting the vitamins, minerals, proteins, and calories you need (see Chapter 2). If you acquire the habit of eating well now, you will find that after giving birth you will have more energy and a better disposition, both of which are vital to the nursing mother. Clinics and HMOs sometimes offer nutritional counseling, which is worthwhile if you feel uncertain.

FITNESS

During pregnancy, childbirth, and lactation, you will have an easier time of it, enjoy yourself more, and be more of a help and pleasure to those around you if you are fit. Staying fit, strong, and supple can be fun, rather than a duty, and it is never too late to start; the smallest effort will bring some improvement. Half an hour of brisk walking outdoors or swimming a few laps every day will do a lot.

The benefits of looking after your body's well-being are many: You don't get as tired, you don't get winded, you feel more cheerful—all especially valuable during pregnancy, but definite benefits at any time. It's nice to know, too, that the fitter you are, the brighter your eyes and the better you feel.

A CHANGE OF PACE

A mother often has the feeling, especially with a first baby, that after the pregnancy is over everything will get back to normal. The housework will get done again; she will wear her normal clothes again, and return to normal life. The trouble is, this doesn't exactly happen. As Jean Kerr says, "The thing about having a baby is, from then on, you have it." If you already have small children, one more may not make too much difference. But if this is the first baby or if it has been a number of years since you had an infant in the house, the usual tendency is to try to fit the baby's care and feeding into your life and still do all the things you used to do. You may especially look forward to doing the things that were difficult in the last months of pregnancy—keeping the floor waxed, going out at night often, entertaining, and volunteering for extra work on the job. This attempt to lead two conflicting lives at once, that of busy woman and that of new mother, is exhausting for anyone and frequently causes breastfeeding to falter. You will find your life is easier if you can postpone the return to "normal." In a way, you can look at these early months of nursing and "tuning in" to your baby as your reward for the hard job of pregnancy and childbirth.

Especially in the first weeks, your baby will want to nurse often and for long periods. This may be the first time in your adult life when you can legitimately sit down, occasionally in the day-time, put your feet up, watch television, or read a mystery novel, because you are also feeding the baby. Perhaps this is nature's way of ensuring not only that the baby gets enough milk, but that you get enough rest for an easy convalescence. The housework and the world's work will always be there, but the nursing relationship is soon over. It is worth taking time off to see it well begun.

In the Hospital

THE HOSPITAL

Hospitals' labor and birth policies changed a great deal in the 1980s and '90s. Fathers now stay with their laboring partners at all times, even during a cesarean section. Lactation-suppressing drugs are no longer given routinely. And breastfeeding immediately after giving birth, even after a cesarean section, is widely allowed and often encouraged. You may even be able to bring your doula with you into the hospital, whether an experienced supportive friend or a professional doula, to ease your labor. Some hospitals have 100 percent "rooming-in" for new mothers and babies, so that they never need be separated from birth onward. However, policies vary from hospital to hospital, and from doctor to doctor. What is promised in the hospital's marketing materials is not always what happens on the maternity floor. Do not assume your desires and plans will fit in with the hospital's protocol. Discuss them with your obstetrician ahead of time; if necessary, make prior arrangements with the hospital administration. At every step, ask questions and make your preferences clearly known to all.

It is important to protect your birth experience and ensure

you have strong support during it. Studies of women in labor have shown that the quality of labor and delivery can affect a woman and her baby in myriad ways and for weeks and months afterward. Having a doula with you during labor, as well as your loving partner, can make an enormous difference in your stress level, even if labor is extended or becomes complicated at any point. Research has shown that the presence of a doula, either an experienced, informed person who helps a mother after delivery or one who guides her through her labor and delivery, decreases the need for medications and anesthesia, and results in fewer complications. A 1992 study by researcher John Klaus showed a decrease of cesarean-birth rate by 50 percent, the length of labor by 25 percent, pitocin use by 40 percent, pain medication by 30 percent, the need for forceps by 40 percent, and requests for epidural anesthesia by 60 percent among women who labored with a doula. A positive birth experience has been shown in separate studies to create confidence and calm in a new mother, qualities that underlie a good start to breastfeeding and mothering.

A widespread improvement in maternity care is the availability of birthing rooms in which you may both labor and give birth to the baby, rather than move to a sterile delivery room in the last stage of labor. These rooms typically have been designed to be as homelike as possible with pretty wallpaper, a comfortable chair for your partner or labor companion, and a bed, rather than a delivery table, for you. An increasing number of hospitals offer labor-birth-recovery rooms in which you may labor, give birth, and rest with your baby for several hours. Birthing centers affiliated with hospitals may even have labor-birth-recovery-and-postpartum rooms, so that you need never change rooms from the time you arrive until you go home.

Although birthing rooms can signify a family-centered

approach to childbirth and a supportive attitude toward breast-feeding, they can also be the result merely of the hospital's public relations department realizing they will attract patients. (One hospital advertises "Homelike rooms complete with entertainment systems for Dad!"—clearly not an innovation designed to support Mom during labor.) An attractively decorated labor-and-birth room doesn't guarantee a positive birth experience or a good start to breastfeeding. It is the education and the attitude of the staff, and those of your own family-practice physician or obstetrician *and* pediatrician, that will make the difference. Of course, even women cared for by supportive and flexible obstetrics staffs may have difficult labors and cesarean sections. The sensitivity of the staff, however, can lessen the stress of a complicated labor and enhance the joy of an easy one.

In addition to discussing your labor and birth in advance, you should speak to your family-practice physician or your baby's pediatrician beforehand. Tell him you plan to breastfeed. Ask him to *write a note on your chart and the baby's chart* that you will be breastfeeding, and that no bottles of water, sugar water, formula, or pacifiers are to be given to your baby at any time. He can also instruct the staff via the chart to let your baby room-in with you, or be brought to you as often and for as long as you wish, and not to skip nighttime feedings. If it is written on the chart, it is an order and has more force than verbal reminders.

GIVING BIRTH AND THE FIRST NURSING

When you first arrive at the hospital, a resident doctor or nurse will probably examine you to see how far along in labor you are. Tell her that you intend to nurse your baby as soon as he is born. Healthy newborns, unless sedated by medications given to their mothers during labor, are usually alert for an hour or so after birth. During this time, your baby will make eye contact, turn toward your voice, and enjoy being touched and held. This is the ideal time to begin breastfeeding.

While lactation-suppressing drugs are no longer administered routinely, other drugs given to you during labor can cause your baby to be sleepy when born and weaken his sucking. When your own obstetrician arrives, remind him that you intend to nurse the baby as soon as he is born. Repeat that you wish to avoid taking any drugs that might make the baby too sleepy to nurse. However, you may desire pain relief, and you have a choice of drugs to provide it. Ask the staff to keep in mind that you plan to nurse soon after birth; your partner or doula can continue to alert them as your labor progresses.

The medical world is now aware of the many protective and nourishing qualities of colostrum, the "first milk," and will not suggest that water is preferable for the first feeding. Most doctors these days also will agree to delay putting silver nitrate drops or antibiotic ointment in your baby's eyes for a few hours. Required by law in most states to prevent eye infections in the newborn in case the mother has venereal disease, silver nitrate especially can cause the baby to squint and his eyelids to swell for a while, keeping him from making the eye-to-eye contact so important to you both in the first hour or so. However, don't assume that all doctors, nurses, or hospitals have changed their policies about giving water or administering silver nitrate drops. Ask the hospital staff ahead of time and make arrangements if necessary. If the staff discourages you from nursing immediately after birth because the baby "might get cold," have your partner or doula remind them that one of the warmest places a newborn can be is skin-to-skin with his mother, her arms around him. Recent research on

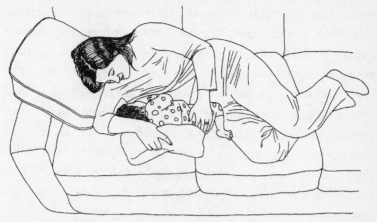

Figure 9.1 Nursing the newborn while lying down: The baby is propped on his side with a rolled-up towel behind his back; thus his body faces his mother so he does not have to turn his head to nurse. His head is level with the breast and free to move. The mother has put a pillow behind her own back for extra support and comfort.

Kangaroo Care, the practice of putting premature and full-term babies against their mothers' chests, skin-to-skin ear-to-heart, has produced remarkable evidence of the power of mother-baby contact. Babies who are allowed to stay on their mothers' chests, skin-to-skin, for an hour or more after birth, cry less and show fewer signs of stress overall than babies who are wrapped up and taken off to the nursery after a half-hour or so of greeting. The soothing effect lasts many hours afterward, and research is under way to examine the long-term effects of this early, extended skin-to-skin contact. Your partner should also remind the health-care staff that your requests have been approved by your doctor, and he or she can remind your doctor to write these orders on your chart and the baby's chart (so all the nursing shifts will be following the same instructions).

When your baby is born, if all is well and you are feeling up to it, the doctor will probably place him on your chest or beside you so that you can have a good look at him. In the excitement after birth, you may have to ask to hold your baby. Your partner can be in charge of remembering to say that you want to hold your baby right away, and that you would like to keep your baby with you for the next sixty to ninety minutes before he is dressed or given treatments of any sort. The nurse will help you get comfortable so that you can begin to breastfeed. If she doesn't, you can manage by yourself. Your partner may already have had a chance to hold and get to know the baby; this first hour of life is exhilarating for all of you, and the perfect time to get acquainted.

PUTTING THE BABY TO THE BREAST

When you are given your baby, turn onto your side (if you can) so that you will face the baby with your whole body, with his mouth directly in front of your nipple. He should be on his side, facing you, so he doesn't have to turn his head to reach your nipple. Put your arm around him and bring him close. Babies' little snub noses are designed so that they can breathe

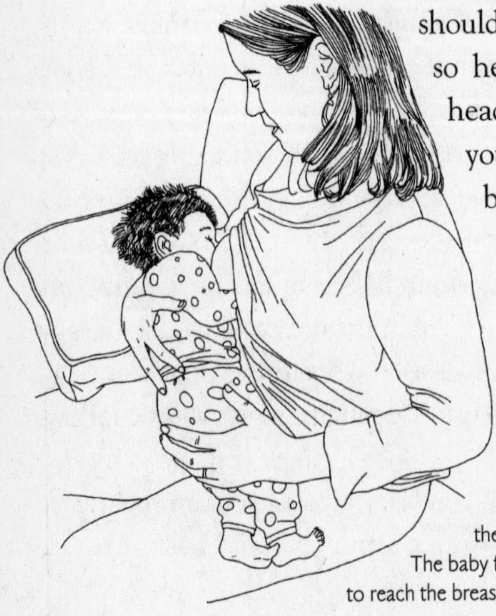

Figure 9.2 GOOD POSITIONING
A good position for nursing while sitting up: The baby's body is flat against the mother's, rolled toward her and held close in. Mother and baby are tummy to tummy. The mother supports the baby's head in the crook of her arm. The baby feels secure and does not have to strain to reach the breast.

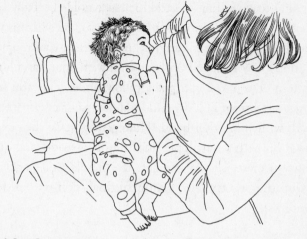

Figure 9.3 POOR POSITIONING
A poor position while nursing sitting up: The baby is flat on her back so she must nurse with her head turned, making it hard to swallow. The nipple will not be placed deeply enough in the baby's mouth, leading to soreness.

even when pressed close to their mothers' breasts. Get as close as you can be (see illustrations).

Hold your breast with your other hand, thumb on top and fingers below. Touch the center of the baby's lower lip with your nipple, and he will open his mouth wide. Then pull him in close, so that he takes the nipple and all or most of the surrounding areola into his mouth. (Don't be concerned if you have a large areola; just let the baby take as much as he can into his mouth.) If the baby's lower lip has been drawn in along with the nipple and areola, gently pull down on the lip to draw it out, after he begins to nurse. For the first feeding, don't offer both breasts to the baby. Cuddle your baby and let him get to know your touch and scent and taste. Some babies don't want to actually nurse at this first feeding, but just to taste and be held and explore this new experience. That's fine; it's good practice.

To nurse sitting up, don't lay the baby on his back as if you were going to give him a bottle; instead, hold the baby on his side, across your midsection, so that he faces you with his whole body and does not have to turn his head to reach your nipple (see illustration). Lay his head on your arm, with your hand holding his bottom or leg. You can put a pillow under your arm so you won't get tired from holding him. Support your breast from underneath with your other hand. Then gently tickle the center of his lower lip with your nipple until he opens wide, and quickly pull him in close, so that he gets the nipple well back in his mouth on the first try (see additional discussion on positioning on page 258).

IF YOU HAVE A CESAREAN SECTION

If you have had a cesarean section, you may not feel strong enough to do anything, even feed the baby, until several hours after birth. Or you may well be able to hold and nurse your baby, with the help of your partner and doula, in the recovery room before the anesthesia has worn off. If so, ask the nurse to place pillows between your knees and behind your back so that your abdominal muscles will not be stressed. Once you are comfortable on your side, ask the nurse to put your baby right up next to you, facing you with his whole body and with his mouth directly in front of your nipple. If you wait to breastfeed until you are settled in your room, the nurse will help you in the same way.

If you have active genital herpes at the time of giving birth, you will probably have a cesarean section to avoid exposing the baby to lesions in the birth canal. This doesn't mean you can't breastfeed; you just have to be careful, while the infection is active, not to carry the virus accidentally to your baby on your hands. Pediatricians advise that you scrub your hands before you hold the baby, and then avoid scratching yourself. A simple way to remind yourself to be careful is to spread a blanket over your lap from the waist down while you are nursing.

IN THE HOSPITAL NURSERY

While keeping your baby with you in your room all or most of the time you are in the hospital, if your baby must spend some time in the nursery, remind your doctor to leave orders that your baby receive no formula, sugar water, plain water, or pacifiers. Your baby is born with extra fluids in the body, which will see him through until your milk supply is well established. He will lose a little weight as he gradually loses these fluids. This loss need not be made up with formula or sugar water, which will ruin his appetite for your milk. Sucking on a rubber nipple may make him a poorer sucker at the breast and will reduce the amount of comfort sucking he does at the breast; pacifier use in the first week has been shown to be associated with early weaning.

FIRST FEEDINGS

In the hours and first days following your baby's birth, try to use both breasts at each feeding, alternating the breast you start with, and letting the baby nurse as long as she wants. The nurses may give you other advice, but this really does seem to be the best system in the early weeks. (If someone tells you to limit the amount you nurse in the beginning to five minutes a side, increasing by two minutes each time, politely nod and ignore them. This is a

certain method of developing sore nipples and delaying the production of mature milk.) You can change sides, if you want to,
without sitting up, by hugging the baby to your chest and turning
over with him. Use your leg muscles, rather than your abdomen,
to shift yourself across the bed and over. You can attach a safety
pin to your bra or move a ring from hand to hand to remember
which side you started with the last time. Later, you will want to
nurse longer on one breast, and the baby may prefer to take one
side only at a feeding; but for now, offer two. The sucking stimulation is good for you, and many small feedings are good for the
baby.

If your baby doesn't want to stop nursing on the first breast,
don't worry. Some babies hate being interrupted. Nursing on one
breast at a feeding will work as long as feedings are *frequent* (every
two hours or so) so that the un-nursed breast doesn't overfill and
become engorged. Hold the baby just as much as you like; nursing
and cuddling, particularly in the simplicity of the first days, are
inseparable, and should flow undisrupted from one to the other.
The baby *won't* be spoiled by this; after all, you've been
cuddling him constantly for nine months.

Keeping the baby with you most of
the time is particularly handy if you
have had a cesarean section. You and
the baby can doze together, and

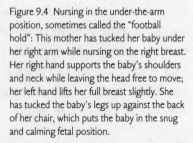

Figure 9.4 Nursing in the under-the-arm
position, sometimes called the "football
hold": This mother has tucked her baby under
her right arm while nursing on the right breast.
Her right hand supports the baby's shoulders
and neck while leaving the head free to move;
her left hand lifts her full breast slightly. She
has tucked the baby's legs up against the back
of her chair, which puts the baby in the snug
and calming fetal position.

you won't have to rouse yourself and get up every time you nurse; you can nurse lying down, rolling the baby to the other side by hugging him to your chest as you turn (remember to use your leg muscles, not your stomach muscles, to turn over) and thus get up and down far less often than if you were bottlefeeding.

If you feel like nursing sitting up, but the weight of the baby bothers your incision, try using the "football" hold (see illustration). This position is fun, anyway, because it allows you to look right into your baby's eyes and talk to him while he's nursing.

If you feel self-conscious because you do not have a private room, and your roommate can watch and hear you, ask the nurse to put a screen around your bed while you are feeding the baby. This is not false modesty. Most of us need time to get used to breaking a lifelong taboo against showing the breasts. Your baby will nurse better and get more and richer milk if you are not feeling embarrassed, and if that means you must have privacy, by all means ask for it. Or consider paying the extra cost of a private room. It may be well worth the benefits of nursing comfortably. It's also more likely your baby will be able to room-in with you twenty-four hours a day in a private room, while it may not be permitted in a shared room.

BREAST CARE

Remember: Soap, alcohol, and most other medicines and ointments are actually harmful to your tender skin. If you keep your clothes clean, nature will keep your breasts clean. A daily bath with plain warm water is plenty. If your hospital still believes in scrubbing or sterilizing the nipples before nursing, you don't have to obey rules that you *know* are inappropriate. On the other hand, you don't need to flood your body with adrenaline by arguing the case with nurses. If a nurse insists, do a lackadaisical job, and follow up later with a note to the hospital concerning unsuitable breastfeeding advice you received, so that the matter can be corrected for mothers coming after you.

SCHEDULES

Rooming-in mothers usually nurse a baby eight to nine times or more during the day, and often nap with the baby at the breast at night. Each feeding may last half an hour or more, or just a few minutes. Such liberal nursing is the best way to avoid breast soreness, engorgement, and infection, because it establishes an abundant, free-flowing milk supply from the beginning. Frequent feedings also reduce the incidence of newborn jaundice. In a few weeks, the baby will settle down to fewer feedings, but for now, ten to twelve nursings—or more—in twenty-four hours is appropriate.

If a hospital insists on a three- to four-hour schedule for feedings, or suggests that more frequent nursing is unnecessary, simply accept that this hospital is not current on its breastfeeding advice and politely ignore the directive. Keep your baby in your room with you, and nurse, and cuddle him without restriction. The more your baby is with you in the first days after birth, the more quickly you will learn to read his hunger cues (instead of the clock) and his other signals and signs. The more you learn about your baby, the more your confidence will grow in all the ways you care for him, including breastfeeding.

CLUSTER FEEDINGS

Sometimes a new baby has periods of wanting to nurse over and over for a few hours, every twenty to forty minutes or so; researchers call this "cluster feeding." It usually happens at night, during the first week or two of life, and an episode of cluster feedings is usually followed by a period of profound sleep (for both of you) lasting several hours. These frequent feedings do not mean you don't have enough milk; the baby may be getting lots of milk. And she's growing, and showing a healthy appetite. Remember, these episodes of frequent feedings help you lose weight, help the baby learn to breastfeed, and help your milk supply. This is nature's way of getting breastfeeding off to a strong start.

NIGHT FEEDINGS

Newborn babies are often night owls, feeding more often during the night hours; perhaps because they are used to being lulled to sleep in the uterus by Mom walking around in the daytime, they arrive still on "uterine time" (see Chapter 5, page 155). So your baby may be especially interested in nursing during the night, just at first. You need to plan on napping along with him during the day, as well as sleeping at night. If your baby is in the nursery, don't let the nurses talk you into skipping feedings between midnight and four in the morning by letting them feed the baby in the nursery with a supplement. If they forget to bring the baby, ring the buzzer and remind them. Your breasts need this feeding as much as the baby needs it.

If you are not allowed to room-in and must leave the baby in the nursery all the time, ask to have him brought to you for an hour at each feeding. If this is impossible, ask that he be brought to you every two and a half to three hours. "May I have my baby?" should become a familiar refrain in your room.

TIME LIMITS, POSITIONING, AND PREVENTION OF SORE NIPPLES

It is a custom in many hospitals to tell nursing mothers to limit the amount of time the baby is on the breast. For example, the hospital staff may tell you to nurse only three minutes per side to begin with, then five minutes the next day, then seven and ten. They are trying to prevent your nipples from becoming sore; sore nipples for the first week used to be considered by many an inevitable part of nursing a baby, so limiting nursing time to brief periods in the first days has been the standard advice for years. No one really took note of the fact that limiting nursing time doesn't seem to prevent soreness at all; in fact, it is a major cause of sore nipples. Time limits, for example, force mothers to take their babies on and off their nipples very frequently, sometimes just as things are going well; this upsets the baby and contributes to more soreness for the mother and less milk for the baby.

Let the baby make the decisions on how long he sucks. If your nipples are going to get sore at all, limiting sucking time to five minutes, or ten minutes or, worse yet, one minute, will simply postpone the peak of soreness. A sucking time limit will also keep the baby from getting as much milk as he needs.

Researchers have reexamined the problem of sore nipples to see what really does cause it and what can be done about it. Kittie Frantz, director of the Breastfeeding Infant Clinic at the University of Southern California Medical Center, studied breastfeeding difficulties in the first days after birth. Her close observations and interactions with mothers and babies led her to conclude that sore nipples are usually caused not by too much nursing, but by incorrect positioning of the baby at the breast. If the baby has to reach for the breast, or takes the nipple only partway into his mouth, abrasion occurs. Frantz found that when babies are properly positioned and allowed to nurse as long and as often as they wish, most new mothers experience discomfort only for a moment, when the baby first latches on, and even that discomfort is over within two or three days. Sore nipples are a brief or nonexistent problem.

If you have acute discomfort when the baby first latches on, you can use the breathing exercises taught in childbirth classes to alleviate the pain; slow, deep breathing can also be helpful if your uterus is contracting uncomfortably during nursing. (Remember, those uterine contractions are helping to flatten your stomach and are also a sign that your letdown reflex is working.)

If your nipples hurt and continue to be painful while the baby nurses, make sure that he is facing you with his whole body, that he does not have to turn his head to reach the breast, and that he has as much of your areola in his mouth as possible. Make sure his lower lip is flanged outward, not tucked in over his gum. Make sure the baby is high enough, in relation to your body, so he is not pulling down on the breast; look at your breast to see if there are "pull" lines toward the nipple as the baby nurses. You may want to put a pillow under your arm or under the baby to raise him a little; or, if you are lying down, just move him up the bed a little farther toward your head. Meanwhile, please see Healing Sore Nipples, pages 267–69.

GETTING THE BAY TO LET GO

A nursing baby can suck with remarkable strength. If you try to pull the breast away, he will just hang on harder. To get him off without hurting yourself, stick your finger into the corner of his mouth to break the suction. Then you can take him off without any trouble.

BURPING AND SPITTING UP

Doctors usually advise "burping" babies after feedings by patting them to bring up any air they may have swallowed. You can also burp the baby before you switch to the other breast. The idea is to coax any swallowed air up out of the stomach before it moves into the intestines and causes discomfort. The nurse will show you how if you don't know. You can hold the baby on your shoulder, with your shoulder gently pressing into her abdomen as you pat her back. You can sit her up on your lap, lean her forward slightly, supporting her with one hand across her chest, and pat her back; or you can lay her across a thigh, using the pressure of her stomach on your thigh to gently massage her stomach. Some babies never seem to have gas in their stomachs, and some often do; some are easy to burp and some hard—you'll just have to find out what kind of baby you have.

All babies spit up sometimes. In the first days, the baby may spit up a little of the yellowish colostrum. Occasionally, a baby burps so heartily that he spits up a great gush of milk. This is nothing to be alarmed about. Spit-up milk can appear to be an enormous quantity, but if actually measured it's usually less than a teaspoonful. To see if your baby wants to replace the milk he lost from a particularly juicy burp, just offer the breast again. If he doesn't want to nurse, he won't.

HOW TO TELL WHEN YOUR BABY IS HUNGRY

Already your baby has many ways to show you how she feels and what's going on with her; by studying her you will learn to understand these communications. For example, try to notice when she is beginning to be hungry; you don't need to wait until she is actually crying to pick her up. Offer her the breast when you see signs of being ready, such as rooting, turning the head, sticking the tongue out; such movements signal that the baby is looking for the breast.

People sometimes talk about "demand" feeding, meaning that the baby should be fed whenever she wants; maybe a better term is "request" feeding, meaning that you don't need to wait for something as severe as a demand. Also, requests work both ways; you can wake the baby and request the baby to feed, too, if you are feeling full or uncomfortable; breastfeeding, after all, is a partnership.

HOW TO TELL WHEN YOUR BABY IS FULL

He signals satiety by relaxing his clenched fists, by a cute little grimace of a smile, sometimes by arching his back and growling in a gesture of refusal, and of course by falling asleep. You can burp him and offer the other side, but after that don't try to prod him into nursing longer. Sometimes a baby will wake up and nurse again when he is switched to the other breast. If not, take his word for it. He alone knows how hungry he was. If your let-down reflex was working well, he may have gotten a huge meal in four or five minutes. One researcher points out that the stomach of a newborn baby is about the size of the baby's fist—not very big—and holds only about an ounce. The baby may be hungry again in an hour, but he knows when he's full now.

THE "LAZY" BABY

Lots of babies are casual about nursing at first. If the baby does not seem to want to nurse, don't be discouraged. Don't try to force him into nursing or to keep him going once he's started, by tricks some nurses may use, such as shaking or prodding him, blowing in his face, tickling his feet or his cheek, and so on. Efficiency may be on your mind or the attending nurse's, but it's not on his, and this kind of treatment just upsets and stresses him. It may make him retreat even further into sleepiness and lack of interest. The sleepy baby needs and appreciates your warmth and voice and nearness, especially if he does not yet nurse vigorously. Let him doze on your chest or stomach, while you doze, too. Babies seem to love this, and perhaps he draws strength from being so near and will wake up to nurse later on. The sleepy baby is a peaceful companion, warmer and dearer than any childhood teddy bear; if he spends some of his feeding periods just being held and cuddled, that's doing him good, too.

If there is concern about whether a sleepy baby is nursing sufficiently to bring in his mother's milk and to avoid developing newborn jaundice, the baby can be fed breast milk with a cup or an eyedropper until he wakes up enough to nurse more eagerly at the breast. Ask the lactation consultant on the hospital staff about this option to avoid falling into a cycle of supplementing with a bottle and hindering the establishment of breastfeeding.

GETTING ACQUAINTED

It is amazing how much personality tiny babies have; each one is an individual, responding to his mother in his own way. Some babies are hearty nursers. When put to the breast, they vigorously and promptly latch on and suck energetically. These babies have been nicknamed "barracudas," and are the easiest of all to breast-feed. Some babies procrastinate. These babies often show no particular interest in nursing, at first. It is important not to prod or force them when they seem disinclined. They do well, once they start. Some babies are "gourmets." They insist on mouthing the nipple, tasting a little milk and then smacking their lips, before starting to nurse. If this infant is hurried or prodded, she may become furious and start to scream. Otherwise, after a few minutes of mouthing, she settles down and nurses very well. (Mothers who have nursed gourmet babies seem to think that this early dallying and playfulness at the breast often turns out to be a sign of a lifelong humorous turn of mind.)

Some babies are "resters." These babies prefer to nurse a few minutes and then rest a few minutes. They often nurse well, but the procedure takes much longer than with a hearty feeder. Small and preterm babies may be resters, interspersing bouts of sucking with periods of remaining latched on but either resting or making the little jaw movements called "nonnutritive sucking." These babies cannot and should not be hurried; they know what they need to do to gather strength.

There are many babies who fall among these groups and others who fall into groups not described, because they are less common. The groupings serve merely to emphasize the fact that each baby nurses differently, and the course of the nursing will depend on the combination of the baby's nursing characteristics, the mother's personality, and the quality of the help the mother receives.

YOUR MILK SUPPLY

When you were eight or nine months pregnant, you may have begun to notice a pale yellow liquid secretion from your nipples. This is colostrum, the "first milk," and it is a wonderful substance. Colostrum, once thought to be worthless, is now known to be the ideal first food for babies. When colostrum changes to mature milk, the breasts start producing more abundantly, sometimes too abundantly. Long and frequent nursing can bring this change about within twelve to twenty-four hours after giving birth, as is usual in many home births. Nursing on a hospital's four-hour schedule postpones this shift to mature milk and the rise in milk production to three to five days after the birth (and increases the likelihood of a baby developing newborn jaundice).

The baby's appetite usually increases wonderfully, along with the milk supply. Still, she may not be able to keep up with the burgeoning supply. Your breasts, in addition to being full of milk, may be swollen as blood circulation increases. Lumps, bumps, and swellings are to be expected as the glands fill up with Grade AA mother's milk. Some areas of the breast do not drain as freely as other areas at first, and may feel lumpy even after a feeding. All this fullness is an unusual feeling and may make you uncomfortable; don't worry, it is normal and it is only temporary. Rooming-in mothers have a real advantage during this initial phase of milk production. They can pick up the baby whenever they feel too full, and in any case the baby usually wants to nurse so often that the breasts don't get too overloaded.

If you find yourself getting too full for comfort, and you don't have your baby nearby, perhaps you can express milk manually (see Chapter 12, page 376). Try to get the hang of this when the breast is not too full, perhaps just after a feeding. At first, the milk will come in drops, and then in a dribble, and then in a fine spray. Sometimes it is easier to do this while standing in a hot shower with the water hitting your back. The hospital can also provide you with a breast pump to reduce your fullness somewhat; the lactation consultant on staff will help you to do this.

Sometimes it is hard for the baby to grasp the breast when it is very full, because the areola is distended and tense. It can hurt you like the dickens when he tries, too. If this happens, express or pump some milk before the feeding to make the areola more flexible. When hospital rules enforce long separations, new mothers sometimes get so full of milk that they become engorged, with the breasts painfully distended, hot and hard to the touch; this should and can be avoided entirely with frequent, unrestricted nursings.

LEAKING, DRIPPING, AND SPRAYING MILK

When this happens, it is wonderful news. It means that your letdown reflex is starting to work. The letdown reflex must work if the baby is to get the milk he needs (see Chapter 2, pages 31–39). Letting down milk is a separate process from making milk. Successful breastfeeding mothers have established a good letdown reflex; they not only have milk but can give milk. At first, unless you have nursed babies before, you probably won't feel the letdown reflex working. But you can recognize the signs of it: milk leaking or dripping in between nursings, or during nursing from the other breast; afterpains or uterine cramps while nursing (these are caused by the same hormones that make the milk let down); sore nipples just at the start of nursing; or a feeling that the baby is biting, which fades away as he nurses (the discomfort stops when the milk starts letting down). You may also feel a great sense of relaxation or sleepiness as the milk lets down, or even find yourself dozing off; that, too, is a good sign that the lactatiom hormones are beginning to do their job.

The milk may let down several times during a single feeding. Some mothers are able to feel the letdown reflex as a sort of pins-and-needles sensation; other mothers never feel it. However, you can tell when the milk lets down because you can hear the baby begin to swallow and breathe—"suck-hah"—with every suck. If you'd like good evidence that your milk is letting down, tuck the forefinger of your free hand under the baby's chin and gently lay it on her throat. You will be able to feel her swallowing heartily, a very convincing demonstration that *something* is getting inside her, if you were wondering.

As your milk supply increases, you may be warned again by the nurses about sucking time limits. But it is bad for your letdown reflex to be fussing about how many minutes you nurse. Babies nurse in different ways, some in one long burst, some intermittently, with little rest periods in between. Your breasts will actually adapt to the rhythm of your particular baby, with the milk letting down strongly at first, and then repeatedly or intermittently, adjusting to the baby's patterns. You can see that this kind of interaction could not easily be developed if you were trying to limit feeding durations according to the clock.

Besides, time limits often do not reflect what is actually going on. The baby may need a few minutes to settle down, you may need a few more to let down your milk, and the feeding may not really start until many minutes have passed. Even if every other mother in the ward is obediently taking her baby off the breast according to whatever system the hospital fancies, you must put your watch away in a drawer and continue to let the baby decide how long to nurse.

SAFEGUARDING YOUR COMFORT

If you feel sick, or uncomfortable from stitches, hemorrhoids, af-terpains, or for any other reason, be sure to tell the doctor and the nurses. Any kind of discomfort makes it harder for you to relax while you are nursing the baby. You are justified in asking for something to relieve discomfort. Pain relievers will not pass through your milk in sufficient quantities to affect the baby (see Chapter 3, page 107). If you are being given antibiotics or other medications, these will not harm your baby. You can minimize the presence of all medications in your milk by taking them just after a feeding, not before.

HEALING SORE NIPPLES

Sometimes, even with proper positioning of the baby at the breast, the occasional mother will still develop sore nipples. Usu-ally, this soreness consists of a pain that makes you wince (or even brings tears to your eyes) as the baby first latches on, but that fades away as the milk lets down. Sometimes the nipple looks red and chafed. It may develop a pale crust or scab tem-porarily. Sometimes it looks very sore, or it cracks and even bleeds. The nipple will heal by itself, in spite of sucking, provided no harmful substances such as soap or alcohol are applied and any positioning difficulties are corrected.

Soreness generally starts around the twentieth feeding, gets worse for twenty-four to forty-eight hours, and then rapidly disappears. Limiting sucking or skipping feedings only postpones the peak of soreness. Mothers who nurse every two or three hours will usually get better by the fourth day, while mothers on a four-hour schedule won't be over their soreness till the sixth day or later. Lots of medicaments and treatments, ranging from special lanolin creams to wet tea bags, get undeserved credit for miraculous cures that nature would have accomplished alone.

Keep a sore nipple dry and exposed to the air between feedings. This will help it to heal. Sunbathing or very cautious use of a sunlamp can help, too. If lack of privacy means you cannot go around with the flaps of your bra down to let the air reach your nipples, an old-fashioned but effective treatment is to have someone bring you a couple of little sieves from tea strainers. You can put these in your bra over the nipples, and they will allow the air to circulate and keep you dry. Hydrogel dressings, a relatively new treatment for sore nipples, seem to be very effective at reducing pain and speeding healing; ask the lactation consultant on the hospital staff if these are an appropriate option for you. The worst thing you can do for sore nipples is to wear nursing pads or gauze pads, which get wet and stay wet; they keep your nipple moist and stick to the sore places so that you do more damage every time you remove them.

It is normal to favor a cracked nipple somewhat, but don't give up now. Skimping on nursings can make soreness worse or lead to other problems. To minimize discomfort and speed healing, you can start all feedings on the least sore side; once the milk has let down, you can switch. Wake the baby up and nurse him before you get too full, rather than wait until you are bursting, when it is harder for the baby to latch on. Make sure the baby's mouth is wide open before you pull him close; don't let him "walk up" the nipple. His lower lip should flare out; pull it down gently if you need to. Try not to let the baby chew on the nipple itself or hang on, sucking but not swallowing, for prolonged periods.

One good way to minimize soreness is to nurse the baby in a different position each time; this distributes the pressure more evenly, rather than letting it fall on the same part of the nipple at each feeding. You may hold him under your arm in the "football" hold at your side (see illustration on page 254); you may lie down and let him lie across your chest to nurse. In all positions, make sure the baby comes straight onto the breast and that you are holding him close enough and high enough that he doesn't drag the breast downward or have to tilt or twist his head to nurse, which will make you sore.

Nipple shields, which are very popular in some hospitals, are rubber or plastic shields that fit over the breasts, often with a rubber nipple on which the baby sucks. They keep your areolas from being touched by the baby, but ensure that the baby gets milk by suction alone; usually he gets very little. That is bad for your milk supply, discouraging for the baby, and no help to your nipples. Above all, don't nurse for a brief period and then take the baby off before the milk lets down. It is the putting on and the taking off that do the damage, especially if the milk has not yet let down. If a nipple cracks and bleeds, you may see blood in the baby's mouth. That is an alarming sight, but not too uncommon; try not to worry about it. The nipple will heal by tomorrow or the next day, and the blood will not harm the baby.

JAUNDICE

Sometimes babies develop a little normal (physiological) jaundice while they are adapting to life outside the womb. The baby's eyes may look a little yellow for a few days. This is nothing to worry about; as soon as lactation is going well, the jaundice will clear up. However, some hospitals and some doctors insist on putting jaundiced babies under special lights and giving them formula supplements for a day or two. If this happens, keep in mind that you will soon be home where you can breastfeed without interference, and that your baby is *not sick* and will be fine; it's just that currently there exists a medical custom of overtreatment for this condition. If this happens to you, read the section on jaundice in Chapter 4, pages 132–39.

THE NURSES

A nurse who has happily breastfed her own babies can be a wonderful help to you and your baby. Most hospitals offer new mothers classes in breastfeeding right on the ward, with videos and demonstrations and a lactation consultant to lead the class. The hospital's lactation consultants are also available to assist nursing mothers one-on-one, as well as to education the rest of staff on lactation issues. Some nurses are young, have never nursed a baby, and don't understand the kind of help you need. Some older nurses were trained in the times when almost all babies were bottlefed and subjected to strict regimens; they may be critical of normal breastfeeding procedures. If you think a nurse is being particularly brisk, careless, or domineering, it often helps to ask her for advice, *not* necessarily about breastfeeding. "Please,"

"Thank you," and a friendly smile can coax indulgences such as a longer feeding time from even the strictest supervisor.

In many hospitals, however, the nurses cannot afford the time to coach nursing mothers, even if they would like to. Mealtimes are rushed, and they must sometimes take the baby back to the nursery for a weighing just when he is getting started. This problem is compounded by early discharge; now, instead of having five days to get you off to a good start, they may have as little as twenty-four to forty-eight hours. Listen closely when knowledgeable nurses do have a minute to help you, and ask them to suggest resources for you to turn to when you go home. A hospital with a solid plan in place for supporting breastfeeding will provide you with extensive resources and information for nursing your baby after discharge.

Even when all the nurses are supportive and willing to help you, they are apt to have been trained at different schools, in different decades, so each nurse may have rules for managing breastfeeding that contradict what some previous nurse has told you. Also, different doctors may leave differing orders, so the poor nurses must tell one patient one set of rules and other patients another set. Stay calm; don't let the confusion bother you. Luckily, nurses are busy, shifts change, and no one is going to have time to check up to see if you are following her particular brand of instructions. And sometimes you'll run into a wonderful nurse who really makes you feel at ease, and really knows how to help. Let her!

GOING HOME

The amount of time mothers and babies stay in the hospital has been dramatically reduced in recent years. Where a week was once considered a minimum for every mother, now only mothers recovering from a cesarean section stay in the hospital four days or more. Mothers who give birth vaginally often go home the next day, or even a few hours after birth. Theoretically, one stays in the hospital to rest, but many women feel that the supposed "rest" you get in the hospital is a poor joke, especially in a semiprivate room or the wards. One mother, in a private room with her rooming-in baby, counted the number of times someone came into her room during the baby's second day of life. Nurses, dietitians, cleaning women, lab technicians—some stranger interrupted or woke her seventy-two times in one twenty-four-hour period. When a janitor came in to fix a broken closet rod, just as she was putting the baby on the breast, she called her husband and went home.

There are some advantages to going home early to escape this overactive environment: The comfort of your own home and the lack of interfering hospital policies can be a help in nursing. On the other hand, early discharge leaves you on your own in learning to breastfeed. In one study, early discharge was closely associated with the development of jaundice in breastfed babies, indicating that mothers who went home before breastfeeding was well established may not have had enough support to put the baby to the breast and let down their milk sufficiently. If you go home twenty-four hours after giving birth, your baby may not really have done more than nuzzle your breast yet, and you may miss out on the careful teaching of the hospital's lactation consultants. If, once you are home, you stay in bed with your baby and nurse often and leisurely, the two of you may well learn to nurse without more assistance. However, someone who is experienced in breastfeeding, a lactation consultant, or a La Leche League leader, should be available during these early days to answer questions and to support you.

If a midwife helped you through labor, you can probably arrange for her to be there to help you in the first days at home, too. A breastfeeding class may be offered during your prenatal instruction or on the maternity floor after the birth of your baby; be sure to attend it if you know you will be discharged early. You should be able to call the lactation consultant (LC) on maternity floor of the hospital for breastfeeding advice after you get home. More and more hospitals maintain breastfeeding "help lines" and even drop-in clinics for new mothers.

You can contact an LC by going online to International Lactation Consultants Association (see Resources) or by calling the lactation consultant department of La Leche League, for the names of the consultants nearest you. La Leche League International has groups and leaders in many communities throughout the United States. An experienced LLLI leader can provide you with encouragement, information, and good advice by telephone. When the baby is crying, and you don't know why, and you are *sure* it's because of your milk, a friendly listener who's been through it all herself may be just what you need. You can locate the leader nearest you by making a toll-free phone call to La Leche League headquarters: dial 1-800-LA LECHE.

When you leave the hospital, you will probably be given a nice good-bye gift of baby-care pamphlets, perhaps a pair of booties or a rattle, and a can of formula. Go through the package. Take the booties, leave the formula can behind. Giving "formula kits" to all new mothers, including breastfeeding mothers, is a widespread insidious practice funded by the formula manufacturers. They are hoping that even if you start out breastfeeding, you will panic and use their product, thus beginning the cycle of supplementing with bottles that so often leads to early weaning. You don't need to let them do this to you. You won't be exposed to temptation if you leave the bait behind.

Some mothers find that the fatigue of going home causes a temporary drop in their milk supply, but that is no reason to stoke the baby with forumula. Just head to bed to rest, keep your baby beside you and let him nurse more often, and your milk supply will return. Other mothers find that they have much more milk available for the baby when they get home, probably because their milk lets down better in familiar surroundings. Home, where rooming-in and request feeding are yours for the asking—as well as privacy, good food, and the tender care of your loved ones—is the best place to establish lactation.

THANKS TO THE STAFF

Before you leave the hospital, take a minute to thank any nurse who was especially helpful to you. If the nurse who helped you is off duty, get her name and leave a note. Getting mother and baby off to a good start can be almost as rewarding for the dedicated nurse as it has been for you. She won't expect to be thanked for her kindness and skill—and probably hasn't been in years. But she will feel pleased. Maybe it will encourage her when the next nursing mother comes along needing her help.

One to Six Weeks:
The Learning Period

HOMECOMING

It is surprising how tiring the trip home can be. Even if you feel more than ready to leave the hospital, you may be glad to lie down when you get home. Put the baby's bed next to your own, so you will be able to feed her or reach over and pat her without getting up. If you have other small children, arrange for them to be out of the house when you first get home. Then you and your new baby can be settled in bed before the welcoming tumult. Do make sure, before you leave the hospital, that there are enough groceries in the house to last a few days, so that you won't be obliged to plan meals and make lists right away.

THE "FORTY DAYS" RULE

Somehow we in the United States have gotten the idea that in primitive societies women give birth more easily, and recover at once. We imagine the peasant woman giving birth in the fields, tying the baby in her shawl, and going back to the plow. If women around the world, goes the theory, can hop up and get back to work so quickly, well, then, so can we. Furthermore, our Puritan work ethic prods mothers to return to their normal activities and responsibilities as fast as possible; we feel guilty for every extra day we can't get that plowing done.

In fact, most cultures provide for a "lying-in" period after giving birth, in which the mother not only is relieved of her duties, but is cared for by other women in the family. The typical duration of sequestration for mother and baby is forty days. Often the lying-in period is justified by superstition; the baby must wear certain clothes or amulets to be safe; mother and child must stay home to avoid the evil eye, and so on. The net effect, however, is that the mother has time to convalesce, her nourishment is guaranteed and provided by others, mother and infant can establish their breastfeeding relationship without hindrance, and neither of them is exposed to new sources of infection during this vulnerable time. A Chicago lactation consultant who works with recent immigrants from Asia, Malaysia, and India says that the mothers she works with are flabbergasted, and their families are horrified, when the mother is expected to bathe the baby herself a day after giving birth, and when she is instructed upon discharge from the hospital to bring the baby back to the clinic for a checkup a week or two later, which may necessitate a long bus ride and exposure to many people.

Perhaps forty days of "doing nothing" seems a ridiculously long time to you, or an unattainable luxury. But there are many generations of experience behind that widespread tradition. People recover from childbirth at widely varying and quite unpredictable speeds. The hothouse flower who catches every cold that goes around may feel perfectly fit in two weeks, while the marathon runner is still feeling weak six months after giving birth. You may well find that you need a month or so of virtual idleness in order to convalesce completely from pregnancy and childbirth. The more work you do in that first month, the more time it will take you to feel strong again. Doing too much too soon is especially hard on the nursing mother, who is using her energy to make milk as well as to recuperate from pregnancy and delivery.

Even in our own culture, this curtailment or even deletion of convalescent time is a relatively new idea. In the 1930s, mothers spent about two weeks in the hospital and then went home and spent another two weeks or so in their bedrooms, with orders not to go up or down stairs. (Certainly, forcing the mother to stay flat in bed all that time would have weakened her, but few mothers did that; a mother could care for her baby, and move around, but a "no stairs" rule effectively eliminated any chance that she would take over the housework too soon.)

Even a few years ago, mothers were kept in the hospital five days. Today, many hospitals send mothers and babies home in one day, and the typical hospital stay is two and a half days, or four days after a cesarean section. While mothers have been persuaded that this is good for them, the main impetus has been cost reduction for the insurance companies. As a result, it becomes the mother's own responsibility to see that she gets enough rest to convalesce quickly after going home.

Taking it easy is especially important if you have to go back to work fairly soon. If you overdo now, you may find yourself paying for it later, with weeks, even months, of fatigue that could have been mitigated by a little more early rest. While home can and should be more restful than the hospital, to make certain that happens you must deliberately stay in bed and curtail your activities as much as you can. Don't worry about finishing the birth announcements. Don't read, however interesting the book, when you feel like sleeping and have a chance to do so. Limit your visitors to a few minutes. Don't drink too much caffeinated tea or coffee, which may make you restless so that you can't nap. (More than a cup or two a day can make your baby very jittery, too.)

Other people in the household, even the baby's father, may be so glad to have you back that they begin relying on you right away—to find the can opener or tell them if the chicken is cooked yet. Resist that urge to get up "just for a minute." Nursing the baby can be your best excuse to stay out of circulation for a while.

A FEW GOOD TIPS

Dr. E. Robbins Kimball, who helped hundreds of mothers to nurse their babies successfully, sends each patient home with a list of three rules.

1. *Spend the First Three Days in Bed.* This does not mean lying down whenever you get a chance; it means staying in bed, getting up only to go to the bathroom. Keep the baby near you or in your bed. Let your partner get breakfast and dinner and bring them to you; let whoever is helping you with your housework fix lunch. Don't even rinse out a diaper; use disposable diapers during this period if possible. Stock up on books and magazines, or move the TV into the bedroom. Remember, you don't have a baby every day, and when you do, you deserve to enjoy life for a little while.

Naturally, when you come home from the hospital, you can see all sorts of things that have been neglected in your absence. But don't even plump up a pillow; instead, plan on doing it after your three days in bed. Three days from now, you may find that the things left undone don't seem quite so important to do as they did at first.

Because you are in bed, visitors will not overstay their welcome or expect you to serve coffee or drinks. Feel free to tell people that the doctor instructed you to stay in bed, even if he didn't. If you have another small child, and there are hours in the day when there is no one to watch him but you, just shut the bedroom door and keep him in your room with you. Even an eighteen-month-old can amuse himself with books and crayons and likes to be read to, and he will soon learn to take his nap on your bed.

2. Take Three One-Hour Naps a Day. During your first three days in bed, pull down the shades and sleep. For the rest of the month, use your ingenuity to get into bed and sleep for each one of these naps. Sleep while the children sleep, sleep before dinner while your partner takes the baby for a walk in the fresh air, sleep after breakfast while a neighbor watches the toddler. Don't read; don't write notes; you can do those things while you nurse the baby. *Sleep.* These three naps a day will do you more good, and do more to make breastfeeding a pleasure and a quick success, than anything else in the first weeks.

3. Remember That It Takes Two or Three Weeks to Learn How to Nurse and a Couple of Months to Become an Expert. Don't regard every little event as a signal for panic. Sure, there will be days when you don't have enough milk. There will also be days when you have too much. There will be days when the baby seems to go on a four-hour schedule, and days when the baby wants to eat all the time, every two hours or more often. These "frequency days," as lactation consultants call them, are nature's way of making your milk supply increase to keep up with your fast-growing baby's needs. You, too, benefit from these days. Research has shown that the more frequent the feedings, the faster the breastfeeding mother loses any extra weight she put on in pregnancy.

Researchers have found that the first two "frequency days" are apt to occur around the sixth and fourteenth days of life. The experienced mother hardly notices them, but the mother who is still clock-watching and counting each feed is very conscious of them. All the events that take place in the early days of nursing your first baby loom very large, just like the events of your first pregnancy. Just remember that you (and your baby) are still learning. Breastfeeding will be easier and easier as you go along.

CONDITIONING THE LETDOWN REFLEX

Sometimes a new mother's letdown reflex doesn't work very reliably and she loses a lot of milk through leaking, or she may never seem to have quite enough, so that her baby does not gain very fast and sometimes cries at the breast. Such a mother needs to make a deliberate effort to induce her letdown reflex to function smoothly and reliably; nursing will be much more satisfactory once this happens. Here are some suggestions:

1. *Concentrate on the Baby While You Are Nursing.* Nursing "etiquette" means that you don't have to make conversation with someone else or answer the telephone while your newborn is at the breast. Go into another room, turn your back, and "retire" a little, mentally; while you are still learning to breastfeed, your body needs a chance to work without distraction.

2. *Cut Out Extraneous Effort,* such as dinner parties (don't accept invitations yet, and don't extend them), *The Late Late Show,* and so on.

3. Monitor Your Own Schedule, taking two or three one-hour naps, no skimping on meals or staying away from the house too long, no long car rides.

4. During the Day, Wake the Baby and Feed Her Every Two to Three Hours, rather than let her sleep for long periods; your breasts need regular stimulation to condition the letdown reflex. At night, waken the baby if you wake up feeling full. Don't let her sleep five or six hours while your milk production slows, or your milk leaks and goes to waste.

5. If Your Milk Suddenly Lets Down, Pick Up the Baby and Feed Her, even if you just fed her. A sudden letdown after or between nursings doesn't mean that the milk didn't let down during the feeding—it may have let down several times, without your awareness. Extra letdowns just mean that your letdown reflex is working *more* than enough; putting the baby to the breast even briefly will help condition your letdown reflex more specifically to your baby's sucking. Then feed her again in two to three hours, or sooner if she fusses.

6. If You Have a Chance, Take Five Minutes Before Feeding to Sit Down, Put Your Feet Up, Close Your Eyes, and Think About Nothing.

7. Nurse in the Same Comfortable Quiet Spot at Each Meal; Take a Drink of Water Before You Nurse. Your body responds well to routine. Your letdown reflex will associate itself with these habits, as well as the sensation of your baby latching on and beginning to nurse.

8. Remove Distracting Influences. You can't let down your milk well if a neighbor is trying to chat with you at the same time, or if the phone is ringing, or if your three-year-old is getting into trouble in the kitchen. Later on, when you're an old hand at nursing, these things won't bother you. Now, while you're just beginning to get the hang of it, send the neighbor home, take the phone off the hook, and read a story to your three-year-old.

9. *Don't Cheat Yourself Through Perfectionism.* Too often a mother feels that it is more important to get the laundry done, the house clean, the children scheduled and presentable, the yard clipped and raked, the errands done, and the meals ready on time than to get enough rest or a good breakfast for herself. But none of these things is as important to your family—especially to your partner and to your nursing baby—as a relaxed, cheerful mother. Learn to look at taking care of yourself as your duty to your family, rather than as self-indulgence.

10. *Don't Let the Baby Skip Night Feedings,* even though you need rest; get up at least once—or better yet, keep the baby beside your bed in a "sidecar" crib so that all you need do is roll over to her to nurse. And, although you may be fatigued, don't ask your partner to give the baby a bottle of formula in the night. At this point, you may have limited storage capacity; if your breasts get too full, milk production slows down. Don't go so long between feedings that your breasts feel lumpy. Your body actually produces more and richer milk at night, which helps the baby go longer on fewer feedings than during the day, and which also makes those night feedings especially important while the baby is still so small.

NURSING TRANQUILLITY

One of nursing's greatest benefits to mothers is that it brings peace. Sitting down to nurse the baby allows you to withdraw momentarily from your other cares and duties. For a little while, all problems can be answered with the words, "I'm feeding the baby, I'll be there in a few minutes." The plumber on the doorstep, your mother-in-law wanting to know where to put the laundry, the phone ringing, the four-year-old insisting on a trip to the playground—all can wait. Behind the closed nursery door, curled in a rocking chair with the baby, you can restore yourself with the physical feelings of peace and tranquillity that come with nursing. These moments of solitude are a simple but rare blessing in the lives of most mothers.

If you are in the habit of leading a high-geared, active life, you will especially come to enjoy these brief excursions into tranquillity. Later on, at the end of a strenuous day, you'll absolutely crave getting home and sitting down with the baby. If you are sometimes overanxious, you can probably be an extremely successful nursing mother. (Dairymen say that the high-strung cows give the most milk; perhaps these are the cows that are most sensitive to their surroundings.) You will soon get into the swing of relaxing with the baby instead of struggling and fretting; and you have a great advantage in so doing over the bottlefeeding mother. The hormones of breastfeeding will help you, or even teach you, to be more easygoing.

One new mother, who all her life had suffered from a severe rash during periods of emotional stress, described an especially ghastly day that ended with her husband's being painfully cut by the lawn mower. True to experience, she broke out in the rash; then she sat down to nurse her twin babies, certain that she would produce no milk. Instead, the milk let down quickly. As she nursed the babies, she began to feel relaxed for the first time all day. By the time the meal was over, her rash was gone. These restorative moments of complete relief from stress are the reward that nature has always meant nursing to give to the mother.

FEEDING FREQUENCY

Dr. Niles Newton says, in an article on breastfeeding that was written primarily for doctors:

> The advice given by Southworth in Carr's *Practice of Pediatrics*, published in 1906, is still worth remembering, since at that time successful breast feeding was the rule rather than the exception.
>   Southworth's schedule was:
>
> First day: 6 nursings
> Second day: 8 nursings
> The rest of the first month: 10 nursings in 24 hrs.
> Second and third months: 8 nursings in 24 hrs.
> Fourth and fifth months: 7 nursings in 24 hrs.
> Sixth through eleventh months: 6 nursings in 24 hrs.

He assumed the baby would have night feedings until six months of age.

What a far cry this natural feeding schedule is from the four-hour schedule that modern formula-fed babies are put on. Even the baby who is fed formula "on demand" is expected to fall into roughly a four-hour schedule within a few weeks. But the nursing baby should not be expected to do so. Throughout the first four weeks, many a nursing baby eats ten times in twenty-four hours, which means an average two and a half hours between feedings. If he sometimes sleeps four or five hours at a stretch at night, he may well double up in the daytime, and take some meals at even shorter intervals. If it seems to you that your baby is "always hungry," keep track for one day to see if he doesn't fall into the standard ten-nursings-a-day pattern, and if his apparent insatiability isn't a result of your expecting him to go three or four hours between meals, as an adult would, and as a baby fed on slow-digesting cow's milk is expected to do.

Sometimes medical advice makes a concession to a small formula-fed baby, and instructs that he be started out on a three-hour schedule. But the breastfed baby may not work up to a three-hour schedule—one that averages out to eight meals a day—until the second or third month, and Dr. Southworth did not expect breastfed babies to cut down to six meals a day, or a four-hour schedule, until they were six months old! No wonder so many mothers in the previous generation could not nurse their babies, when a four-hour schedule was flatly insisted on from birth, and when it was customary to tell all mothers to nurse from one breast only at each feeding. The woman who produced so much milk that she could feed a baby adequately, despite the limited sucking stimulation given by offering each breast only once every eight hours, must have been rare indeed. Suppose your new baby does not fit Southworth's description? The La Leche League manual, *The Womanly Art of Breastfeeding*, says:

> Occasionally, we see a baby who goes to extremes in one of two ways. One day he may seem to be exceptionally active, fussy and hungry all or most of the time. If we nurse him more often than every two hours, which is what he seems to want, he only gets fussier and more restless, but will go right on nursing! This type of baby is often getting more milk than he really wants. What he wants is more sucking, without the milk.

The solution is to feed the baby on just one breast per feeding, and let him stay on for a while when the milk has slowed to a trickle, or return to that breast if he wants more suckling for com-fort, even when he is probably full.

The other extreme is the too-placid baby. This one will sleep peacefully for four, five, or more hours between feedings, be fairly quiet, and nurse rather leisurely. As time goes on, she may seem to get even quieter, and you think, "Such a good baby. She cer-tainly is doing well." Then comes the shock, when you take her to the doctor for her first checkup and find out to your amaze-ment that she has not gained an ounce, and may have even lost weight.

Here again, remember that the breastfed baby needs to be fed, as Dr. Southworth advises, about every two to three hours, with perhaps one longer stretch at night. The trouble in this case is not a lack of milk on your part or a lack in its quality. It is the baby who needs to be encouraged. The exceptionally sleepy, placid baby must be awakened to be fed more often, and should be urged to take both breasts at each feeding. Sometimes a baby tires easily and almost seems to lose interest; that baby needs to be given the opportunity to learn to nurse longer, as well as more often. During "frequency days," a baby may want to nurse ninety minutes or less after the previous nursing. Watch the baby; you can help her to settle down and nurse by reducing outside stimuli (noise, light), increasing the areas of contact between her skin and yours, rocking, singing, and letting the baby rest at the breast between bouts of active suckling.

By increasing the number of times a baby nurses in a day, and encouraging the baby to nurse longer, you will automatically in-crease your supply, and soon the baby will be gaining as she should. In this case, too, it is important to make sure the baby nurses a long time on the first breast—twenty or thirty minutes, say—to get the last few swallows of high-calorie, fat-rich hind milk into her before you offer the second breast (see Chapter 2, page 35). One side is all some babies will take at first, anyway. Research shows that babies who always take only one side get just as many calories as babies who almost always nurse on both breasts.

Some lactation consultants advise the mother of a slow-gaining newborn to massage the breast, gently, for a minute or two as the baby starts to nurse, using the free hand to make firm, soft strokes from the outermost perimeter of the breast tissue toward the areola. The theory is that doing this mechanically moves fat particles toward the milk ducts, and thus helps to increase the calorie count of a particular feeding. It may be also that massage relaxes the mother or stimulates the letdown reflex or both.

HOW TO TELL IF THE BABY IS GETTING ENOUGH MILK

1. What Goes in Must Come Out. Does the baby have good bowel movements? The feces of a breastfed baby are normally yellowish and rather liquid, with the odor and consistency of yogurt. The new nursing baby may have several bowel movements a day; some may be just a stain on the diapers. Later, he will have one every two to four days, but it should be fairly big. The baby who is not getting enough to eat has consistently scanty, watery stools, which may be greenish in color.

2. Does He Have Lots of Wet Diapers? If you are not giving him extra water, which he doesn't need anyway, those wet diapers are an indication that he is getting plenty of breast milk. (Be aware, however, that modern disposable diapers are remarkably absorbent and can sometimes seem dry even if your baby has wet them once or twice.)

3. Is He Content with Eight to Twelve Feedings Per Day, the typical nursing schedule in the first month or so? If you are nursing him this often, and letting down your milk at feedings, he is probably well fed.

4. Is He Gaining? There is a tremendous amount of emphasis these days on how much weight a baby gains; formula-fed babies sometimes put on a lot of weight and the rate of gain has become the yardstick by which the baby's health is measured, by mothers and often by doctors, too. La Leche League says, "A good rule to follow, in a healthy baby, is that he should be gaining from four to seven ounces a week, but that less than this in a given week or two is not in itself cause for alarm." *More* than this is not cause for alarm, either; some breastfed babies gain very fast in the first three months or so. It is very important for mothers and their pediatricians, however, to understand that exclusively breastfed babies grow at a different rate and pattern than formula-fed babies do—and the evidence is increasing that the slower rate, on average, of weight gain among breastfed babies may be the reason that as adults, their cardiovascular health is significantly better than that of adults who had been formula fed.

As long as your baby is happy and healthy, his color is good, his arms and legs are getting plump, and you nurse him long and often, don't worry about how many ounces he may or may not be gaining each day. You'll find out soon enough at your next checkup with the pediatrician. If you really want to weigh the baby, the scales in the supermarket are usually very accurate, and checkout personnel will probably let you weigh him if they are not too busy. Many supermarkets now have automatic checkouts where you do all the weighing yourself in any case. Take duplicates of what the baby is wearing, weigh the baby, weigh the duplicate clothes, and subtract the clothing weight plus the baby's previous weight to see how much he has gained.

YOUR FOOD

Part of enjoying life in these first six weeks is eating heartily and well. This is not the time to diet; lactation is the best "diet" there is, anyway. Six months to a year of giving milk can strip unnecessary weight from you without the slightest effort on your part. Some mothers think that the most enjoyable thing about lactating is that for a few happy months they can dive into meals with gusto, and take two helpings of everything, yet never gain a pound.

Of course, you will have plenty of high-quality breast milk no matter what you eat; milk is produced independently of diet. But while you can at this point safely eat more calories than you used to, this does not mean that you should fill up on "cheat foods," such as cake and sweet rolls. Sugary, starchy foods provide "empty calories" because they are nutritionally deficient. Meanwhile, the mammary glands draw on your body for the vitamins, minerals, and protein missing from your diet but needed for milk production. You don't lose weight, and you tend to feel tired and "used up."

Right now, your own body needs extra protein and extra calcium (especially important for teenage mothers, who may still be growing themselves). Give yourself food such as beans, meat, chicken, cheese, eggs, and fish. You certainly don't need to drink a lot of milk, or any at all, if it doesn't agree with you. Cow's milk doesn't make human milk. Canned fish such as salmon and sardines are a great source of calcium, and so are most green leafy foods, such as lettuce and all the cabbage relatives.

Try to make sure that whatever you consume is nutritionally complete and unprocessed. The whole grain (dark) cereals and breads provide more protein than refined white bread, as well as extra flavor. Enriched or brown rice is more nutritious than polished rice. Fruit and fruit juices can give you as much "quick energy" from sugar as any soft drink can. Beans and tortillas and chilis and even pizza are "real food"; candy bars aren't. And remember—the baby will be fine, whatever you eat, but you will feel better if you eat good food, and enough of it, during the first few weeks. It's your vacation. Enjoy it.

BABY'S REACTIONS TO YOUR DIET

A normal varied diet should have no harmful effects on your baby; people will tell you that nursing mothers ought to avoid cabbage or chocolate or spicy foods, but in general babies don't care (see Chapter 2 for a full discussion). Some babies, however, can become uncomfortable—suffering stomach pains, passing lots of gas, and crying in obvious discomfort—in reaction to one substance common in mothers' diets: cow's milk protein. This is especially likely if you have any sensitivity to dairy products yourself, or if you consumed a lot of dairy products during pregnancy. (Yogurt is a common exception. Adding yogurt to your diet may decrease the risk of your breastfed baby developing eczema, if you have a family history of the condition.) If your baby has a lot of gastric discomfort, you can easily test whether this sensitivity is the cause by eliminating all dairy products (milk, cheese, ice cream, and processed foods containing dried milk solids) from your own diet for one week, and observing whether the baby seems more comfortable. You can reintroduce small quantities of dairy products later, if you wish, to find out what the baby can and can't handle; usually, breastfed babies become less sensitive to such maternal diet effects as they get older.

Another cause of discomfort for breastfed babies can be iron supplements you may have been taking during pregnancy. If you were taking iron pills in addition to vitamins, stop. You probably don't need them now, anyway. Some mothers feel that consuming sugar substitutes gives the baby diarrhea; soft drinks, especially, can contain large quantities of sugar substitutes, but they are also found in some ice creams and many "lite" or diet foods. Some mothers find that their babies get diarrhea if the mother drinks a lot of fruit juice (a quart or more in twenty-four hours). Occasionally, a baby seems to be gassy and uncomfortable if his mother consumes a lot of carbonated drinks. Solid research is hard to come by on infant responses to maternal diets, but if your baby seems to be reacting to something in your diet, remove that food from your menus for a few days. If your baby's reaction disappears, you may have identified a potential allergen for him. If your baby's reaction was not severe, reintroduce the food for a day to test your hypothesis.

LIQUIDS

You may not really be eating for two, but when you are lactating, you are certainly drinking for two. If you are tired or preoccupied, it is easy to forget about taking enough fluids. There is no need to force yourself to drink copious quantities of liquids, but you do not want to go thirsty. If you drink a glass of water or juice every time you nurse the baby, that will be plenty; taking that much liquid will also help to prevent constipation. You may feel intensely thirsty at the moment the milk lets down; nature is reminding you to drink that glass of water. Many women find it convenient to keep a pitcher of water handy where they nurse the baby. Tell your partner that one of the most helpful things he or she can do in the early weeks of breastfeeding is to bring you a glass of water whenever you sit down to nurse.

You do not need to make a special effort to drink milk. In most parts of the world, nursing mothers drink no milk at all. Cheese, meats, and salad greens provide you with calcium. Although you probably avoided alcohol during pregnancy, light use of alcohol—one glass of wine or beer before dinner, say—is not harmful for the nursing mother or her child. One German baby nurse swore that all her maternity patients succeeded in breastfeeding because of her prescription: a big bowl of sugared and creamed oatmeal for breakfast, and a glass of port wine at 10:00 a.m. and 4:00 p.m.

LITTLE PROBLEMS

There are lots of little events in the early days of nursing that may seem like problems because they are new to you. Three months from now you probably won't even remember them. Here are some solutions:

Leaking:

If you leak primarily during feedings, you can open both bra cups and hold a clean diaper to the fountaining breast while the baby drinks from the other. Or use handkerchiefs, cut-up cloth diapers, or nursing pads you can buy at the drugstore, to wear inside your bra. (Take note: Don't use nursing pads with plastic exteriors; they may cause soreness by keeping your nipples wet. Don't use cut-up disposable diapers; many of them are filled with a plastic gel and are treated with chemicals that can irritate your skin.) Mild leaks can be controlled with the flannel liners that can often be bought with nursing bras. Sometimes you can stop the milk from leaking out by pressing down flat on the nipples with your hands or forearms, when you feel the milk let down. Leaking will diminish as your letdown reflex becomes better established. If you *don't* leak, don't feel you are abnormal; some women seldom or never leak milk.

Low Milk Supply at Suppertime:

The early evening meal does seem to be the scantiest. If you have nursed the baby a lot that day, your milk production may still be catching up to the baby's needs. Even newborns sometimes wake up and act hungry when they smell food cooking, so you can find yourself putting the baby to the breast again when you sit down to eat. Instead of feeding the baby, let your partner amuse her or ask a friend to come by in the evening hours to hold the baby while you take a few minutes for yourself. After a shower and a good dinner, you may find you have a surprisingly ample dividend of milk that will send the baby off to a good sleep.

Too Much Milk:

In the early days of nursing, both your milk supply and the baby's needs fluctuate. It takes several weeks for your supply and the baby's appetite to synchronize, and even then there may be days when you have a little more or a little less milk than she wants.

Baby Oversleeping:

If your baby is sleeping six or eight or ten hours at night, so that you wake up every morning groaningly full of milk, wake him in the night to feed him. The baby would probably feed off and on all night if he slept in your bed. Remember that your body produces milk more copiously, and with higher fat content, while you are sleeping. Sleeping separately, babies sometimes sleep through meals that you both need. Getting too full every morning tends to lower your total milk production. In another month or two, both you and the baby will be able to go longer between feeds.

A Strong Letdown Reflex:

If your milk lets down so vigorously that the baby sputters, chokes, and cries during feedings because he is getting flooded, try sitting him upright to nurse, and try nursing him on one side only, per feeding, but for as long as he wants. Sometimes when a mother has a strong letdown reflex, the baby gets full before he has had enough time to suck and be cuddled, and he frets for the comforting, rather than for extra milk. Try putting the baby back on the same breast, rather than switching him to the other side, so that he can satisfy his need to suckle without getting more milk than he can handle.

Night Feeds:

Just take the baby in bed with you, and doze while he drinks. There's no danger of rolling on him, really. Mothers have slept with their babies since the beginning of humanity. You can put him back in his own bed, if and when you wake up.

Criticism:

If a friend or relative criticizes you for nursing, reread Chapter 7, the section on Prejudice Against Breastfeeding, pages 195–200, to understand why they do it; then turn a deaf ear.

Going Out:

Don't go out socially yet, unless you feel very lively and the four walls of your bedroom are really beginning to get you down. If you do go, take the baby—a nursing baby is so portable! Pleasant adult company is sometimes a real tonic, if you are careful not to overexert yourself in new surroundings. Sometimes just a drive in the car or a walk around the block in the sunshine is a welcome change of scene. Plop yourself on a bench at a local playground. The experienced parents around you won't be able to resist a peek at your new baby, and are likely to follow up with a supportive, informative chat. Go to a movie—your baby gets in free and will probably just doze and nurse through the whole show.

GROWTH SPURTS

Many babies seem to go along comfortably for a time and then have a spurt of growth that makes them suddenly extrahungry, wanting to eat all day long. These so-called frequency days don't mean that your milk supply has suddenly dropped, but just the opposite; the baby is growing and his needs have suddenly risen. Think of it this way: If a bottlefed baby suddenly increased his intake, everyone would be exclaiming about his wonderful appetite, and bragging that he took a whole extra bottle today. When a breastfed baby's appetite increases, we tend to panic, certain that we are not satisfying his hunger, instead of just recognizing it as a healthy sign of growth.

Growth spurts are likely to occur sometime in the second week, at somewhere between three and six weeks, and at three months. If you suddenly find yourself "nursing night and day," check the calendar to see if this doesn't coincide with a likely growth spurt. Your production will adjust accordingly.

SPECIAL SITUATIONS: NURSING A "DIVIDEND" BABY

One mother who may have a hard time sticking to her decision to breastfeed is the mother who already has children and who, when her youngest child is ten or twelve years old, has another baby. Somehow a baby born out of season is always at a disadvantage, whether it is a fall colt or a Christmas lamb, or a child who arrives as a dividend to the family that already seemed complete. Even if the mother breastfed her previous children with complete success, she may find that she doesn't seem to do well with this one. The baby nurses, but he just doesn't gain.

The problem is basically one of practicality. Once you get out of the habit of orienting your life around infants and toddlers, it is very difficult to get back into that habit. Life becomes so different for most families when the children are older that it is difficult to go back easily to a nursery world of long, peaceful feedings, weekends at home, and neglected housework. Other responsibilities have intruded on the hours that were once free for sitting around with a baby. The result is that nursing time is curtailed, so that the milk supply dwindles, or sometimes the letdown reflex is inhibited, so that what milk the baby does get is simply rather low in calories.

If you are in this situation, and you want to continue to nurse, stop to think ahead a little about how many changes this is going to make, temporarily, in your household. This baby deserves his mother's milk just as much as the others did; but making it possible for him requires a special effort not only from you but from the rest of your household, too.

Even if you don't work outside your home, read Chapter 12, "The Working Mother: How Breastfeeding Can Help," for hints on how busy women manage nursing and other responsibilities as well. Let older children (and your partner) get into the habit of doing more of their own cleaning, cooking, transportation, and wardrobe management. Teach them to expect just as much from you in the way of love and kindness, but perhaps a little less in the way of goods and services. Get into the habit yourself of resting more and doing less, so that you can enjoy this baby the way babies were meant to be enjoyed. All too soon this one, like the others, will be grown.

The mother who has her *first* baby rather late in life, paradoxically, may have a very easy time breastfeeding. Just having a baby in a childless household is such a big change that the adjustments necessitated by nursing can be accomplished simultaneously. The nursing relationship is a special blessing for an older mother, making this child doubly enjoyable and helping her to be casual and easygoing about motherhood.

NURSING TWINS

Lots of mothers have nursed twins. It is usually easier to breast-feed twins than it is to feed them sixteen or more bottles every day. It is also much better for the twins, who may be small at birth and need the extra boost of mother's milk. Benjamin Spock, MD, surveying mothers of twins, found that mothers who breastfed twins were better organized and felt better than the mothers who bottlefed twins. Several books by mothers of twins offer helpful advice not only for breastfeeding twins (and triplets!) but for managing their care (see Resources).

Most mothers of twins nurse them simultaneously, at least when they are both awake at the same time. This appears clumsy at first, but the fact that both breasts are nursed at once when the milk lets down seems to benefit the necessary high rate of milk production. In the old days, professional wet nurses probably increased their production, in order to feed two or even more babies, by this method of simultaneous feedings. For comfort, try tucking one twin under each arm, supported by pillows or the arms of a big chair. Or put one twin in your lap and use its stomach as a pillow for the other twin. Most mothers have enough milk for twins without adding cereals or anything else, at least until the combined weight of the twins is twenty or twenty-five pounds. That is usually when they are around five or six months old, when one would begin adding solids anyway, but it may occur earlier.

It is customary to advise mothers of twins to rotate the babies, that is, to nurse each baby on each breast, not to always keep the same baby on the same side. The theory is that the stronger sucker will then be able to stimulate both breasts to higher production. However, in all animals that have multiple young, scientists have found that each baby has its own favorite nipple, and after some confusion in the early days soon learns to go to the same place for every meal. In this way, each gland adjusts its secretion of milk to the needs of the particular baby that nurses on it. It may be that human twins can regulate their milk supplies individually and that keeping them always on the same breast would simplify matters. An extreme difference in

needs may make you look a bit lopsided; on the other hand, production may differ without any difference in appearance. It is
also possible that the production level and even milk content
may differ on each side. One mother pumping milk for a sick
twin produced thirteen ounces regularly from one breast, and
seven from the other, each morning, and yet her breasts were
the same size.

The mother nursing twins may have to make a special effort
to get enough calories. With supermarket shelves full of unnour-
ishing products, such as corn flakes and Jell-O, it is easy to eat a
lot without actually getting much food. To nurse twins (or to
nurse one baby and give milk to a milk bank) without losing too
much weight, a mother may need to eat one or even two extra
meals a day, with emphasis on meat and potatoes, beans, or rice,
and perhaps some hearty snacks as well. Like any nursing mother,
if she finds herself losing weight or feeling tired or depressed, she
may need additional B-complex vitamins.

Mothers of multiples agree that one should hunt before birth
for a cooperative pediatrician. As a rule, twins can gain just as
well as singles on mother's milk; some, however, do need supplements as they grow, especially on days when the mother is overtired. A mother nursing twins or triplets runs a higher-than-normal
risk of breast infection if she lets herself get overtired.

NURSING THE DISADVANTAGED BABY

The baby who is born with a serious abnormality, such as Down syndrome or a cleft palate, can still be fed his mother's milk. Nursing a
disadvantaged baby may take patience and dedication. An infant
with neurologic damage may have little or no sucking reflex. An ill
or preterm baby may be separated from you by hospitalization. You

will need the strong support of your health-care team. A lactation consultant can be very helpful in establishing and maintaining lactation under challenging circumstances.

The worried mother of a disadvantaged child is often exceptionally willing to make the extra effort. It is one thing she can clearly do to help, and it brings profound emotional relief to her. The mother of a Down syndrome baby, healthy and nursing at eight months, said, "It is the best I can do for her, to make her feel close and happy, and to give her the best start toward growing up that she can have." One mother who nursed a normal baby and simultaneously expressed enough milk for his cleft-palated twin put it this way: "I believe Steve needed the nutritional advantage of the milk, and I wanted very much to give it to him. The day I took him home from the hospital and began to express my milk for him, I experienced a great sense of relief and my anxiety over his condition seemed to dissipate. The act of providing breast milk for him in the unconventional way of a bottle provided me with a great peace of mind and a feeling of usefulness. I felt I had climbed Mt. Everest when I succeeded."

THE PRETERM OR SERIOUSLY ILL BABY

It is always a shocking experience for both mother and child when a very small baby has to stay in the hospital while the mother goes home. Here again, the maintenance of a supply of breast milk is the most useful thing a mother can provide for the child. Small preterm babies do well on expressed breast milk (see Chapter 2, pages 44–45), showing significant differences in IQ, motor development, and other assessments from their formula-fed counterparts months and years later. The field of preemie care has evolved in recent years, and many developments are based on breastfeeding and Kangaroo Care (see Chapter 6, page 176), as high-tech medicine recognizes the advantages only the milk, warmth, and scent of a mother can provide a very tiny baby.

Feeding of breast milk rapidly corrects the chemical chaos in the bodies of infants who have undergone surgery. Many mothers have expressed milk and carried it to the hospital daily. In one case, an infant with a heart anomaly had to undergo major surgery in a military hospital; the mother's milk was picked up every day in an ice chest by an air force ambulance. Pediatric hospitals have come a long way in supporting parents of young patients, including providing pumping rooms and refrigerators for mothers of nursing babies.

PUMPING MILK FOR THE HOSPITALIZED BABY

To develop or maintain a milk supply while you are separated from the baby, you should plan on pumping your milk; even if the milk cannot be given to your baby, pumping it will keep your supply going until the baby can come home. Information about manual expression, pumping, and kinds of pumps is given in Chapter 12, pages 371–79.

To develop a milk supply or keep production going, you will need to pump an average of every three to four hours (and most definitely, you must pump at nighttime), or six to eight times a day, with no interval longer than five or six hours between pumpings. You should also be prepared to pump in between if you suddenly feel the milk let down. Use the hints in Chapter 2 (page 36) and in this chapter (pages 280–82) for conditioning your letdown reflex, which will help to develop and maintain your productivity.

Hospitals today usually allow parents, especially nursing mothers, to stay with their infants at all times, except of course during surgery. Policies change, however, from hospital to hospital, and even from floor to floor. Find out exactly what your hospital's policies allow you to do and not do. Can you stay overnight with your baby? Can you be with your baby in the recovery room? How soon will you be allowed to nurse your baby after surgery? If the hospital bars you from caring for your baby in ways you feel are necessary for your baby's well-being, speak with your baby's doctor. Call the hospital administration. Find out what the laws are in your state regarding the treatment of families in hospitals. Some states require that parents have access to their hospitalized children at all times. And remember that all rules can be bent—and usually are when the parents express their preferences clearly and forthrightly.

La Leche League International offers experienced support and advice for mothers of seriously ill or disabled nursing babies. Nothing can help so much as talking to someone who has been in the same boat. The league can also guide the mother in ways to get along with members of the hospital staff, and to enlist their support without harassing them. If, in the course of your baby's hospitalization, your milk production ceases, LLLI has several pamphlets on relactation, or reestablishing a milk supply.

THE NURSING MOTHER AND
THE REST OF THE FAMILY: YOUR PARTNER

One of the rewards of breastfeeding for women in married or otherwise committed relationships is the approval of their adult partners. Your partner's pride and confidence in you can keep you nursing while you are a novice at the job. He or she can dispel your doubts, reassure you, and steady you. Your partner can save you from rushing for the bottle just because the baby has had an extrahungry day and your supply hasn't caught up with her need, or because your breasts seem soft, the baby is fussing, and someone remarks, "You can't just let that child starve!" Your partner can brighten the time you spend at home, by bringing news and anecdotes from the outside world. He or she can make you rest when your conscience is urging you to overwork. It is your partner who, in the middle of night, may bring the baby to you to nurse in bed, barely waking you or the baby.

What your partner may need, in return, is appreciation. It's sometimes a shock for the adult who has not gone through pregnancy to have this new person in the household—right in your bed, in fact—a person who occupies so much of your time and attention. You can reassure your partner with praise and verbal thanks, of course, but more effectively, by your attention, even passive attention. For example, if your partner is cooking dinner, or mowing the lawn, you can sit down and nurse the baby while watching him or her do it. You are still resting, and your partner feels appreciated. That feeling is a powerful reinforcement.

YOUR CHILDREN

If you have more than one child, but this is the first you've breastfed, you may feel strange initially about nursing in front of the others. However, children soon get accustomed to the sight and take it for granted. The child closest in age to the baby sometimes wants special attention while you are nursing. Make the baby's mealtime a special time for your older child, too, in which you read to him and cuddle him. A nursing baby makes a very good book rest, and you can quite easily hold two children in your lap, or put your free arm around the older child. You can enjoy your peaceful private nursings alone with the baby now and then, when the other child is asleep or outside playing. Don't let yourself resent the older child's intrusion; if you seem to enjoy his company when you are nursing, and perhaps give him a special half-hour of play or attention at some other time, he won't think of nursing as disadvantageous to himself, and will be less likely to cause intentional interruptions.

Of course, you don't have to let the older child tease or annoy you or the baby at feeding times; just tell him firmly that that is not acceptable behavior. After all, you have a right to breastfeed, and your new baby has a right to his mother's milk, regardless of how the older child feels about it. Most toddlers and older children learn to regard nursing as just what it is: a nice, friendly, and very convenient way to feed the baby.

An older child who sees the baby at the breast may want to try nursing, too. The best way to deal with such a request is to let the child try. He won't be very successful, and he'll find that, after all, it's just milk and not the ambrosia the baby seems to think it is.

GRANDMOTHERS

The sensitive grandmother is usually very pleased that her grandchild is being breastfed. Watching the new baby at the breast, she remembers her own days of new motherhood, and she feels fonder than ever of her daughter or daughter-in-law for being such a good mother to this new member of the family.

But it is not given to all of us, even grandmothers, to be sensitive all the time. A grandmother may well be more skillful at first with the baby than is his inexperienced mother. While experienced with children, she may have ideas about breastfeeding that date from days when it was widely assumed that formula was superior. She may secretly be anxious to have her son or son-in-law see what a good mother she is, and therefore dispense more advice, not always accurate, than is welcome. However experienced a grandmother is at baby care, there is one thing she cannot do for the baby (in our culture, at least) and that is nurse him. So she may be a little jealous because you are the only person who is really indispensable to the baby. Or it is possible that a grandmother can feel conflicted because she is jealous of this little newcomer who takes you away from her. Especially during nursing, the closed circle of rapport between mother and baby may make a grandmother feel excluded. In her anxiety to regain her closeness with you, she may break in with remarks that are more thoughtless or even cruel than she realizes. The cure is simple; seek privacy during nursing, and at other times make a special effort to make your mother or mother-in-law feel welcome and appreciated. Ask for help you really need in areas where she excels, such as cooking your favorite foods, and be sure to show appreciation for this truly needed assistance.

GUARDING YOUR OWN WELL-BEING

Even if you have doting grandmothers and grandfathers and a loving partner and a great medical team, *you* must take responsibility for your own health; nobody else can do it for you. Your baby's pediatrician may be primarily interested in your baby's

health, and not in yours. Your obstetrician may be primarily interested in your pelvic organs, and not in the rest of you. All
too often, a new mother drags on for weeks with anemia or
bronchitis or some other ailment that neither her obstetrician
nor her baby's pediatrician notices, although she may see both
of them during that time, and that she herself tries to ignore,
often because she feels too tired to bother going to another
doctor.

Seeing a family-practice physician may be more useful at this
point than going to two specialists. Either way, you know your
body best, and you need to take primary responsibility. Watch
your nutrition. Get enough rest. If you are coughing, running a
fever, bleeding vaginally more than slightly or with fresh blood
rather than a brownish discharge—if you are pale and have blue
circles under your eyes—see a physician. Get treatment; don't
just try to tough it out if you are not well. Your baby needs you to
be healthy.

THE "BABY BLUES"

No doubt, pregnancy, birth, and lactation are hormonal hurri-
canes and can cause emotional earthquakes. Feeling weepy now
and again is a reasonable response to both the tides of hormones
and the magnitude of the life event of becoming a mother. Most
women, in fact, experience mild, temporary depression around
the third day after giving birth. Generally, physical and emotional
support from family and friends—especially when you talk to
other mothers who have been through it, too—helps a new
mother bounce back.

For 10 to 15 percent of new mothers, however, the baby blues
do not lift, but dip into enduring depression. Signs that a mother

may be facing more than a spell of the blues, and require treatment, include:

- Feeling consistently irritable, restless, anxious, lonely, or sad for more than a week
- Having no energy, or having insomnia despite being very tired
- Overeating and gaining weight, or undereating and losing weight
- Having trouble focusing or remembering
- Being frantically concerned about the baby, or being disinterested in the baby
- Being afraid of hurting the baby or herself
- Feeling worthless and guilty
- Experiencing headaches and chest pain
- Taking no interest in activities that once gave pleasure
- Being unable to function and perform day-to-day tasks, such as showering and interacting with others

Postpartum depression (PPD) can appear in the first weeks of motherhood or months later. The sooner it is treated with counseling and medication, the easier it is to resolve. Left untreated, PPD can continue for a very long time, even years after birth, and become much more difficult to heal. (It can even reach a degree of psychosis, in which hallucinations occur.) Infants of depressed mothers are also affected by the disease and can be delayed developmentally. Don't hesitate to ask for help if you ever feel you need it. Much has been learned in recent years about PPD, and much can be done to make it go away.

IF SORE NIPPLES PERSIST

The likelihood of nipple soreness diminishes after you have left the hospital and the early days of nursing are past. Occasionally, however, a nipple can get sore once you are home. Check the baby's positioning, and make sure the baby is latched on well, with the lips flanged out and the nipple well back in the mouth, out of harm's way. Rotate the positions you hold the baby in from feeding to feeding. Allow your nipples to air-dry between feedings. Let a little breast milk dry on the sore nipple; it has healing properties. If these suggestions do not result in improvement, a lactation consultant can evaluate the situation in your home or at a clinic and provide additional remedies.

Sometimes a new nursing mother gets into trouble because she does not know how to treat a sore nipple and does not want to ask her doctor for fear that he will insist she wean the baby; so she goes on nursing despite the nipple's getting worse and worse, until it is really injured. Where damage is severe, you can nurse on one breast only and let the sore nipple heal, if you have to. Again, a lactation expert can help.

Sore nipples that persist for many days may be caused not by poor positioning but by a yeast infection. Symptoms may include pain that persists or gets worse during the feeding rather than peaking at the beginning, red or weeping spots on the nipples and areolas, and pain within the breast. Typically, a yeast infection, or thrush, starts in the baby's mouth after the baby has been given antibiotics. You may see white patches on the baby's tongue or inside the mouth that look like milk but don't wipe off. The infection can be passed back and forth between mother and baby repeatedly. Even if one or the other doesn't have any overt symptoms, both need to be treated.

OTHER BREAST AILMENTS

Plugged ducts—little areas of the breast that don't drain milk well—are a relatively common problem that can be resolved with a little attention. Left unattended, a plugged duct can lead to a minor infection within the breast that may make you feel ill, and a minor infection, if you are fatigued, can turn into a more serious and painful infection. If you begin to feel feverish and sick all over, check your breasts to see if you can find a "hot spot" that is tender to the touch and perhaps looks reddened. You can treat this yourself with hot moist compresses and frequent nursing; lactation consultants recommend positioning the baby so that his nose is pointing toward the sore spot, "even if you have to stand on your head to do it." That will help to drain the blocked area. Rotating the baby to a new quadrant of the breast at each feeding will drain all the ducts thoroughly. Plenty of rest and fluids for you are also vital. A plugged duct, if not tended to promptly, can lead to mastitis, or a breast infection.

If you do not feel better within twenty-four hours, or if you start running a higher fever, see a doctor immediately and get some antibiotics. Mastitis usually responds well to antibiotics. As a rule, antibiotics will not harm your baby through your milk; tetracycline, however, should not be taken by nursing mothers because it can stain the baby's newly forming teeth.

CONFIDENCE BUILDERS

All of us have doubts sometimes about our nursing ability, even if we have nursed babies before. When the baby is fussy, or the doctor is noncommittal about whether the baby's doing well, or a friend criticizes, it is hard not to worry. You can't see the milk going into the baby, so there's no way to tell exactly what he's getting. You start to concentrate so much on the fear that he's getting no milk that you become tense at feeding time, and lose the easygoing sense of teamwork and friendship with the baby. When these good feelings are there, the milk is there, too, automatically; you don't have to worry about it any more than your happy nursing baby does.

If you are having doubts, try these suggestions:

1. *Find Another Nursing Mother,* past or present. If you don't know one, ask your neighbors and acquaintances. Now is the time to pack up your baby and visit someone who has had more experience. There may be a La Leche League group in your own town; LLLI will notify you of the nearest group leader if you call, toll-free: 1-800-LA LECHE. Or you might ask your doctor for the name of some other patient who is an old hand at breastfeeding. One phone call to another, experienced, nursing mother can boost your morale for a week.

2. *Even Your Pets Can Inspire Your Own Confidence.* One nursing mother wrote about her cat having kittens: "While the actual birth was a bit of a surprise to the cat (the first kitten was born on the back doorstep), by the time the others arrived, she was already confident in her new role of mother. During the first week, Domino was with her babies constantly. She didn't seem to mind their continual nursing. No one suggested that the milk of Cindy Lou, the cocker spaniel next door, might be more nourishing for newborn kittens or at least would help them to sleep all night. And when Domino did leave them for a while, it took only the

tiniest meow to bring her leaping back into the box. Watching Domino raise her family is a continuing delight and inspiration."

3. *Listen to the Baby Swallowing—"Suck-Hah"—Each Time the Milk Lets Down* if you can't believe the invisible milk is there. Or you can tuck the forefinger of your free hand under the baby's chin as she nurses, so you can feel her swallowing. Or try expressing a little milk manually, after a feeding (see Chapter 12, pages 376–77) to reassure yourself that it exists.

4. *Remember That Breast Milk Is an Efficient Source of Nutrients* tailored to the needs of your baby. One way you might look at it is that *two* ounces of breast milk contains as much and more of the needed nutrients as *four* ounces of formula provides, even if your milk looks "thinner" and bluish. And when the fat-rich hind milk is added in, your milk probably has as many calories, per ounce, as light cream. So your baby is getting plenty of nourishment even when the amount of milk he takes seems meager compared to with the bottleful after bottleful that a formula-fed baby may take.

5. *Don't Judge How Much Milk You Have by How Full Your Breasts Seem.* Often we feel very full in the hospital; then, when we get home, the breasts are no longer burstingly full, and it seems as if the milk has gone. However, the fullness you experienced in the hospital is only partly caused by milk; some of it is due to increased circulation and some swelling in the tissues, which quickly dissipates. The breast is never, in fact, really empty, but continually makes milk. And once the letdown reflex is working well, much of the fluid content of the milk is not drawn from the bloodstream into the breasts until it is needed. Thus, there may

be several ounces of milk available to the baby in a breast that feels quite soft nearly all the time.

6. *Remember: The Primary Treatment for a Fussy Baby Is More Rest for the Mother.* Write that out in big letters and stick the note on the refrigerator, to keep it in front of others in the household as well as yourself. A nursing mother, especially in the first weeks and with her first baby, needs to cut back on anything else that takes energy, such as work, phone calls, conversations, reading, cooking, and whatever she may think she ought to be doing. She needs to persuade her loved ones to give her some peace, in whatever way she can manage. Leave the dinner table, and go to bed early. Take the rest you need.

7. *Give Your Baby Lots of Skin Contact If He Cries Often.* Sometimes babies need to be cuddled more than anything else, and feeling the warmth of your skin can have a magically calming effect. A rocking chair is also a great tool for relaxing mother as well as baby, not just during feedings, but between and after feedings when a little cozy time is in order. Some babies need extra suckling; if the baby will not nurse on the breast longer, you could offer him a pacifier, but pacifiers are a nuisance and usually end up on the floor. Instead, try letting him suck on the tip of your little finger, the pad turned up against the roof of his mouth. Sometimes a fretful baby is overstimulated by playful parents or siblings, by too much going on for his young nervous system to cope with; try skin contact and peace and quiet.

8. *Practice Unrestricted Breastfeeding.* Read the section on unrestricted versus standard-care babies in Chapter 5 (pages 166–67).

By three months, standard-care babies on the average cry 35 percent *more* than do unrestrictedly breastfed babies. Are you giving yourself (or is someone else giving you) a lot of reasons why feedings are being curtailed, delayed, or interrupted? Could you change some of that? Maybe your baby would like to have fewer rules in her young life.

9. *Accept That Some Babies Are Just Fussier Than Others. Take Comfort from the Thought.* A pair of breastfed twins supplied a good example, reported in the La Leche League newsletter for mothers, *New Beginnings:*

> "Chatty Cathy," the smaller twin, is a little "fuss pot"— squirming and spitting, sleeping only in short hauls, and gaining rather slowly. Charlotte nurses peacefully, lives life in an easygoing way, and is gaining much faster than her sister."

The same mother, the same supply of milk—no supplements, no solids—and two very different babies.

10. *Don't Permit Yourself to Worry in the Evening.* When you are tired, little worries become big ones. You are especially likely to worry about your milk in the evening, or in the middle of the night. Force yourself to think about something else, to put the milk question out of your mind until morning. Let your partner walk the baby or rock him. Take a shower, have a glass of wine, walk around the block. Call someone who can reassure you. Remember that the best prescription for a fussy baby is not a bottle—bottles bring problems of their own—but more rest for the mother.

11. Remember That the First Six Weeks Are the Learning Period. Good, easy times are ahead of you, when you won't even remember how worried you once were. And if you ever get to feeling that nursing "isn't worth the bother" of learning, try rereading Chapters 1 and 3.

CHANGES AROUND FOUR TO SIX WEEKS

Some babies get weaned to a bottle around the age of one month to six weeks, not because their mothers don't have enough milk, but because the mothers *think* they don't. Why? First, a one-month-old baby is often a rather crabby soul. He is far more aware of things than he was at two weeks, and that means he is more aware of cold, heat, wet diapers, loneliness, and his not-very-grown-up insides. So he cries. Second, around a month or six weeks after delivery, you may begin feeling pretty good. You do more. You don't take those naps. You deal with more of the housework, and you are more and more tempted to take up your social life and outside interests again. You may be returning to your full-time job. So you get tired; and the immediate result of your fatigue is a fussy baby.

Once again, hang this rule up someplace where you can see it often: *The best treatment for a fussy baby is more rest for the mother.* When the baby is not happy or does not seem to be getting enough milk, you need to slow down and spend more time peacefully nursing him.

Many of the mothers who quit around the one-month mark do so simply because they are discouraged. They feel as if they are going to spend the rest of their lives with a baby at the breast, constantly nursing. There will never again be a time for getting the house clean or spending an evening out; they will never sleep through the night again; the idea of breastfeeding presents a picture of endless months of being tied to a constantly fussy baby, just as they've been tied in the past four or six weeks.

But this is not the time to get discouraged. This is the turning point. From about six weeks onward, breastfeeding becomes quite different. The baby rather abruptly drops about two meals a day, so that he is nursing eight times in twenty-four hours, instead of ten or more. You begin getting one six-hour stretch of sleep at night, and your ever-improving letdown reflex works so well that some feedings are over in five or ten minutes; you hardly notice that you had to stop whatever you were doing to feed the baby. (Perhaps you didn't stop, but kept on talking on the phone or reading the newspaper.) Going out becomes easy; you can take the baby or leave him with a bottle of breast milk. The little problems such as leaking and overproduction are beginning to disappear. And you begin having the strength to come and go as you please, without detriment to your milk supply.

These first six weeks have been trying, in some ways. You and your baby have been learning to breastfeed; your baby has been adjusting to the strange and not always pleasant world she has been born into; and you have been gradually recovering from the prolonged demands of pregnancy and from the effort of childbirth: If this is the first baby, you have also been making the emotional transition to becoming a mother. These have been demanding tasks, but most of the effort is behind you now. Now, at the six-week mark, you can expect a major change; now begins the "reward period" of nursing.

The Reward Period Begins

TWO TO THREE MONTHS

A new baby is fascinating, but a two-month old baby is more fun. By two months, a baby is pert and pretty, instead of blotchy and strange-looking. She can "talk" with her delicious coos and smile her wonderful smile. She looks at people, takes an interest in colors, and obviously enjoys the company of your partner and any brothers or sisters she is lucky enough to have. She is a lot easier to care for than she was a few weeks earlier; she is more content, and when she does want something, you can often "read" her cries and tell if she is hungry, or uncomfortable, or tired, or simply needs to be held close for a while.

By the time two months have passed, you probably feel pretty good yourself. Any physical discomforts of the early days after giving birth have passed. The little problems of the learning days of nursing—leaking, milk fluctuations, nipple soreness—no longer exist. You are beginning to take the reins of the household in your own hands again. You may be ready to go back to work, having learned to pump and store your milk for your baby's meals with the sitter (see pages 371–79).

You are beginning, too, to sense the nature of the nursing

relationship, the warm spirit of mutual affection that unites the nursing couple. A brand-new baby is having such a time trying to get fed that he hardly has attention for anything more. But a baby of two months looks at you with his bright eyes as he nurses; he knows you from all other people, and he loves you. He enjoys your company; he waits trustingly for you to feed him, and he wants to be sociable before, during, and after meals. He is no longer a perplexing bundle of contrariness, or a cute but frighteningly helpless doll, to be dressed, undressed, bathed, and fussed over; he is your own little friend, and caring for him is second nature, like caring for yourself. Perhaps you used to feel a sense of relief whenever the baby went to sleep, and of apprehension when he stirred; now, you find you enjoy having him around and don't worry about him, whether he's asleep or awake. In fact, you may miss him, sometimes desperately, if you are away from him. You are becoming a happy nursing couple.

CONTINUING THE HOLIDAY

Ideally, a mother could comfortably go on staying home with her baby for as long as she wanted to after giving birth. Today, the demands of supporting a family and returning to work or school often cut short the time at home once considered every mother's due. Now, it seems as if women are expected to give birth and then continue with every activity exactly as before.

If you can possibly extend the time you stay at home without any responsibilities other than being a mother, to four months at the very least, you will find your return to the outside world much less taxing than at two months. Six months to a year is even better. Nursing can be the excuse you need in order to say, "No, my one and only responsibility right now is nursing and caring for my baby."

Even if you are not returning to work, you may continue to find yourself becoming overtired at this time. You are still convalescing, a fact that friends seem to forget. People who wouldn't dream of imposing on someone in late pregnancy sometimes completely overlook a mother's need for rest after the baby is born. Once the two-month mark is past, you may find yourself being considered available again for business trips, volunteer work, babysitting swaps, and so on. One excuse—"I'm so sorry, the doctor has told me not to accept any additional commitments in the early months of nursing the baby"—will take care of most of these demands.

If you absolutely cannot take more than two months away from your job, don't despair. Read Chapter 12, "The Working Mother: How Breastfeeding Can Help." Breastfeeding will maintain the special closeness between you and your baby as long as you nurse, whether you return to work or not.

PICKING UP THE BABY

Sometimes babies cry because they are lonely and frightened. Just because the baby stops crying when you pick her up doesn't mean she's "spoiled." That's an idea based on outdated theories, and many people, including some health-care providers, still champion it. It's very unfair. Of course the baby stops crying when you pick her up, if picking her up was what she needed. She's not "testing" you at this age; she really needs comforting. Behavioral scientists have shown that plenty of human handling and body contact are as important to babies' emotional growth as plenty of good food is to their physical growth. Isn't it convenient that breastfeeding supplies both!

Grandparents and partners, and even (or perhaps especially) brothers and sisters, can carry and hold and rock a new baby when she needs comforting and you are busy; they don't have the pleasure of feeding her, so they like to share her in other ways. When you are all alone and your baby is fretful, and yet you are too busy to sit and rock her, you might try that time-honored device, the baby sling or backpack, that puts the baby in touch with your body, your heartbeat, and your breathing, even while you continue doing whatever you need to accomplish.

NIGHT FEEDINGS

You can expect a breastfed baby to go on needing at least one night feeding, plus a late evening or very early morning feeding, for five or six months; many babies (and mothers) cherish that predawn cuddle and nursing throughout the first year. Your milk supply may need this feeding, too.

The mother who at this point feels exhausted because she has to feed in the night isn't getting enough rest in the daytime. If you simply can't nap during the day, consider keeping the baby in bed with you, at least for the second half of the night, so that you can doze as he nurses.

CLOTHES

Depressing, isn't it? For months you looked forward to getting your waistline back so that you could wear your own clothes again; and now that your waistline is normal, you still can't get into any of your clothes because you are more bosomy than before. If there are one or two things in the closet that you can manage to get into, they probably button up the back or zip up the side and are very inconvenient for nursing. The woman who has been small-breasted all her life may enjoy this predicament; in fact, her clothes may fit and look better when she is lactating than when she is not. But even she may have the problem of finding something to wear that enables her to nurse the baby without getting completely undressed. This can be crucial when the baby suddenly decides in the middle of a morning of shopping that it is mealtime, and you then realize that you can't nurse him without taking your dress off. (Emergency solution: Find a dress shop and nurse him in the fitting room.)

The problem of finding clothes that can easily and discreetly give nursing access has always been with us. Paintings of Madonnas and other mothers from various periods and countries show all kinds of solutions. Some simply take advantage of a rather low-necked dress, perhaps using a shawl for modesty. Others have been portrayed in dresses that unbutton or untie in the front, or that have slits concealed in drapery. The most elegant solution is perhaps that shown in a Flemish painting in which the Madonna wears an elaborate, high-necked gown with two rows of gold ornaments down the bodice that on close inspection are found to be hooks and eyes holding closed an opening on each side.

Things are easier nowadays. It's easy to find clothes that pull up from the waist or button down the front: cardigans, skirts, shirts or overblouses, shirtwaist dresses. Since you'll be nursing for quite a while, it's worth buying a couple of unbuttoning drip-dry shirts or blouses to wear when you and the baby go out of the house. Pick print material that won't show dark wet spots if you should happen to leak. To nurse discreetly, unbutton the bottom buttons rather than those at the top.

The most convenient and least revealing kinds of tops are those that do not unbutton, but that can be lifted from the waist for nursing; overblouses, jerseys, sweaters, and so on. Some kind of pull-up-able top is invaluable if you want to nurse the baby while you have visitors—and hate to miss the conversation—or while traveling, or at a movie, or indeed anywhere away from home. The baby covers your slightly exposed midriff, your sweater or blouse conceals your breast, and you will find that no one can tell whether you are nursing the baby or just holding him. In fact, the more confidently and calmly you put your baby to the breast, the less likely people are to notice what you are doing.

You do not have to wear a nursing bra, although they are convenient. You can nurse in an ordinary bra by unhooking the back or slipping a strap off your shoulder. If you wear wireless bras, lifting up can be done almost as easily as with a nursing bra. In fact, you do not absolutely have to wear a bra at all, unless of course you are uncomfortable without one. A good bra can improve circulation by lifting a drooping breast and it can keep you comfortable when you are very full. But a bra that hikes up in back and sags in front doesn't do either, and a bra that is too tight may impede circulation and milk flow. How much a bra does to protect your figure is a matter of opinion, and perhaps heredity. One woman who wears bras night and day, massages the skin of her breasts with lanolin during pregnancy, and forgoes nursing lest she damage her figure, may still wind up with striations and loss of shape; while another mother who can't stand bras and never wears them may bear and nurse three or four babies without losing the upstanding bosom she started with. Most women, in fact, find the shape of their breasts to be fuller and firmer after nursing a baby or two.

FRESH AIR

Try to spend at least half an hour walking outdoors every day, even in the winter. Take the baby; it's good for him, too. Being indoors all day tends to make you concentrate too much on your indoor work and the imperfections of your surroundings. You actually need sunshine, in any case, for vitamin D. A short walk in the late afternoon improves your appetite for dinner and lifts your spirits, too. And it may help your milk supply. Dairymen say that cows give more milk at the evening milking if they are turned out of the barn for an hour or so in the afternoon.

NURSING AWAY FROM HOME

Many nursing mothers dislike leaving their small babies behind, no matter how competent the babysitter; often the happy nursing couple hates to be separated, even briefly, during these early months. So take the baby along. It is just as easy to take a nursing baby with you as it is to leave him at home and then miss him all evening. All you need is a blanket and a couple of extra diapers; the bottlefeeding mother may have to portage half a drugstore. Nursing babies are usually cheery and quiet if they are near their mothers; you can take a small nursing baby on a camping trip, to a dinner party or a restaurant, a football game or even a formal dance, with complete aplomb. Feed him before you leave or in the car once you are there. (Please don't feed him while driving; he be-

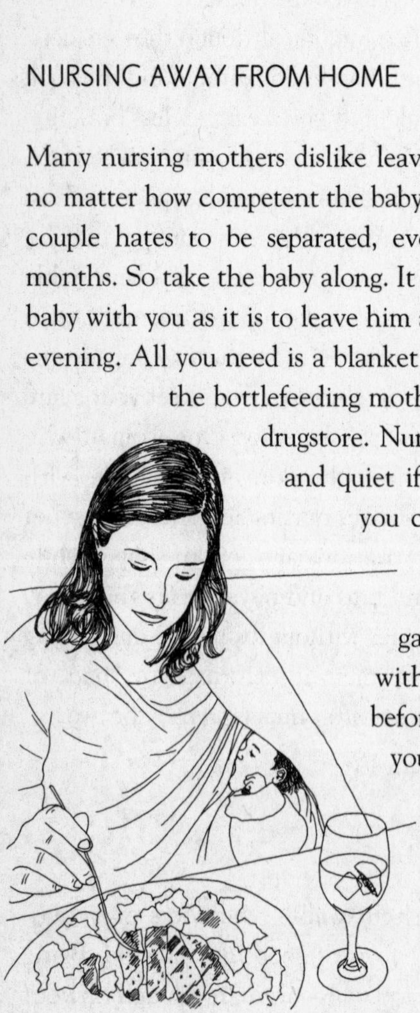

Figure 10.1 Nursing in public can be discreet and comfortable with a little practice.

longs in his car seat. If necessary, pull over and park to nurse—carry a shawl or blanket in the car to put over the baby and your shoulder to ensure privacy.) If you are out visiting and the baby is hungry again before it is time to leave, take him to some quiet corner, such as your hostess's bedroom, and feed him again; that will usually hold him until you are back in your car or at home again.

To take the baby shopping or to the park, feed him just before you leave the house. (Plan on taking time to do it: Don't hustle him, you might hurt his feelings.) Or you can feed him in the car after you get where you're going. That will give you a reasonable amount of time before he is hungry again.

If you must feed the baby before you get back to the car, the most comfortable place to do so is in a ladies' lounge. Usually, there is a chair or couch where you can sit. Buy or take something to read, if you don't want people to talk to you. Don't feel self-conscious about other women noticing you; you may find that most will go by without noticing, except for an occasional woman who will be delighted to see a mother nursing, and an occasional mother who will look at you longingly and then tell you how she tried and failed to nurse.

In emergencies you will probably find that you can nurse quite unnoticed even in a public place, such as a park bench or a restaurant booth. You will feel conspicuous, but you won't be nearly as conspicuous as you would be with a screaming, hungry baby in your arms.

BREASTFEEDING AND SEX

The closeness of a mother and her nursing baby, while it brings joy to the baby's other parent, sometimes partially eclipses the mother's need for additional close relationships, including sexual relations. That may be due in part to the temporary abeyance of the menstrual cycle, with its mood swings and peaks of desire, and its high levels of estrogen. The nursing mother may feel compliant about sexual relations without actually being eager. Perhaps, too, nursing a baby provides some of the fringe benefits of sex, such as closeness with another person and a feeling of being admired and wanted; so a mother may turn less often to her partner for the balm of touching and physical closeness. A mother who notices a reduced need for lovemaking in herself during lactation should take thought to be generous and affectionate to her lover, who needs to be touched and to feel wanted, too.

Some women, on the other hand, find that the experience of lactation intensifies their physical affection for their partner. The hormonal patterns of sex and lactation are very closely allied. One mother, having nursed her first child, found that from then on, when her partner kissed and fondled her breasts, she was swept by a palpable wave of deep affection, almost adoration, such as she had felt for her infant. The play of hormones can be downright startling. Oxytocin, the hormone responsible for the letdown reflex, is also released during orgasm; lactation researcher Niles Newton calls it "the hormone of love." Many a couple has been astonished to discover that, as the woman reaches climax, her milk may let down so sharply that it sprays into the air six inches or more in twin tiny-streamed fountains, sometimes catching her unwary mate full in the face. This phenomenon, like accidental letdown in other circumstances, generally abates as lactation becomes more fully established and the letdown reflex more controlled.

Some men, because of our culture and their own upbringing, feel conflicted about a nursing mother's breasts. Some men worry that they shouldn't touch their wives' breasts as long as they are lactating. In fact, there is nothing in mutually agreeable love play that should be avoided during lactation; a couple can be as free with each other's body then as at any other time, and if a little milk comes into the picture one way or another, it's harmless, and the baby won't miss it. There's always more where that came from.

Babies seem to have an aggravating tendency to wake up and fuss and want attention precisely when their parents are making love. Letting the baby sleep in another room with the door closed, at least some of the time, may help.

In our culture, some parents and more than a few grandparents feel a little uneasy about a boy baby nursing at his mother's breasts for more than a few months. Nursing is such an intense physical pleasure for a baby that it is not uncommon for boy babies to have erections as they nurse—they often do so before urinating, too—and the thought of a male child still nursing when he is "old enough to know what he is doing" (at whatever age that might be!) seems to have disquieting sexual overtones. While it is rather difficult to demonstrate scientifically, the practical experience of many families suggests that male and female nursing babies alike take their mothers' bodies for granted in a healthy, accepting way, no matter how long they nurse. One might speculate that the fetishistic attitude of many American men toward the female breast is at least partly the result of having been deprived during infancy of the experience of long nursing, and of that natural awareness and acceptance of the female body.

DON'T RUSH SOLID FOODS

The American Academy of Pediatrics does not recommend introducing "solid" foods into breastfed babies' diets until they are four to six months old. Formula-fed babies, however, often receive a little cereal in their bottles long before then, often because someone has advised their mothers that it will help them "sleep better." While there is no evidence that this old trick lengthens infant sleep, new research reveals that giving cereal before four months of age increases the risk of developing juvenile diabetes in infants with a family history of the disease. We already know that breastfeeding decreases the risk of diabetes for a lifetime; avoiding cereal and other solids until a baby is ready increases that protection.

Your breastfed baby does not need cereal or any solid food to be "satisfied," no matter how big and husky he is. An extra nursing on a fussy day will do just as well. Every mouthful of cereal or fruit you put into him simply substitutes for the more nutritious breast milk. Young breastfed babies often act as if they know this. They cry and struggle when getting their solid foods, or they take only a mouthful or two. It is a sad sight to see a mother trying desperately to get two tablespoons of applesauce into a frantic, crying baby because someone told her he should be eating "real food by now."

So forget about solid foods right now, despite the brochures and free samples from baby food companies that are arriving in the mailbox. (Of course those companies are interested in seeing you start solids early!) At somewhere around five to seven months, your baby will let you know he is ready for solids, probably by grabbing a handful of mashed potato off your dinner plate and eating it! You can safely wait until then.

VITAMINS

Your healthy nursing baby does not really need vitamin drops, especially if you take vitamins yourself and eat a well-rounded diet. Most nursing babies hate the strong taste of vitamins; why make them suffer? The one exception is vitamin D, which is manufactured in the body upon exposure to sunlight. You and your baby should both get a little time outdoors every day, if you possibly can; even on cloudy days, ten or twenty minutes' exposure to the open sky will help. If you cannot get outdoors because of the climate, especially if you and your baby have darkly pigmented skin, you should take a vitamin D supplement and discuss with your pediatrician whether your baby should receive one, too. If you live in the desert, near the equator, or in any area where sunlight is very strong, you should be careful the baby doesn't get sunburned (there are several sunscreens that are safe for children on the market; put a touch on his nose and cheeks as a precaution.) Several brief exposures to sunlight are safer than one long one. Also, be thoughtful about shading the baby's eyes; when you are holding him or he is in the stroller, he can't choose which way he is facing, as you can. Turn his back to the sun or adjust the stroller top so he doesn't have to squint and fuss at the glare.

EXPECT FLUCTUATIONS

Babies grow and mothers recuperate somewhat in the style of the algebra problem involving the frog in the well that jumped up two feet and fell back one. Sometimes a three-month-old baby goes on a four-hour schedule for a day, like a much older baby; sometimes he falls back to eating like a much younger baby for a while. You, too, may find you gain strength in spurts, as it were, and occasionally fall back to needing that extra nap or rest period you had been doing without.

Your milk production will fluctuate to some degree in relation to sucking stimulus. If your baby is a steady, hearty eater who wants the same big meals day after day, you may experience very little fluctuation; with the "gourmet" type of baby who may want a banquet today and only hors d'oeuvres tomorrow, your milk supply may often be in a state of change. Also, you can continue to expect occasional frequency days, when your baby nurses extra hungrily, thus stimulating milk production to rise over a period of a day or two until supply again equals need.

At three months, your baby will probably get his first immunization shot, the DPT shot, which protects him against diphtheria, tetanus, and whooping cough (pertussis). This may make him fussy and feverish, and he may want to nurse off and on all day, purely for the comfort of it. The mother who has raised both bottlefed and breastfed babies can really appreciate what a blessing it is to have such a surefire way of comforting a fretful baby.

MEDICATIONS AND ORDERS TO WEAN

Most nursing mothers need very little medication. And most of the drugs that are prescribed for transient illnesses are perfectly safe for a nursing couple. They include antibiotics and pain relievers. Occasionally, however, a mother whose lactation is going beautifully is ordered to stop breastfeeding because she must take some prescription drug that the prescribing physician says is not safe for the baby. Too often, this judgment is made, however, not because of clear evidence that the medication shows up in the milk and is ingested by the baby, but because no research has been done on its action in lactation at all. Better safe than sorry, is the usual justification for weaning a baby. What do you do if this happens to you?

It is difficult, of course, to confront or even question the physician on whose help you depend; but this may be the time to go politely toe-to-toe. Here are some things you can say: "I would prefer not to take this treatment, since I intend to keep breastfeeding my baby. Can you suggest an alternative that would be less of a problem? Can we postpone this for a few months?" If an antibiotic is in question, ask if it is ever given orally to babies; if so, the 1 percent dose the baby might get through your milk is far lower than the amount the baby would get directly. One of the problem areas that perhaps can't be avoided or postponed is a radioisotope scan. Some of these chemicals have a very short half-life, and you get rid of them in four days or less; others hang around in the system for months and would definitely be hazardous. Request that isotopes with a short half-life be used, so that you can pump for a few days, discarding the milk and giving formula or milk from a human milk bank (there are six in the United States; see Resources) to your baby, and then resume breastfeeding. Contact a lactation consultant for current information on medications that are considered safe during lactation, and alternatives to those considered unsafe.

Often the physician ordering you to wean is in a specialty that doesn't normally deal with nursing mothers or babies. If you are at odds with any physician over medication, bring in a lactation consultant to be your professional ally, one with whom the physician can work comfortably. If you must deal with the matter by yourself, here is a summary of the advice given by Jerry McKeagan, MD, director of pharmacology at the Williamsport Hospital in Pennsylvania, who is the father of seven breastfed babies and an authority on medication and mother's milk:

First, explain that you intend to continue breastfeeding, as you feel that it is important. Ask if you might get along without that drug, or if some other, safer drug or therapy might be used instead. It's rare that there is no acceptable substitute. Second, ask how long you are going to have to take the drug. Drugs that will be administered only once, or for a few days, are a different matter from drugs that must be taken for months. Third, tell the doctor how old your baby is. If you are nursing a jaundiced newborn, your medication might add significantly to the baby's load of toxins; if you are nursing a lusty ten-month-old, it's quite a different matter. As for the newborn, even a drug that you must take for some chronic condition can often be safely suspended for two or three weeks, right after childbirth, so your infant gets off to a good start.

If the question remains unresolved, ask your physician to look up the drug in the *current* (no earlier than 2002 for the tenth edition, as of this writing) edition of *Medications and Mothers' Milk*, by Thomas W. Hale, PhD, for comprehensive and authoritative information on the topic. Refer your physician to the discussion in this book on what kinds of drugs can pass into the milk and what kinds cannot (Chapter 3, pages 107–11).

If none of this works, you can get a second opinion from another physician, perhaps one more in tune with lactation. Or you can call La Leche League's Board of Medical Advisors for the latest information (see Resources). Be prepared. Write down the information they will want to know: the name of the drug, the size and frequency of the dose, and the condition you are being treated for; this last is very important. Sometimes the drug may not even be the right choice for you. And stay cool, this is not a hard one to win.

LUMPS AND BUMPS

It is less likely that a woman who is lactating will develop breast cancer than a woman who never lactates. However, the breast is apt to be full of strange lumps and bumps during nursing, especially in the first weeks. Usually, such lumps are simply enlarged lobes of alveoli that swell and dwindle and that feel very hard and distinct when the milk has just let down. A lump that does not change in any way is often a lacteal cyst, or milk-filled pocket within the breast. These cysts are harmless. If you are worried about such a lump, it's wise to have it checked out, but be sure to find a physician who is really familiar with lactating women. She is the only one who has the experience necessary to tell good from bad in these matters. General surgeons and obstetricians whose patients do not usually breastfeed have been known to recommend surgery for conditions that are actually part of the normal range of breast changes during lactation.

THREE TO FIVE MONTHS

While the growing baby can now get a full meal in five or ten minutes, he sometimes likes to nurse on and on until he falls asleep at the breast, now dozing, now and then sucking, until you finally lay him down, still dreaming of sweet milk and sucking in his dreams. To get the baby to bed without wakening, take him off the breast, and if that partially wakens him, hold him until he subsides again. Then take him to his crib and lay him down, but keep your hand on his tummy, if he stirs, until he sleeps once more. It is sudden desertion that makes him roar. (Laying a nightgown you have worn across his crib sheet may work like a charm. Your scent is one of the things he knows best and finds most calming.) If you use a sling and "wear" your baby, he is likely to fall asleep to the motion of your walk. You can put him down sound asleep, then, by simply slipping out of the sling as you lay him down in his crib, still draped by the sling. (See

The Baby Sling, on page 333, for more on this age-old convenience.)

Around four months, the baby develops a new trick. He interrupts himself. Suddenly he is very interested in noises. If someone in the room starts talking, or if you speak suddenly while nursing, the baby may drop the breast and jerk his head around to locate the voice. He may jerk his head around without letting go, too! The TV distracts him, and you may find you can't even read a magazine because he is interrupted by the rustle of the turning pages. An exceptionally alert baby may be unable to start nursing again when interrupted by noises, or may cry at such interruptions.

Fortunately, in about two weeks the baby will have learned to nurse and listen at the same time. Meanwhile, keep your own voice down while nursing, put your hand over the baby's ear to keep sounds out, and sit so that the baby can see the source of any disturbance and continue nursing while studying the event. If he does break away from the breast, you can usually coax him back with soothing words and a gentle pat.

Once the baby has learned to look, listen, and drink at the same time, she takes a genuine interest in her surroundings, watching the faces of others as she nurses. By five months, if you cover her ear, she will reach up and pull your hand away; she wants to hear everything. She may also play at the breast, waving her free hand about and watching it, playing with your clothes, patting your face. A five-month-old baby is apt to get hold of a button on your blouse and try to put it in her mouth, while she is nursing. She loves to watch your mouth as you talk to her while she eats, and her biggest problem is trying to smile at you and nurse at the same time.

Another feature of the four- or five-month-old baby's awareness of the world is that she may refuse to take a bottle. Although you may have left her with a sitter before, and she may have taken bottles occasionally in the past, she suddenly refuses them. Now, apparently, she would rather wait for her own warm, good-smelling mother, and her sweet milk, than drink that same milk from a cold plastic and rubber contraption while in the arms of a babysitter. Luckily, by this age she can wait three or four hours between daytime feedings, which is long enough for you to get errands done without her. And in the evenings, many babies are willing to eat at 5:00 p.m. or 6:00 p.m., and then sleep through until 1:00 a.m. or 2:00 a.m. This gives you enough span for an occasional night out. By contrast, mothers who work nine-to-five often find that the baby at this age shifts her own schedule so that she sleeps most of the time her mother is gone, and wakes to nurse and socialize in the evening when Mom is home again.

If your baby is going through a spell of refusing the bottle, you may be able to get around her persnicketiness by having the sitter offer milk in a spoon or a cup with a spout. In a month or two, the baby will accept the bottle again. You can even skip using a bottle altogether. A baby as young as three or four months can learn to drink from a cup with a spout, if it is held for her, and she may never need a bottle at all.

THE BABY SLING

The oldest labor-saving device in the world is probably the baby sling. Every human society seems to have some version of it, some way to carry a baby comfortably and safely on your body instead of in your arms. Psychologists point out that the backpacked baby, in addition to feeling loved and secure from body contact, meets the world at your eye level and facing forward, which is better for his confidence and morale than seeing everything from your knee level in a stroller.

Many families nowadays backpack the baby when out and about, instead of using a stroller. But have you ever thought of doing it at home, when you have a thousand things to do, and the baby is fussy and fretful with a stomachache or tooth coming in, or plain lonesomeness? Mothers who have tried this are astonished at the tranquillity it produces. There is something extremely soothing to a baby about being closely, snugly wrapped on his mother's warm, loving back, looking over her shoulder at the interesting things she is doing, or being lulled to sleep in a front pack simply by the rhythm of her breathing and moving. A half-hour of being carried may tranquilize the baby all day. One mother says that when she has company coming for dinner, she always carries the baby for an hour or so while she is cleaning up and getting the meal started; then the baby is quite happy to be alone in the playpen or on a blanket with some toys while she cooks and talks with her guests.

Carrying your baby properly on your back (or on your chest, if he's tiny) is far less tiring than carrying him in your arms. You can carry quite a heavy baby that way for hours and never notice it. Did you ever see pictures of children in India or China, carrying heavy baby brothers or sisters on their backs, and wonder how they do it? The answer is that the weight is properly located. Your legs are doing most of the work, rather than your easily fatigued back and arm muscles. Carrying the baby in a sling can actually make you feel better because it improves your posture; countering the extra weight in front that keeps you from slumping and slouching. Meanwhile, you have both hands free to scramble an egg, use the telephone, or work at the computer. And you can get more work done because you aren't being interrupted to soothe a fussy baby. Errands out of the house are easier (and safer) without wrestling a stroller in and out of stores and over curbs. Some working mothers find they can even sit at the computer or talk on the phone with the baby content and slumbering in a front or backpack.

Fathers can backpack babies, too, of course. This is especially handy if the family wants to go on a long excursion, sightseeing or hiking or cross-country skiing. A tall man who is backpacking a baby should try to position the load so the baby's head is no higher than his own; that way, he can judge more easily the height of doorways and other overhead obstacles, and duck low enough for both of them.

TRAVELING

Traveling is much, much easier with a nursing baby than with a bottlefed baby. In the first place, your baby doesn't care where he is as long as he's with you. Nursing is such a comfort and reassurance to him that your lap and your arms make even the strangest places quite acceptable. He doesn't cry for his familiar crib, or get thrown off schedule because he happens to be on an airplane or in a car; you, not cribs and schedules, are the center of his world, so he is completely nonchalant about travel. You can go on a business trip, or go hiking with your spouse or friends in the wilderness, and take your baby along—and all of you will enjoy yourselves.

Nursing is infinitely more practical than bottlefeeding while you are on the move. The logistics of supplying a baby with sterile formula during, say, a car trip from New York to California or a camping trip are formidable. Pity the poor bottlefeeding mother, with her insulated bottle of formula (how long will it stay cold, how long will it be safe to use?), heating the bottle under hot water in the motel sink while the baby screams; or, several days from home, mixing dry milk powder with tap water in a far-from-sterile bottle and hoping the baby "won't mind." The breastfed baby is the only baby who can be safely taken traveling in Africa, rural Latin America, the South Pacific, or other spots where sanitation may be poor. If you are likely to be sent abroad on business, or if you have a chance to travel for some other reason, this is a real point in favor of making breastfeeding a success.

If you plan to fly with your nursing baby, you may want to choose a night flight. Darkness, with fewer passengers moving up and down the aisles, means more privacy for you. Ask for a seat on the bulkhead row, so that you have more room to put a bassinet or baby basket at your feet. Many airliners have fold-down bassinets for babies built into the wall in this bulkhead row. If possible, purchase a seat for your baby and bring along your infant car seat so your baby can sleep safely and your arms and lap can be free for eating and reading. You aren't, at this writing, required to purchase a seat for a child under two, but the FAA advises doing so. Request a seat at the window or farthest from the aisle, when booking your flight, and wear a two-piece outfit that can be lifted from the waist on the day you fly. Nurse your baby on takeoff and landing so as to equalize the pressure in his ears and prevent earaches and the tears that accompany them.

If you are traveling with your partner or a friend, let him or her do the work of carrying the bags and managing the check-in procedures. Your baby depends on you not to get exhausted, and if you do get overtired, he will respond by being fussy. You can keep rested if you stay cool, don't rush, and let your partner do all the driving and cope with the tickets and baggage. If you must travel alone, plan your schedule reasonably, so that you will have adequate time between planes and before boarding to avoid stress and to relax. It's not impossible; one management consultant took her five-month-old nursing baby on a three-week business trip, along with a sitter to watch the baby during her meetings, with complete success.

IF YOU EVER FEEL LIKE QUITTING

Sometimes when you are feeling tired or your milk seems skimpy or a relative is pressuring you to do things her way and put your baby on the bottle, it seems easy to say, "Well, I've nursed this baby three months—or four, or five—I'll put him on a bottle now, and perhaps I'll have better luck and be able to nurse the next one longer."

Don't kid yourself. First, you'll never again have as much time or leisure as you have with the first baby in which to learn this womanly art. Second, it is a common fallacy to assume that breastfeeding becomes less valuable as the baby grows older. From the nutritional standpoint, this may be so as the baby adds other foods to his diet. But breastfeeding continues to provide protection against illness for as long as it is continued; this can be extremely valuable for a baby of eight months or even eighteen months, just as it is for one of a few weeks. Nursing continues to be practical, too, saving time, easing stresses, and keeping the baby happy, healthy, and close, for as long as it continues. Experienced mothers would also tell you that the nursing relationship changes as your baby grows. Your older baby won't nurse as often, of course, as he did when he was new. Fewer nursings become more important nursings; quiet points in the day when you connect with each other. Unless you would really prefer to stop, keep on nursing; you'll be glad you did.

HOW TO UNWEAN A BABY

Suppose sometime in the last few weeks you lost your confidence, or your doctor or partner came out strongly against continuing breastfeeding, or you suffered some discomfort, such as mastitis, and you are now giving your baby supplementary formula. There is no reason why you cannot gradually build up your milk production until your baby is entirely breastfed, especially if he is still small—the younger the baby, the more cooperative he is likely to be—and not yet receiving a lot of solid foods. If you don't make the effort to eliminate formula-feeding entirely, your milk supply will almost certainly continue to dwindle until the baby is entirely bottlefed.

Before you begin, take a couple of days to keep track of how many ounces of supplement your baby is actually taking in over twenty-four hours. Write that down, and stick the note on the refrigerator or someplace where you'll see it. Then pick a day when you can count on peace and quiet, nurse the baby as often as possible, and offer her one ounce less of formula per feeding than she has been getting. You may worry that she'll be hungry; you are more likely to discover that she doesn't even seem to miss it.

Wait a day—or two or three—then drop another ounce out of the supplement feedings. Your milk supply will be increasing, meanwhile, especially if you increase the frequency of feedings; giving *more* feedings is more important than giving longer feedings. Nurse the baby several extra times during the twenty-four hours. (Extra feedings at night should be compensated for by an extra nap in the daytime if possible).

After a week, write down how much supplement the baby is still getting; see the difference from where you started? Depending on how much formula your baby was getting at the beginning, over a period of three weeks or more, you should be able to feed the baby all by yourself again. You will know you can trust your body, and that it is making enough milk, because the transition has been made without misery or hunger, and when the bottle was gone, the baby didn't miss it.

One circumstance can upset mothers no end, during a period of rebuilding a milk supply: a growth spurt. When a frequency day—a sudden increase in appetite—occurs during this period, instead of recognizing it for what it is, you're likely to despair and think your production is at fault. Stay calm! Remember, a sudden increase in the baby's needs happens repeatedly to any nursing mother, because the baby is growing. It happens to bottlefed babies, too; we just notice it less when they're on the bottle—and we interpret it differently: We don't say, "Oh no, the baby's hungry again," we say, "Wow, what a wonderful appetite." So take care of yourself; remember the first prescription for a fussy baby is more rest for the mother. Get some rest, nurse a lot, and the supply will keep on growing.

Sometimes a baby who is accustomed to a bottle can be very unpleasant about being asked to nurse when your milk production is still low. He sucks for a moment and then screams and wrenches away. Try squeezing a few drops of milk out so that he will taste it as soon as he latches on; once he is nursing, you can soothe him so that he stays on the breast, by rocking, patting him, and talking or singing to him.

If your baby is far along the road to being weaned to the bottle, and you are nevertheless eager to bring him back to the breast, you might find a nursing supplementer helpful. This is a device designed to speed the process of relactation, or reestablishment of the milk supply; there are several on the market. The device has a container for formula—either a little bottle or a plastic bag—that hangs around your neck; a slender tube can be taped to your breast so that it fits in the baby's mouth as he nurses. Some supplementers drip milk in by gravity; some—the Medela company's SNS, for example—let the milk flow only when the baby actively nurses; that, of course, reinforces the suckling, so that milk production is stimulated even during supplementary feedings. A nursing supplementer can be obtained through any board-certified lactation consultant, who will also coach you in its use; or you can order one through La Leche League or a local lactation consultant.

It is always worth making the effort to reestablish your milk production for a young baby, if only for the pleasure and convenience of being able to nurse him for as many months as he needs you to do so; but it is especially worthwhile if you have a family history of allergy, or if your baby is exposed to colds at a day-care center or babysitter's home.

CHANGES BETWEEN FOUR AND SIX MONTHS

A five-month-old baby has probably settled down to two naps a day. He may sleep ten hours at night, especially if his mother is well rested, so that daytime nursings are ample (with temporary exceptions: See Sleep Changes, page 341). He has learned to anticipate, and he whimpers or calls for meals instead of crying. He is well aware of the difference between you dressed and you undressed, and will lie quietly in your arms while you uncover the breast. However, he will roar with indignation if you answer his whimper by picking him up and then putting him down again before feeding him! This age is probably the peak of the nursing cycle. Soon your baby will be taking more and more nourishment from other sources. Now he is still growing fast, may already have reached twice his birth weight, and may be taking one and a half pints or even a quart of milk from you every day. You find this reflected in your own larger appetite and greater thirst. You may find, too, that some of your physical energy is definitely being given to milk-making. Even though you feel strong and are getting plenty of rest, new or recently resumed physical exercise—such as playing sports or attending an aerobics class—may leave you breathless and drenched with perspiration. If so, build up to strenuous activity slowly over the next few weeks; you will have more stamina when your nursing baby is seven or eight months old.

A baby of five or six months has a characteristic gesture in coming to the breast. Arms are raised and fists are clenched; when he nurses, the baby hugs his mother, one arm on each side of the breast; he may or may not hold on to her clothes. This gesture enables him to home in on the breast almost without help from her, and is especially useful at night; it also helps to keep him in the nursing position even when his mother, carrying him on one arm, gets up to answer the phone or turn down the stove. You can see this gesture in a bottlefeeding baby of the same age who raises his clenched fists up on either side of his head while he drinks, but in his case the utility of this apparently instinctive gesture is lost.

Around five months, a baby may suddenly become extremely efficient at the breast. He hardly gets started before he's all through, and wants to get down and play; and you can't believe he got any milk in that brief time. Actually, the baby nurses so strongly and the milk lets down so well that he may easily nurse both breasts and get a full meal in five minutes or less. Don't interpret this speed as a sign that he is losing interest in the breast. It is still the source of all his nutrition and an important part of his emotional life.

SLEEP CHANGES AT FIVE MONTHS

Five to six months is a very exciting time in a baby's life; she is beginning to creep, to explore, to handle things; every day is full of discoveries. One result is the self-interruption of daytime nursings; the baby sometimes seems almost too busy to nurse, especially if there are older children around. As a consequence, babies at this age sometimes go back to wanting a *lot* of nursing at night; maybe that's the only time when they can relax and really concentrate on being close to Mom.

For a week, or even several weeks, the baby may want to nurse longer or more often at night than she has been doing. If this happens to you, have patience; soon the baby will mature just a little more, and will be able to handle these event-filled days and mealtimes, too; then she will go back to sleeping more soundly. One lactation consultant points out that at any age a sudden increase in nighttime nursing is often a signal that the baby is getting ready for a big developmental milestone. Watch her; within a week or two, chances are that she will do something she's never done before—crawl, sit, or stand, perhaps. When the change has been accomplished, the feeding pattern will revert to normal.

SOLID FOODS

You can tell that a baby who is nearing the six-month mark is ready for solid foods. Her first teeth are coming in and with them an urge to put everything she gets hold of into her mouth (this urge, of course, may begin much earlier). This mouthing and tasting is a baby's way of getting to know the universe. It may soothe her gums, and it also serves to teach her the difference between food and nonfood. By five or six months, a baby can put finger and thumb together and pick up a crust of bread. She can creep about. If the adults of the family sat on the ground and ate with their hands, as our ancestors must have done, this baby would be ready to join right in and help herself. In preliterate societies, adults—men and women both—often share food with creeping and toddling babies, either by scooping up something soft on a fingertip and putting it in the baby's mouth, or by kiss-feeding (passing the baby a little food that has already been partly chewed); the idea may be repugnant to us, but sensible in a world without strained baby food—or spoons.

Doctors usually recommend that you start the baby on mashed bananas and cereal, which are both digestible and tasty. Since your baby is not used to spoons, he may bite down on the spoon or try to spit it out. Put a bit of food on his lips and let him lick it off. He'll catch on quickly, and will soon be leaning forward with his mouth open like a baby bird. You may have received free samples in the mail from baby food companies or your doctor's office may have given you samples it has received from such companies. Since your baby has been thriving on nature's menu alone, you have probably put all the little cans and jars on the shelf; now, when you do try them out, you may find that your baby regards these preparations as pretty insipid, and is much more interested in sitting at the family board and helping himself with his fingers to everything that looks good.

Fine. A baby of six or seven months can manage anything she can mash up with her tongue and gums, and will enjoy scrambled eggs, cottage cheese, ripe avocado, cooked carrot or sweet potato, pieces of soft pear or melon, bread, rice, and so on. One baby's very first solid food was a mouthful of blackberry pie; her face made it clear that this new sensation was a world-class thrill. Babies also like something fairly firm to hold in the hand

and chew on. A cube of cheese will be relished, as well as a hard old heel of bread for trying out those teeth. A rib bone with nothing left on it but the flavor is fun to chew. Some babies are crazy about dill pickles. In any case, don't bother with the packaged teething biscuits; they make a sticky mess and contain a lot of sugar, to start your baby on the road to the dentist. (Stay away from peanuts and foods that contain peanut oils for the first few years of life. The cause of the rapidly escalating rate of peanut allergies among children has not yet been identified, so it is common sense to keep this complex protein out of young children's diets for now.)

The most useful of the prepared baby foods are the meats, which provide the protein and iron your baby is beginning to need. Prepared "dinners" seem to be mostly starch; they are handy for traveling or other emergencies if your baby likes them, but are less nutritious and more expensive than good fresh food from your own table. You can make your own fresh pureed meat, too, by putting a little cooked lamb or chicken in your food processor.

The principles to follow in choosing your baby's foods are the same principles of good nutrition that you follow in feeding the rest of the family. His meals should be high in meats, vegetables, fruits, whole grain bread or cereals, brown rice, beans, and potatoes, and low on sugar, fats, and calories-only foods such as puddings. You can puree just about anything you make for the rest of the family, and share it with your baby. If you have other small children, he can probably eat almost anything they eat with hardly any processing. Both he and your other children will enjoy being together at mealtime.

THE CUP

A baby of five or six months may enjoy drinking water and juice from a cup, or he may refuse it. If you offer regular cow's milk in a cup, chances are your baby won't take it. The breastfed baby's usual reaction to his first cup of milk is to taste it, and then laugh and push it away, as if that were the most ludicrous place to find milk. By nine or ten months, when he can manage a cup more or less by himself, he will take more pleasure in drinking from it. Hand him a cup with a lid and spout and nothing but water in it, or a cup without a lid whenever he's in the bath, for splashy practice sessions.

BITING

About this time, your nursing baby may try out his teeth on you. Usually, he will do this at the end of a meal; so if he shows an inclination to bite, don't let him dawdle, but take him off the breast as soon as he seems to be through. If he does bite, tell him firmly that he may not do so, and take him right off the breast. After one or two tries, he'll get the idea. Occasionally, a baby of six or eight months may bite deliberately if you try to feed him—perhaps because you are planning to go out—when he isn't hungry.

REFUSING A BREAST

Occasionally, a baby will develop a predilection for nursing from one breast but not the other. A baby may reject one breast temporarily because his mother has tried to slip him vitamin drops or medicine while he was nursing on that breast. You can fool the baby into taking the "wrong" breast by holding him under your arm instead of across your lap, so that the breast he has been rejecting is on the same side of his face as the one he likes would normally be. Of course, you could nurse him on one breast only, if you had to.

Sometimes the baby is taking so much solid food, as well as milk in a cup, that he is actually weaning himself without your knowing it. One can, without noticing it, favor one breast for convenience, so that the baby nurses longer and more often on that side. Then the other breast will produce less and involute more rapidly. As the milk supply wanes, it changes, becoming less sweet and more salty; the baby may come to reject the breast because the milk in it really does taste different to him.

FATIGUE

Around five or six months is another vulnerable period similar to that around one month or six weeks, when a great many mothers wean their babies. The reasons are the same: The baby is bigger; the mother is going out more, doing more, and getting too tired. The baby responds by being fussy and wanting to nurse more often, and it seems as if the milk supply is waning. Or the baby is doing well, but the mother feels tired all the time and the convenience and pleasure of nursing no longer seem worthwhile.

Fatigue starts a vicious cycle. It is only when you are tired that dust clusters under the bed or dirty windows or cluttered toys seem unbearable. Perhaps your obligations at your job hang over you, so that you drive yourself to do more and more work just when you most need the rest. Poor nutrition also contributes to fatigue, and the fatigue kills your appetite, so that your nutritional state becomes worse and you lose weight; that, too, makes you feel tired.

VITAMINS AND FATIGUE

Look to your diet. Despite the wide availability of good food in the United States, some women's diets are very poorly balanced; mild vitamin deficiencies are common among pregnant American women. When you are lactating, you need calcium and you need protein. Vegetarians especially need to be very careful not to become protein-deficient. Remember, the baby will do fine if your diet is deficient to a certain degree in any way. *You* are the one whose energy levels and resistance to infection will take a dive. When the baby is over four months old, or when he reaches a weight of twenty pounds or more, your milk production may be at its peak. On a Western diet of refined flours and processed foods, some mothers begin to suffer from deficiencies in the B-complex vitamins. Again, vegetarians are particularly susceptible. One symptom seems to be fatigue. If you wake up in the morning as tired as you were when you went to bed, so tired that you feel like crying at the thought of having to get up at all, you may be suffering from a B-vitamin deficiency. You may be so depleted that replenishing your B vitamins from food sources, such as liver and whole grains, would take quite a while. A natural supplementary source such as fenugreek herb tea or brewer's yeast (both available in health food stores) will give you the rapid boost you need.

Synthetic B-complex vitamin pills will also help, but in our experience they don't seem to be as effective over a long period as is brewer's yeast, which you take by mixing it into milk or juice. Start with a tablespoon a day and work up to three or four; or take natural-source vitamin tablets. Start with a normal day's dose and then double it in a day or so. (Too much, too fast, may give you diarrhea.) You may feel the difference after the very first dose. With a little experimenting, you will be able to tell yourself how much is ideal, and you may benefit from this daily supplement as long as you are nursing.

Tearful exhaustion in the nursing mother is often attributed to poor time management—"Stop trying to do too much!" she is told—or to psychological depression. The role of possible B-complex vitamin deficiency in lactation, which could also be related to thyroid activity, has not been the subject of extensive research, and extra B-complex-rich supplements are not needed by most nursing mothers. When the need is there, however, the supplement's effect can be a blessing, as a previously exhausted mother abruptly cheers up, gets her appetite and her energy back, and finds that her milk supply simultaneously increases from merely adequate to abundant.

HOUSEKEEPING SHORTCUTS

It's not the dirt and dust that get us down, it's the mess and clutter and disorganization in the house. What we need are a few quick ways of producing the appearance of neatness; then we feel calmer about the state of the house, and there is more time and strength left for enjoying partners and babies, working at your "other" job outside the home, or doing a few things for yourself.

Take a few tips from the newspaper columnist Heloise Cruse: When you first get going in the morning, quickly make the bed; then at least something's done. Put the breakfast dishes (all right, and last night's dinner dishes, too) in the sink, and cover them with hot soapy water. That gets them out of sight, and meanwhile the grease and food are soaking loose. Then take a very big paper bag and walk around the living room and bedrooms, putting everything into the bag that needs to be disposed of: crumbs, newspapers, magazines, opened envelopes, toys, and all the other clutter a room acquires in a day. You can put pillows back and gather up toys as you go. Don't put everything away separately; never walk down a hall or up the stairs with just one or two things in your hands. Put things that belong in other rooms in a pile at the door, then take them along when you're going there anyway.

Then take a pad of toilet tissue, wet it with rubbing alcohol, and quickly wipe the bathroom fixtures. Alcohol is a cheap disinfectant, leaves no odor, and makes chrome shine. Then with a broom or carpet sweeper, quickly clean up the middle of the living room and kitchen.

You've worked for about fifteen minutes, and your house is clean and neat-looking. If someone drops in, you won't be embarrassed. If you never get a chance to do another thing all day, you're still ahead because the depressing, overwhelming mess is gone. If you are heading off for the day at your job, you won't have to face a messy house when you return home in the evening; you can relax with your baby and partner instead. Later on, you or your partner can load the dishwasher or just rinse off those dishes—that's about all they need, after all that soaking.

Now start the laundry. Then plan what you're going to have for dinner. That way, there will be no last-minute scramble in the cupboards at six o'clock, only to find out that you don't have some ingredients that you need, or that the dinner you do have available should have been started an hour ago.

To Heloise's advice, we would add: In the late afternoon, take a walk in the sunshine. Then just before the rest of the family comes home, quickly tidy the living room and set the table. Everything is nice and neat. If the table is set, everyone feels optimistic about the chances of getting dinner pretty soon—even if it won't be ready for an hour, or even if your partner or some other member of the household is going to cook it. Then you have time to sit down, nurse the baby, hear the day's news, and relax.

If you have returned from your own job, skip neatening the house and setting the table. Put your things down as soon as you walk in the door, pick up the baby, get something nutritious to eat and drink (a few chunks of cheese and a glass of water), and sit down. Nurse the baby and rest; let your partner set the table and get dinner started. You must attend to the baby and yourself before anything else. If you are a single mother, don't skimp on making yourself a real meal, but see to it after you have rested and nursed the baby.

Shortcut cleaning is more important than all the other housework, such as vacuuming under the beds and washing windows, because that is what soothes your nerves and takes away that feeling of pressure and futility. To make it even easier:

1. Go through every room in the house and throw out or give away everything that you haven't used in a year. (Heloise Cruse suggests that you do this when you're angry; you'll be more ruthless.) That dress you were planning to make over but never will; the waffle iron that always burns the waffles; all the old clothes that no one is wearing (which fill up your closet and drawers and crowd and wrinkle the clothes that you do wear); that ugly chafing dish you don't use; and all that stuff in the kitchen drawer that you might want sometime. Have you wanted it in the past year? No! Then throw it

out. Give it to the Salvation Army; they will be glad to have it. It's much easier to keep half-empty closets and shelves clean and orderly. Do you really use those hand towels? Will you ever mend that old sheet? The fewer linens and clothes and possessions you can get along with, the fewer things you will have to wash and clean and sweep around.

2. Before you acquire something in the way of furniture or interior decorations, stop and think: Will this make my life easier or harder? Will it have to be cleaned or guarded from scratches? As La Leche League leaders suggest, before buying something for the house, ask yourself: Wouldn't I rather have that nice empty corner or bare tabletop?

3. Confine the children's toys to one room. Concentrate on toys that are discarded after use, such as paper dolls, or on activity toys that are sturdy and can be used by several children, instead of clutter toys with a hundred parts for you to pick up. Big baskets or even cardboard boxes are good for keeping toys—and boots and sporting equipment—in one spot and out of sight. Convenience is more important than style. And by all means, give your children the message that their toys are their responsibility. Even a three-year-old can learn to put his own toys away.

4. As La Leche League leaders advise, order before prettiness, convenience before style, and above all, people before things. Sure, it would be great to have the floors waxed all the time, like those on the TV commercials, and to have interiors with that unlived-in look, like the cover of a magazine. But it is far more vital that you get a nap and a walk in the sunshine, and time to nurse

your baby. It is far more vital to do just a little jiffy top cleaning and save your strength and good humor for smiling at your family and listening to what they have to say. Your partner may care about a certain amount of neatness, but most of all wants your good company. Your children need clean clothes and hot food, but most of all they need a cheerful, loving mother. People—including yourself—before things.

BREASTFEEDING AND CREATIVITY

A creative woman, an artist or a scientist, may find that her work flourishes during lactation, or she may be inclined to give up creative work entirely during the months when she is breastfeeding. While loss of interest in one's work can be exasperating, it is only temporary. Psychiatrist Helene Deutsch suggests that breastfeeding can bring its greatest benefits to the woman who is usually immersed in serious creative work. Nine months or more of a happy nursing relationship can provide a rare interlude of peace and satisfaction in a demanding lifetime. In her classic *Psychology of Women*, Deutsch describes women who set their creative work aside to nurse their babies and then returned, reinspired, to their callings.

EMERGENCY SEPARATIONS

What can you do if you are suddenly separated from your nursing baby for a few days? What if one of you has to go to the hospital, or you must make a sudden trip to a dying relative, or keeping your job depends on your attending an out-of-town business meeting?

First, do what you can to prevent the separation. You can take your nursing baby with you, even to a distant funeral, and that will be less trouble than trying to dry up your milk and worrying about the baby while you're away. If you have to go to an out-of-town meeting, perhaps you can hire a nanny when you get there to take care of the baby in your hotel room when you must work; or perhaps you can take a friend or relative with you to babysit—someone you trust, who will actually get pleasure from the trip.

When a nursing mother must be hospitalized, it is sometimes possible to let her baby go with her, if she is in a private room. If the baby is the patient, he needs his mother's milk more than ever. It is the rare hospital today that does not allow parents to be with their hospitalized children twenty-four hours a day; in many cases, this relaxation in rules was first made so that nursing mothers could stay with their babies.

If the separation is unavoidable, pump your milk while you are gone and discard it if you must. The important thing is to keep the supply going until you can be home again. If the separation takes place when the baby is at the stage where he likes mother's milk only from the breast and will not take a bottle, try having him fed with a cup or spoon. In emergencies some nursing mothers have solved the problem by leaving the baby with another nursing mother who was willing, temporarily, to breastfeed two. Babies, of course, can tell the difference; some don't mind and some do. The baby who objects to nursing at the breast of a stranger can sometimes be induced to nurse if his face is covered with a handkerchief so he cannot see the unfamiliar mother's face.

SCHEDULE CHANGES AFTER SIX MONTHS

Your baby may drop the 2:00 a.m. feedings at six months, but chances are he may still want one very early morning feeding, around dawn. Some nursing babies never give up this feeding voluntarily until they are weaned. During the day, the baby of eight months or more will probably eat three meals of solid food with the rest of the family or just before they eat. But he may still want four or five nursings in each twenty-four hours; these feedings still provide a useful excuse for you to get off your feet for a while. Sometimes he'll be through with the breast in five or ten minutes. Sometimes he'll want to linger. When you can give him the time (perhaps after lunch, when both you and he are planning on a nap, or when you first come home from work, or at his bedtime), you can get a good deal of vicarious enjoyment out of letting him nurse for half an hour or more until he nurses himself to sleep.

BEDTIME NURSING

Falling asleep at the breast would certainly appear to be one of life's most satisfying luxuries; just watching your baby as he blissfully relaxes is enough to make you fall asleep yourself. And it certainly makes it easier to put him down for the night without tears or fuss.

Bottlefeeding mothers use the bottle in the same way. However, leaving the bottle in the baby's mouth means that he goes to sleep with the front of his mouth awash in a sugar solution; this situation contributes to the development of cavities when a baby's teeth begin to emerge. Physicians, therefore, are apt to warn bottlefeeding mothers against letting the baby fall asleep on the bottle. On the same basis, they may tell the breastfeeding mother that she should never let the baby fall asleep at the breast. What they often don't realize is that in breastfeeding the nipple is well back in the mouth, not near the teeth where the bottlefeeding baby holds it. Also, breast milk doesn't go on flowing after the baby falls asleep; the breastfed baby does *not* sleep with a mouth full of sugar solution, and you don't have to worry about cavities if you nurse your baby to sleep.

Some physicians also forbid mothers to let the baby fall asleep on the breast because they believe it will cause a sleep disorder; the baby will wake in the night and be unable to fall back asleep on his own without nursing again. This currently popular theory is disputed by many mothers who sense that nursing their babies to sleep helps them to sleep more peacefully than making them learn to fall asleep without the comfort of their mother's arms and breasts. In fact, the security you give your baby now, suggest studies in the field of attachment and developmental psychology, will help him to be more confident and independent when he is older. Depriving him right now would upset both of you. If someone tries to lay down the law to you on this matter, be kind but firm, appreciative of the concern but unmoved. Don't let this misguided hypothesizing interfere with your family life.

Another controversial question is where you will put your baby down to sleep at night. Our culture prizes independence: the earlier, the better. This belief may be at the heart of our insistence that babies should sleep alone in cribs in separate rooms. Many other cultures find this custom bizarre and unnatural, as they keep babies near their mothers at night. There is a story that the Samoan mothers who met Margaret Mead during her anthropologic fieldwork in their islands ask her if, "it was really true the American mother kept their babies in cages at night." While the American Academy of Pediatrics discourages co-sleeping—bringing a baby into the parents' bed at night—nursing mothers find this arrangement to be the most convenient. With your baby beside you, night nursings happen without either of you waking fully; both you and your baby sleep more soundly—and more safely, according to anthropologist James McKenna. director of the Mother-Baby Behavioral Sleep Laboratory at the University of Notre Dame. McKenna has produced a body of evidence that co-sleeping may well protect babies against sudden infant death syndrome, or SIDS. He and his research team measured the physiological differences between solitary and co-sleeping mother-baby pairs. They found that babies who sleep next to their mothers breathe better, sleep more, feed better, and maintain more stable body temperatures. Could it be that a mother's breathing and warmth and breasts help regulate a young baby's immature physiology during deep sleep? McKenna thinks so. It is true that in cultures where co-sleeping is the norm, SIDS is nearly unheard of.

If you don't sleep well with your baby next to you, or you sleep in a waterbed, or you are worried about your partner rolling on the baby (you, however, are very unlikely to, unless you are under the influence of alcohol or drugs), consider setting up a "sidecar" crib next to your bed. A crib designed for this purpose is ideal, but a regular crib can be made into a sidecar crib by dropping down one side and bringing the crib next to your bed. Make sure that there are no gaps, not even a tiny one, between the crib mattress and the adult bed mattress. With this arrangement, rolling over and reaching out for your baby to nurse is easy and peaceful. After nursing, you can put your baby back in his crib, an arm's reach away.

THE PERSISTENT NIGHT FEEDER

By the time a baby is seven or eight months old, he doesn't need a night feeding as a rule, although he may still need a predawn snack. You are now lactating steadily without the stimulation of night feeds. If you feel you would like to give up feeding the baby at night, there are three methods to try. You can let him cry it out, which may be ghastly for everyone; for some babies, an abrupt desertion is very frightening, but for others, this works like a charm.

You can try rocking or singing to him, without feeding him; sometimes company and reassurance are what he really wants, and forty minutes of singing the first night becomes twenty minutes the second, a back rub from cribside the third night, a called-out reassurance the fourth, and peace and quiet from then on. Or you can let the baby's father take over. Amazingly enough, some babies will go right back to sleep because their fathers have told them to.

Don't think that you can have uninterrupted nights by weaning to a bottle. Your baby may give up his midnight snack if it no longer consists of breast milk, but then again he may not. There are plenty of bottlefed babies who go on demanding a bottle in the night well into their second or third year. Several papers in pediatrics journals demonstrate that sleep patterns in infants are individual and utterly unrelated to whether they are breastfed or bottlefed. This does not mean that you must tolerate the behavior of a fifteen-month-old baby who wakes you up for company once an hour all night; you have some rights, too. But some babies just can't bear to give up that last night feeding. If you can't break the habit, resign yourself. Something so terribly important to him isn't worth fighting over. Take a nap in the daytime, if you are able, and try again in a month or two.

CHANGES AT EIGHT MONTHS

By now the reassuring nature of breastfeeding as a sign of love is almost more important to your baby than the fact that it satisfies her hunger. She may want to nurse for comfort, if she bumps her head or has been very frightened. A baby of this age can be very bossy about feedings. When the flow from one breast has slackened, she may fling herself across your lap and indicate that you should make the other available, and pronto. If you are carrying her, and she decides to eat, she may pull at your clothes, wriggle and wrench down to breast level, and all but help herself. Her purposefulness is hilarious, but it can create problems; she is no respecter of privacy and may all too obviously decide to have a snack when you are standing at the supermarket checkout counter, or talking to your minister's wife or your father-in-law. Fortunately, people who are not used to breastfed babies sometimes don't realize what she is doing.

Now that your baby can sit up, and perhaps creep and stand, she likes to nurse sitting up, too, straddling your lap and regarding the world as she eats. She is quite dogmatic about this; you may wonder what's wrong as you try to make her lie down on your arm and nurse, and she wriggles and complains, until you discover she has a change in mind. She may also like to hold on to the breast that she is not drinking from, as if it might go away before she gets to it.

MENSTRUATION AND PREGNANCY

Because you are a successful nursing mother, you are probably finding that your menses continue to be suppressed. You will probably not menstruate until the baby is eight to eighteen months old. Until you have had at least one period, and probably two or three, you are unlikely to conceive again.

Don't count on it, though! People have conceived before that first period; one doctor feels that this can often be traced to a few very busy days, or perhaps an illness of mother or baby that led the mother to nurse less frequently, so that lactation was reduced or suspended "long enough to let an egg slip through." If you do not wish to get pregnant, use a contraceptive. It is not a good idea to take birth control pills—even the mini-pill—as long as you are lactating. Use a barrier contraceptive—such as the sponge, a con-dom, or a diaphragm—together with spermicidal jelly. If you used a diaphragm in the past, you will probably need to be refitted for a new one after pregnancy and labor.

When your periods do resume, they will not affect your milk supply. Someone might tell you that you "can't" nurse on the days when you are menstruating, or that the baby will be fussy on those days, or that the milk will diminish. Not so. In some cases, the taste of the milk does change for a day or two; sugar content goes down and sodium up, temporarily. Sometimes, however, you yourself are irritable during or before your period, and this will be reflected in your baby's behavior; he may be cranky, too, or want to nurse more, for reassurance.

What if you become pregnant while you are still nursing? While it might be a strain on you to nurse all the way through pregnancy, there is no need to come straight home from the obste-trician's office and wean the baby. You can plan on weaning him very gradually over a period of weeks, as described in Chapter 13.

Some mothers never wean when they become pregnant again and thus find themselves, at the end of nine months, with two nursing babies! This event is common enough nowadays to have a name, "tandem nursing." Some mothers find that the taste of the milk changes, becoming "weaning milk"—more salty, less sweet—and the baby loses interest; or their milk supply dwindles to nothing during pregnancy, and the baby weans himself. Some find that their breasts become sensitive in the early pregnancy, and nursing is uncomfortable. Occasionally, a mother complains of pain in the breast while nursing during pregnancy. These dis-comforts are presumably an indication from Mother Nature that nursing should stop, and that the present baby should receive his love and attention in ways other than at the breast.

Nursing during late pregnancy can cause uterine contractions;

in fact, some obstetricians prescribe gentle use of a breast pump to initiate labor when a woman is overdue. If you have any history of miscarriage or premature delivery, you probably should avoid nursing during pregnancy.

CHANGES IN THE LETDOWN REFLEX

After the baby passes the six-month mark and is beginning to get nourishment from sources other than your body, you may find that the letdown reflex no longer operates promptly when he is put to the breast. He may have to suck for fifteen seconds or more before the milk lets down. Gradually, the interval will become longer and longer as your baby grows older and begins to wean himself. This delay in milk flow is reason in itself for some babies to lose interest in the breast, at or around the age of nine months.

CHANGES AT NINE MONTHS

In *A Baby's First Year,* Dr. Benjamin Spock wrote of the bottlefed baby:

> Around nine months of age babies begin to divide into two groups as far as feelings towards the good old bottle are concerned. Of one the mother says: "He's getting bored with it. After a couple of ounces he stops to fool with the nipple and grin at me. He likes milk from the cup." Such a baby seems ready for gradual weaning. Other mothers will say: "She loves her bottle more than ever . . . she usually drains it to the last drop, stroking it and murmuring to it.

She's gotten suspicious of the cup lately." Such a baby seems to be saying, "I'm nowhere near ready to give it up."

Exactly the same things are true of the breastfed baby. Some babies will wean themselves rather abruptly, at or around the age of nine months. You start by giving the baby a cup of milk at breakfast, or perhaps dinner, because you are busy, the baby is too restless to nurse, and it just seems easier. By and by, the baby expects a cup at every meal, and your own milk supply diminishes correspondingly. Without really noticing it, you find he is weaned. He may cling to one favorite feeding, such as early morning, or to a bedtime snack, for a few more weeks—and then, all by himself, he is through with nursing and ready to go on to more grown-up things.

Other babies at the age of nine months don't give up the breast at all. They become even fonder of being cuddled and nursed, and while they may nurse only three or four times in twenty-four hours, those feedings are terribly important to them. Others may come to their mother many times during the day for a quick comfort-nursing. With such a baby, you can plan to continue nursing as long as is convenient for you, and as long as you both enjoy being a happy nursing couple.

The Working Mother:
How Breastfeeding Can Help

If you're returning to work or school after your baby is born, you're not alone. Since 2000, 58 percent of mothers have returned to work before their child's first birthday. In one large sampling of working mothers, 76 percent were back at work before their babies were thirteen weeks old.

The reasons for this vast change in American women's lives are varied. It's the unusual couple, these days, that doesn't need two incomes to make ends meet. Most single mothers have no choice but to work. Many women have their first child after years of education, training, and building a career; they do not wish to relinqiush the work to which they've devoted their adult lives. Whatever your reasons, whatever your job, know that returning to work need not mean an end to breastfeeding. Many mothers have returned to work six to eight weeks after giving birth and have nursed their babies through toddlerhood. With information and the right equipment, you can keep your baby an exclusively breastfed baby, no matter what your job.

While employment outside the home is one of the most common reasons given for weaning, in reality breastfeeding can be one of the working mother's most comforting supports. A working mother's secret torment is that her baby loves her and the day-care provider interchangeably. Never mind that every baby knows exactly who his mother is, and that she is not the babysitter; a working mother may sometimes feel insecure in her place as the center of his world. When nursing mothers have this fear, they can remember that breastfeeding is the one thing they do with their babies that no one else can do. One mother discovered that "it was easier to adjust to being back at work since I didn't feel like I was losing my relationship with my baby." Your nursing baby will reassure you after separations that your bond is as special and close as always. When you see how he wriggles as he hears your voice when you walk in after a day at work, when you feel how his body relaxes against your own, and how he settles down for a long cuddle and satisfying nursing, you'll know that for him you are unique. When you are apart, you'll still feel reassured. The babysitter may be very nice, but you are his mama with the warm breast full of milk. It makes all the difference in the world.

Another huge advantage to breastfeeding if you work is the measure of protection it will give your baby against the illnesses passed around in group day care. Day-care children have an unfortunate tendency to bring home every cold in town. They're simply catching all the bugs in their first three years that children who remain at home usually catch when they begin school. While your baby, breastfed or not, will probably catch a few colds, the protective factors in your milk will help guard him against many serious bacterial infections and secondary complications. Even when you are not exposed to all the germs in your baby's day care, you will be exposed to anything he picks up, produce antibodies in your milk to those pathogens, and increase your baby's immunity to those day care–produced germs.

Cultural obstacles to nursing and working remain, although nursing working mothers have more support socially and legally today than they once did. Not so very long ago, in the 1980s and '90s, nursing mothers fought a battalion of discouraging circumstances, including employers who refused mothers twenty-minute breaks to pump their milk (while breaks for cigarette smokers were considered acceptable), demands that breast milk be pumped in bathroom stalls and not be kept in office refrigerators, embarrassed and amused co-workers, unwilling day-care providers, loss of professional status once one's dedication to motherhood became apparent, and so on. In some industries, companies, and regions of the country, these attitudes are still prevalent.

Nursing mothers persisted, as they tend to do, one woman at a time, in changing the world. They worked with their employers to show them that breastfeeding was not a threat to profits, indeed, that nursing babies have fewer illnesses and therefore their mothers miss fewer days of work. They negotiated gradual returns to work, easing the transition, so that fewer mothers gave up from stress and exhaustion, and employers lost fewer valued employees. Personnel departments have begun to promote breastfeeding-friendly policies. A few states have enacted laws requiring employers to protect the rights of nursing mothers. In 2002, the California Lactation Accommodation Law was passed, requiring employers to provide "a reasonable amount" of break time for women employees to express breast milk and the use of a room other than a toilet stall in which to do so. No longer can a woman be fired for "indecent exposure" if she expresses milk or nurses her baby at her workplace. She may, however, still be discriminated against in subtle or overt ways, depending on the environment in which she works. We are still changing the world.

THE SCHEDULE

Many working mothers, breastfeeding or not, adopt a totalitarian daily schedule. From the moment the baby wakes at his customary hour, whether it is 7:00, 6:00, or 5:00 a.m., the mother's day belongs to the schedule. If she has not showered by 6:15, then her blouse is not ironed by 6:30, and the baby is not fed, dressed, and ready to go to the sitter's by 7:00. In other words, if one stage of the morning's preparations is delayed, the entire schedule falls to pieces. Not only will that mother be late to work, but she will be flustered, will perhaps snap at her partner, and will feel once more that she has not kept her balance atop the tightrope that stretches between motherhood and the workplace.

Breastfeeding can make a working mother's grueling schedule easier. An early morning nursing is a peaceful start to the day. Mother and baby can say a long hello to each other while the rest of the household sleeps. Once done, the baby, satiated and secure, will be far more willing to entertain himself with a few toys while his mother puts the morning events in motion, and she will do so with the calmness that always follows a satisfying nursing. Some working mothers take the baby to bed with them at night to have as much time together—as much skin-to-skin contact and nursing—as possible. If you would prefer not to have the baby in bed with you all night, take him in when he first wakes at 4:00 or 5:00 a.m. Have a long, quiet nursing, lying down while your partner sleeps on. You may all doze off again for another hour or two, your milk supply boosted, and your contact with the baby extended. And you won't have to squeeze a nursing into the harried morning routine.

Nursing can help you prioritize the way you spend your time with your baby. When a mother returns home from a long day

at work, she may see only the dishes still in the sink, the un-
made beds, and the laundry to be done. Tired and anxious to
keep the house in order, she may feel she can't visit with her
baby until the house is neat and dinner started. If she hurries to
get the worst of the mess out of the way, precious time with the
baby is lost. The baby probably is tired, too, and would like
nothing more than a long, quiet cuddle. If his mother forgets
the housework for an hour and nurses him, both will be refreshed. The dinner preparations will seem less intimidating,
the laundry less urgent. It will suddenly be difficult to remember
what was so vexing at the office that day. Some mothers find
that a peaceful nursing—and the accompanying flood of
hormones—replaces the glass of wine they used to relax with at
the end of the day.

Most working mothers never feel comfortable just sitting;
there's always something that needs to be done. But when you're
nursing, the baby gives you a reason to do just that. You don't
have to get the chores out of the way to earn time with the baby.
Breastfeeding will help you remember that what the baby needs
most of all is you.

GUILT

Along with her grueling schedule, guilt may be the working
mother's most difficult hurdle. The stress of meeting the demands of being a mother, partner, employee or employer, house-
keeper, and individual can lower many a woman's self-esteem.
She may feel at times that she is not fully succeeding in any of
her roles. The satisfaction of successfully breastfeeding can restore her confidence and counteract the working-mother blues.
The breastfeeding working mother knows that in the things

that really matter, she is doing a bang-up job. (And remember that guilt can plague any parent, even mothers who stay at home.)

THE SECOND NEWBORN PERIOD

The most important preparation you can make before returning to your job may be in your attitude and expectations. Too often a woman's return to work marks in her and her family's minds the end of her recovery period. Now that her maternity leave is over, everyone assumes that life can get back to normal. Nothing could be further from the truth.

Instead, your emotion, energy, and vulnerability during the first two or three weeks back at work are likely to mimic the feelings you experienced in the first two or three weeks after your baby was born. As in the early postpartum days, returning to work is a tremendous, exhausting transition as you fuse your newly acquired identity as a mother with your established identity as a working woman. You and your baby will need to settle into a new schedule of nursing and sleeping, just as in the early days, that accommodates your working hours and your day-care schedule. Your milk supply may take a few days to catch up and you may feel full of milk when not with your baby, and less full when you are together at times, until your body catches on to your new schedule. You need to sleep and rest whenever you are not at work and not feeding and holding your baby, just as you did in the early days. You need to eat nutritiously (cooking meals in advance for the freezer) and drink lots of fluids to protect your strength and your health. You may feel your confidence falter briefly, and must patiently rebuild your trust in your abilities to manage everything, just as you learned in the early weeks that you could care for your new baby. Family and friends need to understand all of this, too, as their help and understanding will get you through these weeks of transition. You can call on the lactation consultant or La Leche League leader who first helped you establish breastfeeding, to help you learn the techniques of expressing and storing milk. Respect the demands of the early weeks of returning to work, and you will find them far less a trauma than does the mother who sallies back into her job, expecting everything to be as it once was. (For an in-depth exploration of the many-layered experience of nursing and working, read *Working Mother, Nursing Mother: The Essential Guide to Breastfeeding and Staying Close to Your Baby After You Return to Work*; see Resources.)

GETTING READY TO GO
BACK TO WORK: A TIMETABLE

While sixteen weeks of maternity leave would be an ideal minimum, most women find eight to twelve weeks is all their employers will allow. (And if they are paid during those weeks, they are in the minority. As of this writing, just 23 percent of U.S. businesses offer paid family leave. The federal Family and Medical Leave Act requires businesses of fifty employees or more to offer workers twelve weeks of unpaid leave; paid leave is therefore a voluntary benefit for U.S. companies.) If you must return in eight weeks, or even six weeks, don't despair. You can still nurse your baby if you plan carefully.

In the First Four Weeks After Birth, your first priority is to establish your milk supply and become a nursing couple with your baby. Nurse whenever the baby wants to nurse. Don't allow yourself to worry, and don't think about work. Enjoy your baby. Frequent, long, and relaxed nursings will give you the bountiful milk supply you need. If you own a breast pump already, don't bother practicing on it, unless you are doing so to increase your milk supply.

After the Fourth Week, you can begin to learn to pump or manually express your milk and freeze the milk you pump. (Follow Gerry Anne's Recipe for Pumping Success on page 373.) Pumping and expressing are learned skills and require practice, and you will need a couple of weeks to get the hang of them.

At Six to Eight Weeks, have your partner or someone other than yourself give the baby a bottle of expressed breast milk. (You may need to go for a walk outside your house during this first feeding off the breast so that your baby does not see or hear you or even catch your scent.) Before six to eight weeks, the baby is still learning how to nurse from your breasts. Nursing from a rubber nipple requires a completely different sucking motion and can confuse some newborns so that they have difficulty switching back to a breast. Later, your baby may be set in his ways and may not accept a bottle; he can practice without difficulty in the second month.

At Around Ten to Twelve Weeks (or one to two weeks before you return to work), introduce the day-care provider and the baby in your own home, if possible. Spend some time with the provider and the baby so that the provider sees how you care for the baby. Then, when he isn't hungry, leave them together in your home or at the sitter's home for short periods, building to several hours at a time. Increase to the amount of time that you will be away when you are working. Make sure that your care provider understands the importance of breastfeeding to you, and how it will make her life easier as well in that your baby is likely to be content, healthy, and have less offensive stools than a formula-fed baby. (One mother took her sitter to La Leche League meetings so she could share the mother's enthusiasm for breastfeeding.) Teach her how to thaw your stored breast milk (see Storing Your Milk, page 379) and ask her not to feed the baby just before you are due to arrive at home or at the sitter's home or the day-care center.

When You First Return to Work, cancel all activities except working and being with your baby. (Consider returning to work on a Friday. Knowing the weekend is ahead may help you ease into the separation.) Forget the housework; let your partner do it, hire a cleaning service, or don't do it at all. Save laundry and grocery shopping for the weekends. Go to bed early. Eat hearty, nutritious meals. Drink plenty of fluids—don't pass a water fountain at work without drinking from it, keep a bottle of water or juice nearby as you work, and don't sit down to nurse without something to drink beside you. On weekends you can cook the meals for the coming week. It helps to double-batch every meal you make, and freeze leftovers to use during the week.

IF YOU RETURN TO WORK BEFORE EIGHT WEEKS

If you have to go back to work before your baby is two months old, and possibly before breastfeeding is well established, the most straightforward solution is to take the baby with you. When a baby is still small enough to be tucked into a front pack or sling, he is quite portable and content, as long as you are near. It is less revolutionary than it once was for a workplace to allow a new mother to bring her baby to work and keep a portable crib by her desk; often the whole staff enjoys the baby's company. Some working mothers—television and movie performers, for example—bring baby and sitter onto the set with them and nurse during breaks. A few farsighted corporations have their own built-in day-care area, where mothers and fathers can enjoy a lunchtime break with the baby, and where at least a midday nursing can be managed.

PUMPING AND EXPRESSING MILK

If you cannot bring your baby to work with you, you will need to pump your milk every two to three hours until he is five or six months old, and then every three to five hours until he is eight or nine months old. After that point, you may be able to call an end to pumping, while continuing to nurse during the early morning, evening, and sometimes still at night. Some babies of working mothers develop a pattern called "reverse-cycle feeding" earlier than that, which enables a mother to pump very little during the day, and nurse mostly at night (see pages 382–83). Learn to pump (and save the milk you do pump) during the final four weeks of your maternity leave. (See Gerry Anne's recipe for pumping success, page 373.)

Pumps made today will allow you to maintain your milk supply and obtain eight to sixteen ounces of fresh milk every day, more than enough for most babies during an average workday. The essential job of a pump is to mimic the speed and pressure of your baby's suck and swallow, about sixty cycles per minute. The "hospital-grade" electric pumps achieve this. More expensive than other pumps, they are widely available for a nominal rental fee from lactation consultants, La Leche League leaders, hospital breastfeeding clinics, and pharmacies. If you work full time, it is worth the effort to locate and rent one of these high-quality pumps. If you work part time and need to pump only once a day or occasionally, consider purchasing a portable pump, the Medela Pump-in-Style, for example, that comes in a discreet black brief-caselike carrying case with an insulated pocket for carrying bottles of milk. These portable pumps don't quite match your baby suck-for-suck and swallow-for-swallow, but do a good enough job for brief separations.

For the very occasional need to pump, you may wish to throw a hand pump in your bag. While it takes more practice to learn the knack of using them, their convenience can't be beat. If you plan to use a manual pump, look for the cylinder variety or the piston style, rather than a bicycle-horn pump. Bicycle-horn

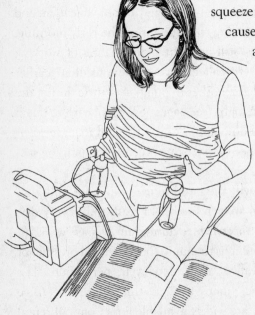

pumps, with a rubber bulb you squeeze to create suction, can cause serious nipple damage and are generally ineffective anyway. Cylinder pumps can create a powerful suction as well, but you can control its strength.

Figure 11.1 Electric pumps enable you to pump both breasts simultaneously while reading or talking on the phone.

GERRY ANNE'S RECIPE FOR PUMPING SUCCESS
(from Gerry Ann Dubis, La Leche League leader)

Before beginning learning to use your pump and saving milk in preparation for your return to work, it is important to understand two things:

Morning pumpings will yield the most milk, whether you're pumping at home or work.

The amount of milk yielded when you pump regularly during the day will decline as the day goes on. This is normal for most women.

Begin to pump this way:

1. Nurse the baby well on one side between 5:00 a.m. and 8:00 a.m. Pump the other side for approximately 10 minutes. Then nurse the baby on the pumped side to further drain the breast.
2. Refrigerate or freeze the milk.
3. Later in the morning, about one and half hours after a feeding or during the baby's nap, pump both breasts.
4. Chill this milk, add it to the milk already refrigerated, and then freeze the container. If you froze the milk you collected earlier, freeze this portion separately, or chill it before adding it to the frozen milk. (Do not add warm milk to chilled or frozen milk.)
5. You have finished pumping for the day. For the rest of the day, just take care of yourself and your baby.

Assuming you collect three to four ounces of milk per day, pumping twice a day for three weeks will put sixty-three to eighty-four ounces of milk in your freezer before you return to work. With practice, you may soon be able to pump as much as eight ounces a day. At that rate, in three weeks you can collect 164 ounces! When you return to work, this frozen stash will serve as your backup supply for the next six months, as the fresh milk you pump each day can be dropped off at your day-care providers' to be saved for your baby's meals on the following day. The frozen milk you've stored is ready in case your baby has an extrahungry day or if you work a longer day than usual or want to go out for an evening.

USING AN ELECTRIC PUMP

Electric pumps come with manufacturer's instructions; pay careful attention to the cleaning process and to the level of suction, which should never be allowed to become uncomfortable. As with any pump, the key to success is learning to let down your milk in response to the sensation of the pump as readily as you do when your baby is at the breast. Choose a pump with a double-pumping capability, so that you may pump both breasts simultaneously. The lactation consultant or other professional from whom you rent the pump will walk you through the steps of setting up, using, and cleaning the pump. See Pumping at Work (page 377) for more information on pumping in the work setting.

HOW TO USE A MANUAL PUMP

Some electric pumps can be converted to a manual pump. To use a manual pump, follow the manufacturer's instructions about assembly and cleaning. Fit the pump over one breast; hold the pump from below so that you pull the plunger out with your palm facing upward; that way your wrist will flex forward. If you hold the pump from above, you will bend your wrist backward on each stroke; this may eventually strain your arm.

Begin pumping, pulling the plunger slowly away from you to create suction, then slide it toward you so the suction ceases. When the letdown action occurs, some instructions tell you to hold the suction of the pump on your breast, rather than continue to pump; however, that is not what your baby does: Your baby sucks and swallows, about once a second, releasing suction with every swallow. If you develop the same rhythm of suction and release with the pump, your breasts will respond well and you will protect yourself from soreness.

Because letdown happens simultaneously in both breasts, once you have learned to pump, you may want to collect the milk that is dripping from the other breast while you are pumping. This is easily done by holding a cup or baby bottle over the free nipple. By the time you move to the second breast, your first letdown may have subsided, but the breast will respond to the stimulation again. You may find that, with practice, you can let down your milk repeatedly in a single pumping session.

The first few times you pump, the whole process may seem clumsy and awkward. Be patient—it gets easier. While you are still learning to pump, be careful that you don't pump so frequently or with such strong suction that your nipples become sore. If you have a spontaneous letdown, grab your pump and practice while the milk is flowing, thereby reducing the chance of making your nipples sore.

Allow your letdown reflex to do the work. Experiment with positions and tricks to help you let down as you pump. Strive to have your letdown reflex as conditioned to the pump as it is to your baby. (Don't worry, you will not interfere with that conditioning; any response can be conditioned to several stimuli, just as we stop the car out of habit when we see a red traffic light, but also when we see a sign that says "Stop.") You may be able to get your letdown started with a couple of pumping actions. If you then use a pump-and-release rhythm, mimicking your baby's nursing rhythm, the milk will spray freely into the pump almost by itself. Mothers who learn this technique do not find pumping so tiresome.

When you've learned to let down as you pump, you may well be producing more milk than the pump cylinder can hold. Also, if the pump cylinder starts to become full while you are pumping, you may want to empty it into a bottle; when there is less air space in the pump, suction is reduced and efficiency goes down. Put one or two plastic nurser bags, supported within nurser bottles, in front of you. Each time you've filled the pump's cylinder with two to three ounces of milk, empty it into the bags. That will also reduce the chance that you might accidentally spill the collected milk as you pump. When you have done expressing your milk, simply extract the plastic bags from the bottles, close them with a twist tie, date them, and put them in the refrigerator or freezer. New bags produced especially for storing pumped milk may make the process even easier.

HOW TO EXPRESS YOUR MILK MANUALLY

Expressing your milk by hand is truly an art, and mastering it may save you the cost and inconveniences of a pump. Even if you rely on the pump, it is always useful to know how to express your milk by hand in case you are ever caught away from home longer than you planned, and without the pump. To express your milk manually, begin with a light, tickling massage to stimulate the letdown reflex. Place your thumb on top of your breast and your first two fingers below your breast. Both your thumb and your fingers should be about an inch behind your nipples so that they are positioned over the milk ducts (see Chapter 2). Then roll your thumb and fingers outward so that the milk in the ducts flows ahead of them.

Achieving letdown as you express is essential to collecting more than an ounce or two. When the milk lets down, rotate your hand around the breast. Repeat this motion until you have drained the ducts or until your letdown has subsided. A rolling motion, rather than a squeezing, pulling, or sliding, will help you avoid bruises or skin burns. Express milk from the second breast and then repeat both breasts. An excellent illustrated summary of this technique can be ordered from La Leche League.

Don't be discouraged if you obtain no more than a few drops the first few times you try manual expression. Practice when the baby naps and your breasts are brimming. Practice when you have a spontaneous letdown (once in the morning—when your letdown reflex is strongest—should be enough in the beginning). Practice early in the morning or during naptime before the baby wakes. Don't worry that you are "using up" your milk before the baby nurses; if you express milk regularly, your milk supply will adjust to the increased need. In addition, your baby is better at stimulating your breasts than the most skilled manual expression or pumping and will be able to draw out milk you have not.

PUMPING AT WORK

More and more workplaces provide a lactation room for nursing mothers—a private room with chairs, electric breast pump, sink, and refrigerator. These enlightened employers understand that supporting nursing mothers makes good sense in business as well as human terms. At CIGNA, the huge insurance and benefits corporation, more than 1,000 women at most of the 250 offices nationwide have participated in a program that encourages them to breastfeed for as long as they can. Recognizing that women make up about 75 percent of CIGNA's 41,000-member workforce, the director of their Working Well program states, "We recognize that, for many women, continuing to breastfeed when they return to work has been an obstacle." CIGNA recognized that "if babies are healthier, the mothers will be healthier and will have less absenteeism. It makes sense from a health and productivity standpoint." If your employer needs convincing that supporting your effort to breastfeed is a smart choice, see the Appendix for a sample letter that explains why.

Meanwhile, if your workplace does not provide a dedicated lactation station, an office with the door closed, a first-aid room, or a women's lounge will do in a pinch. (Don't settle for a bathroom stall. If this is the only choice offered to you, explain to your boss or human resources department that breast milk cannot be equated with other bodily fluids. It is not dirty. You are preparing your baby's meals, and do not want to do so in a toilet.) One mother discovered a locked supply closet to which she obtained the key; when she was ready to pump, she locked herself in, taped up a picture of her baby, and pumped undisturbed.

Set up a routine for pumping; it will calm your mind and help condition your letdown reflex. Wash your hands and arrange your pump, a storage bottle, and a picture of your baby in front of you. Think about your baby and about nursing him. (Take along a sleeper the baby has worn. Your baby's scent can be a powerful letdown stimulator.) Breathe deeply. Lightly stroke your breasts with your fingertips. When you are relaxed and ready, fit the pump to a breast and let the milk flow.

HOW MUCH WILL YOU PUMP?

In time, after three to four weeks, you may find yourself pumping eight to ten, even twelve ounces a day. One mother found that by the time her baby was five months old, she could easily get eighteen ounces! Many mothers, however, never pump more than six ounces. Others find they can manage a great deal one day and very little the next. Regardless of how much milk you can pump, it will benefit your baby and your milk supply. Continuing to stimulate your breasts during separations from your baby, whether you save the milk or not, will maintain production and help you nurse for a longer time. Pumping will also keep you from getting uncomfortably full while away from the baby, which makes you more likely to leak at inopportune times.

STORING YOUR MILK

Breast milk is a remarkably sturdy fluid. Fresh breast milk contains elements that keep bacteria from growing in it for several hours after it's been expressed. (Formula, in comparison, is an unstable substance that spoils quickly.) However, because you will be giving your breast milk to your baby, always chill it and, if you freeze it, thaw it with care.

Breast milk should be stored in sterile plastic nurser bags, baby bottles, or small, sterilized plastic containers. (Glass containers are not recommended because they are bulky and breakable, and because fat particles in the milk and the nutrients they hold tend to cling to the glass.) Refrigerated breast milk must be used within forty-eight hours. If frozen in the freezer compartment of a refrigerator, breast milk can be kept two to four weeks. If kept in a separate freezer at 0 degrees F, it can be kept six months or more. Once thawed, breast milk should not be refrozen.

Freeze milk in small quantities so that if the baby doesn't drink a lot at a feeding, none is wasted. Breast milk is much more fully utilized by the baby than is formula, so your baby will take fewer ounces of your milk than an artificially fed baby would take from a bottle. (Be certain to explain this difference to your day-care provider, especially if she is caring for a formula-fed baby at the same time as your breastfed baby.) Try to estimate how much your baby may take at each feeding; a very young baby may not want more than two to three ounces at a time, a three- to six-month-old may take four to six ounces or more. Remember that the milk will expand as it freezes, so leave some room in the containers. Date the containers, and use them in the order in which they were frozen. To add milk to already frozen batches, cool it in the refrigerator first, then pour it on top of the frozen milk.

To thaw breast milk, run cool tap water over the plastic bag of frozen milk. Very gradually, raise the temperature of the tap water until it is warm, but not hot. When the milk is thawed, insert the plastic bag in a nurser bottle. If you wish to heat the milk after it has been thawed, put the bottle in a pan of warm water on the stove and heat the water, and the milk, very slowly until it is just warm, no hotter than your own body temperature. Thawing milk over direct heat on the stove, however, will heat it too quickly and alter its valuable elements. Never use a microwave oven to heat breast milk; it heats too hot and will eliminate many of the immune factors in the milk, as well as the helpful enzymes and the vitamin C. In addition, milk heated in a microwave will be hotter at its core than at the surface; it can feel just warm to you but be dangerously hot for your baby.

Many companies keep a small refrigerator for their employees' use. Put the bottles of milk in a paper bag and no one will know it's not your lunch. If there is no refrigerator, bring a small ice chest for your milk. If you work far from your home, or if the weather is hot, keep your milk cool or frozen the whole way home—although breast milk, with its living antibacterial cells, can safely go unrefrigerated longer than can cow's milk (see Chapter 3, pages 66–67). There are also insulated bags with shoulder straps on the market, made just for transporting breast milk (see Resources).

Pumping and storing milk at work may raise a few eyebrows, but not nearly so many as you might fear. One mother found that her colleagues reacted with fascination. "They wanted to see the milk, asked if it hurt to pump, and wanted to examine the pump," she said. If someone does react negatively, and lets you know it, brush it off the way you would any intrusion into your private life. You have chosen to do this for your baby and yourself; no one else's opinion matters. It is more than likely that your proud example will enlighten your co-workers and encourage other working mothers to breastfeed, too.

THE WORKING MOTHER'S NURSING SCHEDULE

A typical working mother's day begins when the baby wakes. If your baby is an early riser, nurse him in bed before your partner or other children are awake. If your baby sleeps a little later, express a bottle of milk before the first morning feeding and save it for the baby's lunch. Nurse once more when the baby wakes, just before you leave for work, or at the sitter's house. Then go to work.

At work, if you are free to take a break when you wish, pump your breasts once in the morning and again in midafternoon. Once you are comfortable pumping, you may be able to get eight or more ounces in twenty minutes. In the afternoon, you may find you get half that much, but at the end of the day, you may well have ten to twelve ounces to give to your day-care provider for the next day. If you are able to pump only during your lunch hour, pump a little longer; increasing your demand will increase your supply. Or try to arrange to have twenty-minute breaks in the morning and afternoon in exchange for a shorter lunch hour. Try to pump at the same times each day so that your letdown reflex and peak production periods can become conditioned to those time intervals. Store the milk in a refrigerator at work or in a thermal container.

Nurse again as soon as you get home or at the day-care provider's. If your baby is not being cared for in your home, let the provider know in advance that you want to nurse him for fifteen to thirty minutes as soon as you are reunited. Pay for this extra time if necessary. Many working mothers find this particular nursing creates a crucial sense of being reconnected with their baby. Or if your baby stays at home during the day, lie down in a dark room, with the bare baby against bare you, and rest and nurse; the skin contact is calming for both of you. Nurse again before the baby goes to bed.

Many mothers nurse several times in the evening and once again at night. Some mothers find a night nursing to be the most peaceful and pleasant of all. If you and the baby are just barely awake and shortly go back to sleep, a 2:00 a.m. nursing will not tire you. Keeping the baby near you at night in these early months will make these night nursings even less tiring.

All in all, try to fit in four to five nursing sessions from the end of one working day to the beginning of the next, in addition to your pumping sessions. On weekends, nursing during the day as well as at night will build your supply for the coming week. This amount of nursing will keep your milk production up for as long as you and the baby wish to keep nursing.

TIME-SHIFTING: HOW BABIES FIT THEMSELVES INTO YOUR SCHEDULE

A frequently seen phenomenon of babies with working mothers is the reversal of their waking and sleeping patterns. In studying working mothers and their babies, Irene Frederick, MD, and Kathleen Auerbach, PhD, have found that a baby will sleep for longer periods during his mother's absence and be wakeful when she is present. This adaptation may protect the breastfeeding relationship, ensuring that mother and baby will nurse when they are together. You may find that your nursing baby stays awake longer in the evenings and takes longer naps during the day than the baby of your friend who stays at home. Surely, this time-shifting, or "reverse-cycle feeding," is the highest compliment a baby can give his working mother.

In some cases, mother and baby can get on the same schedule so effectively that by three or four months of age, the baby sleeps while the mother is away: The baby receives no bottles, and the mother doesn't pump her milk either, and yet the baby is fully breastfed and gaining well. Enough nursings are fitted into the hours they have together to maintain lactation and ensure sufficient calorie intake for the baby.

SUPPLEMENTING WITH FORMULA

If you have to return to work while your baby is under five or six months old, and you really can't bear to pump or you haven't found a pump that works well, you will probably be able to maintain a milk supply with frequent nursing at night and on the weekends, letting the baby have formula during the weekdays. Do this cautiously. It can be deleterious to your milk supply, especially in the first months, and it reduces the protective benefits that breast milk has for your baby, as well as the beneficial hormonal effects on you.

Some mothers set a goal of pumping until their babies are six months old, and only then allow the babysitter to use formula or introduce solid food. While one study suggests that mothers who pump their breasts to compensate for missed feedings are more likely to nurse for a longer period than those who do not, many mothers find a combination of formula while separated from the baby and nursing while together to be the best solution for them, especially after the baby is several months old. If you do not plan to save your breast milk and will supplement with formula for one to two feedings during the day, you will probably still have to express or pump a little milk at work in the first few weeks, to relieve discomfort and minimize leakage. Pump or express just enough to be comfortable. Pumping more than you need to for comfort will cause your breasts to continue to produce extra quantities during your working hours. Let your baby nurse liberally, meanwhile, and your milk-production schedule should gradually coincide with your working schedule.

INTRODUCING A BOTTLE

Wait until your baby is six to eight weeks old to introduce a bottle of expressed breast milk. Start any earlier and you may be tampering with your milk supply and interfering with your baby's suckling skills. Six- to eight-week-old babies, experienced nursers that they are, may be less confused when asked to alternate between two different milk sources—their mother's breast and a plastic-and-rubber substitute. Later on, at three and four months, their preferences may be firmly set, and they might refuse any substitution. Lactation consultants consider the eight- to twelve-week period to be the best "window of opportunity" for introducing the bottle. Some babies will take a bottle in the first five or six months and begin refusing it later; by then, they may be very happy with a cup or spoon to sip from.

A week or two before you return to work, have your partner or someone other than yourself give the baby a bottle once or twice every few days. Introduce the bottle somewhere different from the place where you usually nurse. Leave the room; some babies will refuse the bottle as long as they know their mother is near. Experiment with different types of rubber teats. Many babies will gladly accept a bottle, but are picky about the kind of nipple used. If one is rejected, try another type.

Babies' reactions to bottles vary. Some babies will take a bottle, even from their mothers, as happily as they'll breastfeed. One mother said, "I was sure he wouldn't take the bottle from me. Ha! He nuzzled into my chest and acted just as he did when he nursed. He caressed his hair and stretched his legs and happily drank." Or it might take the baby a minute to discover that it's his beloved breast milk in there. Said another mother, "At first, he played with the bottle's nipple and made funny faces at the taste and at the texture of the nipple, but once he tasted the breast milk, he drank almost three ounces."

A few babies will refuse a bottle no matter when or how you introduce it. One mother found that her baby, upon her return to work, would not take a bottle from anyone. She said, "He took it only a couple of times when hunger won out. We eventually gave up trying, and he soon drank from a cup anyway." Occasionally, a baby will drink only from a cup with a spout, rather than accept any substitute for his mother's breast. Some babies refuse a bottle altogether. If you have one of these determined souls, don't worry. Even a very young baby can be fed with a cup rather than a bottle, and "soft cups" made just for this purpose are now available (see Resources). Most babies younger than three months, however, will come around with the gentle persuasion of your partner, the babysitter, and their appetite.

LEAKING

This is not the time for silk designer suits. Leaking is a sign of a terrific letdown reflex, but it's also an inconvenience: One mother's letdown seemed to be triggered by the slight adrenaline surge she felt just before speaking up at business meetings. Cotton pads in your bra will help keep your blouses dry and are available at maternity clothing shops. Putting pressure directly on your nipples with the heel of your hand will stop the flow. To be discreet, cross your arms in front of your chest and press against your nipples with the backs of your hands. Or press against the breast with your upper arm while you touch your hair or an earring. Only another nursing mother will know what you are really doing. As soon as you have a chance, pump to relieve the fullness and to capture the overflow of milk. Spontaneous leaking should disappear as your letdown reflex becomes fully conditioned to responding only to the baby and the pump.

COPING WITH FATIGUE AND STRESS

The fatigue and stress of working full time while your baby is very young can be overwhelming. One mother describes her exhaustion: "I try to get to bed by 10:00 or 10:30 p.m. to counteract fatigue, but sometimes there is so much to do and never any time just for me. Also, there was a period of several months when the baby got up in the night. Those times were very difficult. Sometimes, after I had nursed him back to sleep, I'd lie awake worrying about how tired I'd be the next day. A few times, I was so exhausted I took a long lunch and went home to sleep.

"When my baby was about nine months old, I had a week

when my husband was gone most of the time, and the baby was waking up in the night. I was incredibly stressed, crying when anyone asked me how I was, tired, and feeling very sorry for myself. I talked about my feelings with anyone and everyone, preferably other working mothers. I wanted to know how they managed. I discovered that everyone gets exhausted and stressed and doubts her ability. I also learned that I needed ongoing support from women in situations similar to mine and that I needed to make time for myself."

Fatigue and stress overwhelm nearly every working mother at some point, and not just those who are breastfeeding. Because working mothers have no time "just to talk," they are astonished at the difficulty of combining motherhood and work, and believe that they alone find it so hard. No working mother has time for what she needs most of all—the support of other mothers whose circumstances are the same.

There may be a La Leche League group of working nursing mothers near you that meets in the evenings or on weekends. If not, or if organized groups don't appeal to you, you might find another breastfeeding working mother you can call when you have a question or need encouragement through a rough spot. A lactation consultant is always available by phone. Women at work with whom you've had only a professional relationship in the past may turn into your most valued supports, even if you only have time to chat as you pass each other in the ladies' room.

THE HELPFUL MATE

Your partner can be a deciding factor in your ability to continue working. If he carries at least 50 percent of the household and child-care duties, you are already a long way toward meeting the challenge of working and mothering. Unfortunately, many partners don't comprehend what the full load of caring for a house and children entails. They may support your choice to work and say they'll help out, but may not know how or may not really comprehend what that means.

Even when your partner intends to help and tries to help, he may not be doing things the way you would. Your partner's idea of an adequate meal or a clean room may differ from yours. The constant inadequacy of the help can be infuriating. Expressing your frustration, however, may lead your partner to feel that there is no point in offering to do things, because you always get mad and tell him he's done it wrong, anyway.

One way out of this is to learn to accept what your partner finds adequate, at least for now. So what if the laundry is left in the dryer and it all gets wrinkled. So what if "washing the dishes" doesn't include putting the leftover food away, wiping the counters, and scrubbing the pots and pans. You don't have to learn to tolerate disaster—like the working mother who came home to find her husband and two-year-old son throwing peanut butter at the walls for the dog to lick off—but you can be a bit broadminded. After all, you may not be perfect at jobs your partner takes seriously. One couple have been married for ten years and yet she never remembers to save the gas receipts or write down the car mileage, information he keeps meticulously; another woman reflects that she still can't see why her husband was so upset when he found her stirring a can of paint with a screwdriver.

To keep your peace of mind, you can settle for what your partner does do. You can talk about the most important jobs; and you can also gradually teach your jobs, with attention and thanks, rather than just expecting your partner to know them simply because you've done them a million times.

Another step toward fair partnership is to make a list of every single chore that absolutely has to be done regularly, from picking up the dry cleaning to scrubbing the bathtub. Remember to list nursing the baby as your most important job. Perhaps cooking dinner can be your partner's most important job. There's no need to be inflexible about who does which job, but refer to the list from time to time to see how much is actually being taken on by each partner.

Real partnership comes with sharing what Jeanne Stanton, author of *Being All Things*, calls the "psychological burden." She writes, "Someone has to think about what the family will have for dinner, not just who will cook it and who will clean it up." She advises dividing jobs by project rather than task. "Don't say, 'You cook, I'll clean up.' Instead say, 'You take care of dinner Wednesday night.' That means planning the menu, doing the shopping, cooking, clearing the table, and cleaning up. Then, for one day of the week at least, a piece of both the physical and the psychological burden is set aside." She also suggests giving your partner those jobs he is most likely to do well, such as driving to do errands and shopping or "other jobs that require more physical strength than skill, like scrubbing the kitchen floor and cleaning the bathroom."

The third critical element to managing working and motherhood, along with support from other working mothers and from your partner, is time to yourself. It may seem impossible on some days, but just a hot bath or a walk around the block can make you feel renewed. Some mothers find that extra B-complex vitamins in their diets really make a difference. Get all the rest you can, any way you can. Lie down on the couch to nurse or to play with your older children, take the commuter train to work and sleep on the way instead of driving, shut your office door and nap during your lunch hour. And view each nursing as a small but intense vacation from the world, a moment when you and your baby exist only for each other and the clamoring demands on you are nothing but a muffled murmur.

IT REALLY DOES GET EASIER

Fatigue and stress can affect your milk supply in the early weeks. However, after two to three months, your milk production is established. As long as you continue to drink plenty of fluids, it may well not be affected by a stressful period. One mother found that "regardless of how exhausted I would get, I always seemed to have enough milk. It was as if my body knew what my priorities were."

Even so, when most stressed and exhausted, a working mother may feel that she doesn't have any more to give; that she simply cannot answer another need, another demand. And then one day, perhaps around three or four months after returning to work, life seems a little easier. A day this week, then two next week, run smoothly. She manages to get to the babysitter's on time and doesn't forget to bring extra diapers; she is prepared for her 10:00 a.m. meeting, and that evening, while her partner does a load of laundry, she and the baby peacefully rock and nurse. What's happening? she wonders. Is it actually getting easier, or am I getting better at this? Both, say experienced working mothers. Life does get easier as the baby grows and as your partner learns to help out. But your ability to manage the demands of your life calmly and efficiently will increase more than you thought possible. Make time for yourself, enjoy your baby, and be proud—you are an accomplished woman and a loving mother.

Nursing Your Older Baby

CHANGES AT THE END OF THE FIRST YEAR

The American Academy of Pediatrics urges mothers to continue nursing through the first year; if you do, you're in for a treat. The older baby really enjoys nursing. You can see that it means more to him than just a way of filling his stomach, and that you mean more to him because of that. He wants to nurse for comfort and reassurance as much as for food. If you leave him with a sitter, he welcomes you home by scrambling into your lap for a swig of milk. If he hurts himself, or is frightened, nursing consoles him. When he is tired and ready for bed, nursing is his soothing nightcap. Often, he likes to nurse sitting upright, unless he is sleepy, when he goes back to lying in your arms like a little baby. Often, an older baby likes to play by putting a finger in your mouth while he nurses, stroking your face, or patting your hair.

Many babies do not have a visual association with the breast until they are twelve months old or so. To such a baby, the things that mean "Mother's going to nurse me" are being held in the nursing position, having you raise your blouse, and feeling your breast against his cheek. Perhaps because he does not look at your breast as he nurses, the sight of the breast has in itself no meaning for a surprisingly long time. Some babies, of course, do make the visual association earlier, and may dance up and down in their cribs, anticipating being nursed, whenever they catch a glimpse of Mama dressing or undressing.

TALKING

Naturally, as the baby learns to talk, he can tell you when he wants to nurse, in whatever terms your family uses. This can be disconcerting, as when a toddler climbs into your mother-in-law's lap, plucks at her blouse, and asks, politely, "Mi'k?" Some babies even make jokes with their minuscule vocabularies, like the sixteen-month-old who started to nurse, then pulled away from the breast in mock haste, and said "Hot!" and burst into laughter.

The ability to converse can be handy. The baby, who at eight months imperiously insisted upon being nursed right that minute in the middle of the housewares department, can at twelve or fourteen months be dissuaded by verbal explanations: "Pretty soon," "When we get to the car," and so on. Some families develop a private term for nursing that both mother and baby can use in public.

HOW LONG WILL YOU BE NURSING?

When you are down to one or two or three feedings in twenty-four hours, your baby is not exactly "breastfed" because she is getting most of her nourishment from one or more other sources. But she is still a nursing baby, and those one or two feedings may be very warm and dear moments for both of you. There's no need in the world to cut them off abruptly just because someone says the baby is "too old" to nurse, or no longer "needs" to nurse. Suppose she hangs on to a prebed snack, or likes to welcome you home by nursing, until she's two or more? Why shouldn't she? How many children of two—yes, and three and four—have you seen in the supermarket sucking on a bottle for dear life? Cherish these moments of closeness with your older baby; all too soon she will be a baby no longer. There's no need to stop nursing altogether until you or your baby are really ready to quit.

WEANING CUSTOMS

In the United States, the rigid child-care systems of the 1920s and subsequent decades included abrupt weaning. When a doctor decided that it was time, a patient ceased breastfeeding. He may have instructed the mother to give no more access to the breast whatsoever; the mother should take "drying-up" pills, bind her breasts, restrict fluid intake, and cease producing milk as promptly as could be arranged, while the baby was expected to complete the transition to being fully bottle- or cup-fed with equal speed.

This system is workable only when lactation has been mismanaged to such an extent that milk production is already very inadequate, so the baby gladly abandons the unsatisfying breast for the bottle that fills his stomach. Engorgement and distension are not too much of a problem when feedings are suddenly halted, if the mother has not been secreting much milk anyway.

But such sudden weaning is rough on both parties if it is undertaken when the baby is still nursing happily and the mother is producing well. The mother has to be a stoic indeed to obey orders to cease nursing completely. However, even during sudden weaning, letting the baby drink off enough milk, once or twice, to ease the mother's discomfort probably provides an insignificant amount of stimulation. There is hardly a mother in existence who, in this predicament, hasn't resorted to the forbidden relief of allowing the baby to nurse one last time.

Fortunately, most pediatricians today approach the mothers and babies in their care with more sensitivity. The concept of natural weaning, gradually and with the consent of both parties, is now accepted as a better method. You may find, however, that even if your doctor agrees with the concept of gradual weaning versus sudden weaning, he may pressure you in subtle ways to give up breastfeeding before you or your baby are really ready. He may say, casually, that if a baby is nursing for longer than a year, it is only because the mother is indulging herself. He may imply that you are insecure in some way and are trying to keep your baby dependent on you. He may suggest that nursing is developmentally inappropriate for a child of your baby's age (whatever that age is); that it's time to find another way to communicate with your baby. If you find your confidence shaken by such comments, remember that this is a decision to be made by you and your baby. No one else's opinion—for that's all this type of comment is—matters. You and your baby understand each other completely and know what is best.

Weaning without intervention often takes place very slowly as the baby's interest in the breast wanes; some people call this "baby-led" weaning. The baby who abruptly loses interest at nine months provides the exception; he may go from five meals a day to none in the space of three weeks. However, the baby who goes on to nurse for many months longer is more apt to lose interest in the breast very gradually. Sometimes you are too busy to feed him; sometimes he is not interested in nursing. Gradually, you forget about one meal and then another, until he is nursing regularly only at one time in the day, his favorite feeding, which is apt to be either the early morning feeding, the bedtime feeding, or upon his mother's return from work.

Of course, there are days when he is tired or teething, and he "backslides" to taking two or three feedings again for a while. But the general trend continues. Slowly the favorite meal, too, is abandoned. He sleeps through his early morning feeding or sometimes gives up his evening meal because you are out for the evening, and then begins going without it even when you are at home. A day goes by when you don't nurse him at all; then a week later, two days go by. Now your milk is really almost non-existent. Still, occasionally your baby likes to lie at the breast and recall his infant comfort. Then one day you realize he hasn't nursed in a week. Perhaps he remembers and tries again, but the empty breast is really not very interesting. He may nurse for a moment, and then give up, perhaps with a comment. One twenty-monther suddenly asked for the breast after three weeks of not nursing; he tried it briefly, and gave up, remarking matter-of-factly to his nearby father, "Nope, Mama's mi'k aw gone."

With this kind of weaning, there is no crying, heartbroken child who cannot understand why the dearest person in the world is denying him the thing he wants most; there are no discomforts, no problems. It is so gradual that often a mother cannot remember just exactly when the nursing stopped. Neither can the baby.

Sometimes a mother can't help wishing that the baby would get things over with and give up the breast, much as she loves to nurse him. Without any definable reason, she may just be ready to move on. At this point, a mother may feel restless whenever she sits down to nurse; she may be impatient and even resentful of the baby's demands. Weaning should begin when either party is ready to stop; in this situation, the mother may need to help the baby give up nursing.

You will probably be able to see how to encourage your baby to wean herself without making things hard for either of you. Give her lots of other kinds of attention. Anticipate her needs for food and drink. By keeping an eye on how long she has gone since the last meal, you can forestall her hunger pangs with food. Once she asks to nurse, a battle may ensue if you say no. You can avoid that by offering healthy snacks and juice *before* she notices she's hungry and thinks of nursing.

You can sometimes tell a toddler to wait if you are busy, or even promise to nurse her some other time, at bedtime perhaps. Don't begrudge her the breast if she really longs for it, and don't be too sudden. Let her linger on with the favorite meal for a few days or weeks. When she wants to nurse only once a day, it is hardly a great inconvenience for you, and you can satisfy prying relatives who ask, "When are you going to wean that baby?" by saying, "I am weaning her." One meal a day soon dwindles to an occasional meal, and then to none. What a pleasant, peaceful way to bring to close the pleasant, peaceful experience of nursing your baby.

THE NURSING TODDLER

The nursing toddler is a perfectly normal phenomenon in many cultures. Psychologically and biologically, there is no reason why a two- or three-year-old should not still nurse. Nursing is terribly important to some toddlers; they obviously draw immense reassurance and security—as they begin to explore their world—from being able to return from time to time to the breast.

Mothers are likely to keep the second and subsequent babies on the breast longer than the first. The more familiar one becomes with breastfeeding, the less susceptible one is to fad, fashion, or criticism; so the baby is not weaned according to the customs of others. Also, the very essence of the nursing relationship is to set no rules, to just let it happen; the more a mother becomes attuned to this receptivity, the less likely she is to be arbitrary about weaning; and so breastfeeding, for comfort and affection rather than nutrition, lingers on.

The mother with the nursing toddler must expect some criticism. "What are you going to tell his kindergarten teacher?" is the commonest wisecrack. Interestingly, toddlers can understand this and learn to nurse clandestinely, in privacy only, never asking to nurse or trying to nurse in front of strangers or disapproving relatives. Often, nursing becomes what one researcher has dubbed "the secret bond" between mother and child. One mother and her nursing toddler spent a month visiting in-laws who would have been appalled to learn that their twenty-month-old grandchild was still being breastfed. Without discussion, the mother simply said, "I think I'll put the baby to bed now" (or "down for a nap") whenever nursing was in order. Mother and baby disappeared upstairs, and nursed as they wanted. The baby kept the secret well, never asking for

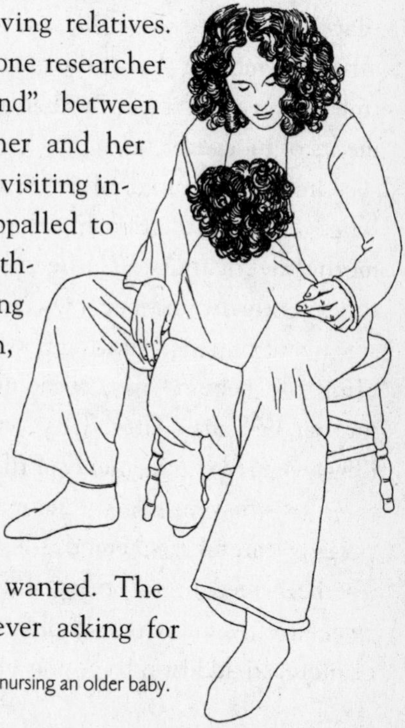

Figure 10.1 Nursing a toddler: Anything goes in nursing an older baby. This child likes to nurse standing up.

nursing except when they were alone, and the grandparents never knew.

THE DEMANDING NURSER

Two-year-olds can be both negative and bossy, and one sometimes sees a nursing toddler who has learned to wield his demand for the breast as a weapon over his mother. Perhaps the mother is intellectually convinced that she must not "reject" her baby by refusing the breast. She gives in and nurses even when she doesn't really want to; when it means leaving her company, or interrupting a shopping trip, or when she has just sat down for dinner. She feels secretly resentful, and she is right! The mother of a two-year-old doesn't have to be, and shouldn't be, the omnipresent, all-giving mother that the same baby needed at two months. Nature decrees that both mother and baby should be feeling moments of independence.

Under these circumstances, a dutiful mother sometimes prolongs a nursing relationship that is really a running battle. The mother resents nursing, at least some of the time; the baby feels the resentment and becomes even more demanding and aggressive about nursing, wanting reassurance more than ever, but also using the demand as a weapon. When he feels angry at his mother, he roars, "Titty! Titty!" no matter how unwilling she is or how awkward the moment, until she gives in.

This situation takes some management. One needs to be especially careful to meet the basic needs of hunger and thirst. Toddlers need to eat every three or four hours when they are awake; yet in many households, regular meals are six hours apart or more. In addition to giving him snacks, you may be better off feeding the toddler his own lunch or dinner ahead of the rest of the family, rather than making him wait past his endurance for something to eat.

Sometimes a toddler asks to nurse just for lack of anything better to do. What do many people do when they're bored or restless? Go to the refrigerator for a snack. A baby, too, will sometimes ask to nurse when he would be just as happy with some company or amusement. It's the mother's job to sense these needs, and to adjust as the baby grows; she is not doing the baby any favor if she allows him to get so hungry he can't think straight, or if she substitutes suckling for a romp on the lawn or being read to, at an age when the baby needs to be exploring and experiencing more and more.

Sometimes a mother clings to the comforting nursing relationship when her baby is ready to outgrow it. A woman who has an unhappy marriage might tend to postpone weaning her child. The youngest child in a big family is sometimes encouraged, and not just by the mother, to cling to his infant ways, including nursing. And late weaning, like early weaning, can become fashionable. In nonnursing circles, the announcement that you nursed the baby for two years has a certain, satisfying shock value. But among some groups of nursing mothers, one can get the feeling that long nursing has become competitive, with the mother who nursed thirty-two months enjoying more status than the mother who nursed twenty-two months.

Finally, some mothers use the nursing relationship aggressively. This kind of mother will snatch up her toddler and put him to the breast almost forcibly, because he is making too much noise or straying too far, and she wants to quiet him; paradoxically, she is nursing the baby so she can take her attention off him. Also, it's not just the mother who can use breastfeeding unfairly. In one family, older brothers and sisters habitually carried the toddler to Mom and told him to nurse, just to keep him out of their way and their toys.

When the nursing relationship has deteriorated to the point where either partner uses the nursing to manipulate the other partner unfairly, then it ought to be stopped. That is not a happy nursing couple anymore; relations between mother and child need to be rebuilt on a more grown-up basis.

TANDEM NURSING

Suppose a mother is still nursing a toddler agreeably when the new baby comes along? Some mothers nurse through pregnancy and continue to let the older baby nurse, at least occasionally, after the new baby has arrived. "It's so important to him," is the usual feeling. This so-called tandem nursing can be reassuring all around, although a mother must be certain that the new baby's needs are being fully met, and that she herself is not being physiologically or emotionally overwhelmed. The main danger is that the mother may begin to feel that nursing the older child is an obligation rather than a pleasure. She needs to listen to her own body and her own heart. If nursing during pregnancy becomes uncomfortable or wearing, she should gently stop. If after the birth she feels resentment, feels that the older baby is taking the newcomer's milk or too much of her attention from the newborn, she should stop. Being resented is much harder on a child than being weaned.

In this case, the resentment is not an emotion over which one should feel guilty; it is a biologically natural phenomenon. Animal mothers urge their young ones on to more mature behavior before the next babies arrive. In wild horse herds, a mare may be followed by her yearling and even her two-year-old, and she will graze with them and keep company with them, but she will kick and nip them if they try to nurse. Viola Lennon, a La Leche League founding mother who had a large family quite close together, was asked how it happened that she never found herself tandem nursing? "Because Mother Vi didn't let it happen," was her sensible response.

Weaning a toddler, when you have had enough of breastfeeding, is common sense, too. How long to nurse is a matter to be decided between you and your baby, and at this point, you both have equal rights. Weaning is part of the baby's growing up, but it is sometimes part of the mother's growing up, too.

TODDLER WEANING PROBLEMS

What if the toddler has been freely indulged in nursing and now, at the age of two or three, is nursing many times a day, often at night, and has a temper tantrum if nursing is denied or postponed even for a few minutes? Weaning such a child by just refusing the breast may be pretty traumatic for the baby, the mother, the rest of the household, and even for the neighbors. Tact and perhaps a little duplicity are called for. In rural Mexico, mothers put a little chili pepper on their breasts. (Angostura bitters, a nonalcoholic flavoring sold in liquor stores, might be gentler and safer.) When the child reacts to the bad taste, the mother feigns surprise, offers sympathy, and agrees that it's too bad the milk has turned so funny-tasting. A few tries over a few days is usually enough to discourage future nursing, and meanwhile the mother can be sure to spend extra time going for walks, playing, and giving the youngster other attention.

In some parts of the Pacific region, women wean late-nursing children by painting their breasts or nipples an odd color with a harmless dye; the changed appearance is sufficiently alarming to discourage the child. Food coloring would be safe to use if a mother wanted to try this dodge. A practice in Europe for weaning two- or three-year-olds is that the mother takes a four- or five-day trip away from home, while other members of the household take care of the youngster. Usually in her absence the toddler will grow accustomed to being happy without nursing. Although he may ask to nurse when she first returns, the firm statement that the milk is all gone now, coupled with lots of affection but the refusal to let him try nursing, should soon finalize the weaning process. Baby-led weaning, however, is the ideal path to weaning, and one in which neither mother nor baby quite remembers when they last nursed. One day the mother may realize it's been several days or more and say to herself, "Oh, I think the baby is weaned."

AFTER WEANING

If a baby is weaned abruptly, the mother's breasts first fill with milk, and then gradually become empty and slack over a period of several days. Slowly, as the breasts change to the nonproductive state, they return to their former, smaller size; this will take about six months. If a baby abandons breastfeeding very gradually, over a period of many months, the breasts return to normal during that period. By the time the baby is nursing once every few days, the breasts are producing almost no milk, and their appearance is pretty much as it was before pregnancy. Long after the baby has ceased nursing altogether, it remains possible to manually express a few drops of milk from the breasts. Gradually, the drops that are expressed change in appearance to the yellowish look of colostrum. Finally, perhaps a year after weaning, even this milk disappears.

When breastfeeding ceases entirely, it's only natural to feel a little sad, especially if this is the last child you plan to have. Some of this reaction is hormonal, but some of it is a very natural regret. Breastfeeding is soothing and comforting to mothers, too, and it brings a special closeness. Sometimes we grieve a little at giving it up.

NURSING AN ADOPTED BABY

The mother who is planning to adopt a baby may well wonder if it wouldn't be possible to give that baby—and herself—the benefits and joys of breastfeeding. Techniques do in fact exist by which a woman who has breastfed in the past can at least partly feed an adopted baby from the breast; this is called "relactation." Even a woman who has never given birth, or perhaps never even been pregnant, can develop a little milk production, using the proper technique; this is called "induced lactation." Both processes are described in detail in Chapter 2, pages 53–54.

Milk production in the adoptive mother is a result of sucking stimulation, and is initiated by nursing the new baby as long and as often as possible, before and after bottle-feedings, during the night, and so on. Some babies are cooperative and some are not; in general, the younger the baby, the more willing she is to nurse without much recompense. There are some physical impediments to developing a truly adequate supply of breast milk for an adopted baby. The mother who has never given birth must develop secretory tissue as well. The mother who has previously lactated may produce milk tailored to the needs of an older baby or toddler, not to a newborn. And, in the absence of a subsequent pregnancy, milk production tends to dwindle over time in spite of sucking stimulation.

A full milk supply is not the aim of nursing an adopted baby; the aim is to facilitate the emotional attachment process, and make the baby a member of the family. Progress is considerably more likely if the adopting mother uses a nursing supplementer, a feeding device worn around her neck that trickles formula into the baby's mouth while he nurses. The new baby is thus fed on formula, but he obtains it by nursing at the breast, which stimulates milk production.

Many mothers who reestablish or induce lactation feel that nursing an adopted baby, even if they can never forgo supplementation, is worth the trouble. One experienced nursing mother who nursed her adopted baby said, "You have to focus on the relationship, not on the quantity of milk. She nursed like any other baby—to go to sleep, for comfort—and she still nurses like any toddler. That is the real payoff; it's a perfectly wonderful way of mothering." Other experienced nursing mothers feel that nursing an adopted baby produces the nursing experience for the baby, but not for the mother. The supplementer can diminish the spontaneity of nursing, and the hormonal side effects of peace and joy may be reduced as well. One experienced breastfeeding mother who also nursed an adopted baby confessed that she resented the process, but added, "She thinks she's a breastfed baby. I can resolve the resentment in my heart." The adoptive mother, however, who has never nursed a biological child is likelier to consider that nursing her adopted baby is a very rewarding experience.

If you are considering nursing an adopted baby, read the section on induced lactation and relactation in Chapter 2. You will benefit from the advice of a lactation consultant and the support of other mothers who have relactated. Information on relactation and nursing adopted babies can be obtained from La Leche League International. It is important, in considering nursing an adopted baby, to have the help of an enthusiastic doctor and a lactation consultant. Many doctors have never heard of such a thing, but may become supportive if presented with some of La Leche League's and other literature on the subject. Tact and discretion are also called for in presenting the idea to social workers and agencies. A foster mother was forbidden to breastfeed her infant charges on the ground that the milk was not pasteurized. One couple were refused as adoptive parents when the agency discovered that the mother planned to try to nurse the baby.

EXTENDING MOTHERING SKILLS

Breastfeeding is not an end in itself, although it may seem so in the weeks and months in which you are learning about it and enjoying it. The goal, of course, is a happy and healthy baby and a fulfilled mother. Breastfeeding does so much to ensure this. The benefits of the nursing relationship linger long beyond weaning. Your baby will be healthier for months, perhaps years. And don't you have the feeling that he is a happier person than he might otherwise have been? Happy nursing babies are all kinds of people—introverts, extroverts, thinkers, or doers—but they tend to share certain basic traits: a generous, affectionate nature, coupled, after weaning, with an almost comic self-sufficiency. Probably your youngster, too, has these qualities, which are typical of the little child who has spent most of his first year of life, or longer, as a happy nursing baby.

And for you, the benefits of being half of a nursing couple continue, too. Looking back over the months of nursing, you remember the big pleasures, not the little problems. Do you sense how much you have learned? Dr. Richard Applebaum says that breastfeeding teaches "receptivity." Think of the difference between "passive" and "receptive." There is a partnership implicit in being receptive, a partnership that is the very nature of the nursing relationship.

The warmth and receptivity one sometimes first develops as a nursing mother doesn't vanish with the milk. It can extend into the rest of your life, *for* the rest of your life. It can become the heart of your relationship to your partner, to your family, to the rest of the world. Our society values achieving; it does not much value perceiving. The nursing mother, however restricted and unfeeling her own upbringing might have been, learns more and more about perceiving, about awareness of others, about reaching goals by means of receptiveness instead of aggressiveness.

We live long lives now, and many women have small families. Women have more education than in the past and more access to the world outside the family. There are many years ahead, and many opportunities, to put the lessons of the nursing relationship to work in other ways. If there's one thing every part of society could use right now—from the crowded cities to the medical establishment, from the arts to big business—it's the receptive way of achieving together instead of being at odds with nature and against each other. The nursing relationship is a glimpse of how things can be. Some of this enlightenment can carry over into the rest of your life. Perhaps in the return of breastfeeding we are witnessing a small but contagious sample of revolution, a humanizing revolution of our own culture.

References

The references given here are by no means a complete list of the sources used in the preparation of this book. From the research literature we have attempted to select for you: (1) studies or authors directly cited in the text; (2) the best and most reliable studies we have found on most topics covered in the text; and (3) major "review" papers, where they exist, that will lead you to a wider range of studies. In this section, each reference is listed only once, under the chapter to which it most directly pertains. The references are cited in abbreviated form for accessibility for a general readership; abstracts for all studies may be located online at the National Library of Medicine/PubMed (http://www.ncbi.nlm.nih.gov/entrez/query.fcgi?db=PubMed).

There are many general books, both scientific and popular, on breast-feeding and related topics. In a separate list, we have selected some we consider interesting and reliable for additional reading. La Leche League International and the *Journal of Human Lactation* are also excellent sources of information on breastfeeding.

References

PART 1

Chapter 1: The Nursing Couple

Bevan-Brown, M., 1950. *The Sources of Love and Fear.* Coulls, Somerville, Wilkie, Ltd., Dunedin, New Zealand.

Bowlby, J., 1969. *Attachment and Loss, Vol. 1.* Basic Books, New York.

Bowlby, J., 1953. *Child Care and the Growth of Love.* Penguin Books, Baltimore.

Brody, S., 1956. *Patterns of Mothering.* International Universities Press, New York.

Labbok; M. H., 2001. Effects of breastfeeding on the mother. *Pediatric Clinics of North America*, February.

Lindbergh, A. M., 1955. *Gift from the Sea.* Pantheon, New York.

Middlemore, M. P., 1941. *The Nursing Couple.* Cassell & Co., London.

Montagu, A., 1961. Neonatal and infant immaturity in man. *J.A.M.A.*, October.

Montagu, A., 1971. *Touching: The Human Significance of the Skin.* Columbia University Press, New York.

National Maternal and Infant Health Survey, 2004. Breastfeeding and risk of postneonatal death in the United States. *Pediatrics*, May.

Newcomb, P. A., et al., 1994. Lactation and a reduced risk of premenopausal breast cancer. *New England Journal of Medicine*, January.

Smith, H., 1765. *Letters to Married Ladies*. Quoted in: G. F. Still, 1931: *A History of Paediatrics*. Oxford University Press.

Thirkell, A., 1959. *Love at All Ages*. Alfred A. Knopf, New York.

Winnecott, D. W., 1957. *Mother and Child*. Basic Books, New York.

Chapter 2: How the Breasts Function

Alho, O. P., et al., 1990. Risk factors for recurrent acute otitis media and respiratory infection in infancy. *International Journal of Pediatric Otorhinolaryngology*.

American Academy of Pediatrics Work Group on Breastfeeding, 1997. Breastfeeding and the use of human milk. *Pediatrics* (http://aap.org/policy/re9729.html).

Andran, G. M., F. H. Kemp, and J. Lind, 1958. A cineradiographic study of breastfeeding. *British Journal of Radiology*.

Andrusiak, M.S.W., and M. Larose-Kuzenko, 1987. The effects of an overactive letdown reflex. *Lactation Consultant Series* Unit 13. Avery Publishing Group, Garden City Park, N.Y.

Asselin, B. L., and R. A. Lawrence, 1987. Maternal disease as a consideration in lactation management. *Clinics in Perinatology*.

Auerbach, K. G., and J. L. Avery, 1981. Induced lactation: a study of adoptive nursing by 240 women. *American Journal of Diseases in Children*.

Ball, T. M., and A. L. Wright, 1999. Health care costs of formula-feeding in the first year of life. *Pediatrics*.

Baumslag, N., and D. Michels, 1995. *Milk, Money, and Madness: The Culture and Politics of Breastfeeding*, Bergin & Garvey.

Bradshaw, M. K., and S. Pfeiffer, 1988. Feeding mode and anthropometric changes in primiparas. *Human Biology*.

Brewer, M. M., et al., 1989. Postpartum changes in maternal weight and body fat deposits in lactating vs. nonlactating women. *American Journal of Clinical Nursing*.

Brun, J., et al., 1995. Breast feeding, other reproductive factors and rheumatoid arthritis: a prospective study. *British Journal of Rheumatology*.

Byers, T., et al., 1985. Lactation and breast cancer: evidence for a negative association in post-menopausal women. *American Journal of Epidemiology.*

de Carvalho, et al., 1983. The effect of frequent breast-feeding on early milk production and infant weight gain. *Pediatrics.*

Casey, C. E., and K. M. Hambridge, 1983. Nutritional aspects of human lactation. In: *Lactation: Physiology, Nutrition and Breast-Feeding.* M. C. Neville and M. R. Neifert, eds., Plenum Press, New York.

Chandra, R. K., 1997. Five-year follow-up of high-risk infants with family history of allergy who were exclusively breast-fed or fed partial whey hydrolysate, soy, and conventional cow's milk formulas. *Journal of Pediatric Gastroenterology and Nutrition,* April.

Chao, S., 1987. The effect of lactation on ovulation and fertility. *Clinics in Perinatology.*

Chayen, B., et al., 1986. Induction of labor with an electric breast pump. *Journal of Reproductive Medicine.*

Centers for Disease Control and Prevention, 2000. *Healthy People 2010 Maternal, Infant, and Child Health.*

Collaborative Group on Hormonal Factors in Breast Cancer, 2002. Breast cancer and breastfeeding: collaborative reanalysis of individual data from 47 epidemiological studies in 30 countries, including 50,302 women with breast cancer and 96,973 women without the disease. *Lancet,* July.

Cumming, R. G., and R. J. Klineberg, 1993. Breastfeeding and other reproductive factors and the risk of hip fractures in elderly women. *International Journal of Epidemiology.*

Dewey, K. G., D. A. Finnley, and B. Lonnerdal, 1984. Breast milk volume and composition during late lactation (7–20 months). *Journal of Pediatric Gastroenterology and Nutrition.*

Dewey, K., M. Heinig, and L. Nommsen, 1993. Maternal weight-loss patterns during prolonged lactation. *American Journal of Clinical Nursing.*

Engelking, C., and J. Page-Leiberman, 1986. Maternal diabetes and diabetes in young children: their relationship to breastfeeding. *Lactation*

Consultant Series Unit 5. Avery Publishing Group, Garden City Park, N.Y.

Ferlay, J., et al., 2001. GLOBOCAN 2000: Cancer Incidence, Mortality and Prevalence Worldwide, Version 1.0. IARC CancerBase No. 5. IARC Press.

Ford, R.P.K., et al., 1993. Breastfeeding and the risk of sudden infant death syndrome. *International Journal of Epidemiology.*

Gdalevich, M., D. Mimouni, and M. Mimouni, 2001. Breastfeeding and the risk of bronchial asthma in childhood: a systematic review with meta-analysis of prospective studies. *Journal of Pediatrics*, August.

Greco, l., S. Auricchio, M. Mayer, et al., 1988. Case control study on nutritional risk factors in celiac disease. *Journal of Pediatric Gastroenterology and Nutrition.*

Gould, S. F., 1983. Anatomy of the breast. In: *Lactation: Physiology, Nutrition, and Breast-Feeding.* M. C. Neville and M. R. Neifert, eds., Plenum Press, New York.

Gwinn, J. L., et al., 1990. Pregnancy, breastfeeding, and oral contraceptives and the risk of epithelial ovarian cancer. *Journal of Chronic Diseases.*

Hale, Thomas W., 2000. *Medications and Mothers' Milk.* Pharmasoft Medical Publishing, Amarillo, Tex. (http://neonatal.ttuhsc.edu/lact/).

Hartman, P. E., and J. K. Kulski, 1978. Changes in the composition of the mammary secretion of women after abrupt termination of breast feeding. *Journal of Physiology.*

Hening, M. J., 2001. Host defense benefits of breastfeeding for the infant: effect of breastfeeding duration and exclusivity. *Pediatric Clinics of North America.*

Hill, P. D., 1991. The enigma of insufficient milk supply. *Maternal Child Nursing*, November.

Hytten, F. E., 1954. Clinical and chemical studies in human lactation. *British Medical Journal.*

Imaginis Web site, 2000. Breast cancer: statistics on incidence, survival, and screening. http://www.imaginis.com/breasthealth/statistics.asp?mode=1.

Johnston, J. M., and J. Amico, 1986. A prospective longitudinal study of the release of oxytocin and prolactin in response to infant sucking in long term lactation. *Journal of Clinical Endocrinology and Metabolism.*

Jorgensen, C., et al., 1996. Oral contraception, parity, breast feeding, and severity of rheumatoid arthritis. *Annals of Rheumatic Diseases*.

Karra, M. V., et al., 1986. Changes in specific nutrients in breast milk during extended lactation. *American Journal of Clinical Nutrition*.

Kippley, Sheila, and J. Kippley, 1989. *Breastfeeding and Natural Child Spacing*, rev. ed. Couple to Couple League International.

Kjos, S., et al., 1993. Effect of lactation on glucose and lipid metabolism in women with recent gestational diabetes. *Obstetrics and Gynecology*.

Koetting, C. A., and G. M. Wardlaw, 1988. Wrist, spine, and hip bone density with variable histories of lactation. *American Journal of Clinical Nutrition*.

Kovar, M. G., et al., 1995. Relation between infant feeding and infections during the first six months of life. *Journal of Pediatrics*.

Gerstein, H. C. Cow's milk exposure and type 1 diabetes mellitus. *Diabetes Care*.

Kramer, F., et al., 1993. Breastfeeding reduces maternal lower-body fat. *Journal of the American Dietetic Association*.

La Leche League International, 1996. *Breastfeeding Remains Best Choice in a Polluted World* (Press release).

Lawrence, R. A., 1999. *Breastfeeding: A Guide for the Medical Profession*, 5th ed. C. V. Mosby, St. Louis.

Lawrence, R. A., 1987. The management of lactation as a physiologic process. *Clinics in Perinatology*.

Layde, P. P., et al., 1989. The independent associations of parity, age at first full term pregnancy, and duration of breast-feeding with the risk of breast cancer. *Journal of Clinical Epidemiology*.

Lucas, A., and T. Cole, 1990. Breastmilk and neonatal necrotizing enterocolitis. *Lancet*.

Lvoff, N. M., et al., 2000. Effect of the baby friendly initiative on infant abandonment in a Russian hospital. *Archives of Pediatric and Adolescent Medicine*.

McTiernan, A., and D. B. Thomas, 1986. Evidence for a protective effect of lactation on risk of breast cancer in young women. *American Journal of Epidemiology*.

Mayer, E. J., et al., 1998. Reduced risk of IDDM among breast-fed children. The Colorado IDDM Registry. *Diabetes*.

Mitchell, E. A., R. Scragg, et al., 1991. Cot death supplement: results from the first year of the New Zealand cot death study. *New Zealand Journal of Medicine*.

Neifert, M. R., et al., 1981. Failure of lactogenesis associated with placental retention. *American Journal of Obstetrics and Gynecology*.

Neville, M. C., 1983. Regulation of mammary development and lactation. In: *Lactation: Physiology, Nutrition, and Breast-Feeding*. M. C. Neville and M. R. Neifert, eds., Plenum Press, New York.

Neville, M. C., J. C. Allen, and C. Watters, 1983. The mechanisms of milk secretion. In: *Lactation: Physiology, Nutrition, and Breast-Feeding*. M. C. Neville and M. R. Neifert, eds., Plenum Press, New York.

Neville, M. C., R. P. Keller, J. H. Secort, et al., 1988. Studies in human lactation: milk volumes in lactating women during the onset of lactation and full lactation. *Am. J. Clin. Nutr.* 48:1375–86.

Neville, M. C., and M. R. Neifert, 1983. An introduction to lactation and breastfeeding. In: *Lactation: Physiology, Nutrition, and Breast-Feeding*. M. C. Neville and M. R. Neifert, eds., Plenum Press, New York.

Newcomb, P., et al., 1994. Lactation and a reduced risk of postmenopausal breast cancer. *New England Journal of Medicine*.

Newcomb, P. A., and A. Trentham-Dietz, 2000. Breast feeding practices in relation to endometrial cancer risk, USA. *Cancer Causes Control*, August.

Newton, N., and C. Nodahl, 1980. The role of the oxytocin reflexes in three interpersonal reproductive acts: coitus, birth, and breastfeeding. In: *Proceedings of the Serano Symposia*, L. Caranza, P. Panceri, and L. Zichelli, eds., Academic Press, New York.

Newton, N., and C. Modahl, 1980. New frontiers of oxytocin research. In: *The Free Woman: Women's Health in the 1990's*, E. V. Van Hall, and W. Everaerd, eds., 1989. Parthenon Publishing Group, Park Ridge, N.J.

Oddy, W. H., P. G. Holt, et al., 1999. Association between breastfeeding and asthma in 6 year old children: findings of a prospective birth cohort study. *British Medical Journal*.

Oddy, W. H., J. K. Peat, and N. H. de Klerk, 2002. Maternal asthma, infant feeding, and the risk of asthma in childhood. *Journal of Allergy and Clinical Immunology*, July.

Olsen, C. G., and R. E. Gordon, Jr., 1990. Breast disorders in nursing mothers. *Annals of Family Practice*.

Oyer, D., and N. Stone, 1989. Cholesterol levels and the breastfeeding mom. *J.A.M.A.*

Paradise, J. L., H. E. Rockette, et al., 1997. Otitis media in 2253 Pittsburgh-area infants: prevalence and risk factors during the first two years of life, *Pediatrics*.

Pederson, C. A., and A. J. Frange, Jr., 1979. Induction of maternal behavior in virgin rats after intracerebroventricular administration of oxytocin. *Proceedings of the National Academy of Science USA*.

Radford, A., 1992. The Ecological Impact of Bottle Feeding, *Breastfeeding Review*, May.

Reid, R., 2002. The skeleton in pregnancy and lactation, *Internal Medicine Journal*, September.

Rigas, A., B. Rigas, et al., 1993. Breast-feeding and maternal smoking in the etiology of Crohn's disease and ulcerative colitis in childhood. *Annals of Epidemiology*.

Riordan, J. M., 1997. The cost of not breastfeeding: a commentary. *Journal of Human Lactation*.

Riordon, J., and F. H. Nichols, 1990. A descriptive study of lactation mastitis in long-term breastfeeding women. *J. Human Lact.* 6:53–58.

Salazar-Martinez, E., et al., 1999. Reproductive factors of ovarian and endometrial cancer risk in a high fertility population in Mexico. *Cancer Research*, August.

Salber, E., et al., 1966. The duration of postpartum amenorrhea. *American Journal of Epidemiology*.

Salmenpera, A. L., 1984. Vitamin C nutrition during prolonged lactation: optimal in infants while marginal in some mothers. *American Journal of Clinical Nutrition*.

Shu, X. O., M. S. Linet, et al., 1999. Breastfeeding and risk of childhood acute leukemia. *Journal of the National Cancer Institute*.

Sinigaglia, L., et al., 1996. Effect of lactation on postmenopausal bone mineral density of the lumbar spine. *Journal of Reproductive Medicine*.

Sowers, M., et al., 1995. A prospective study of bone density and pregnancy after an extended period of lactation with bone loss. *Obstetrics and Gynecology*.

Specker, B., 1991. Changes in calcium homeostasis over the first year postpartum: effect of lactation and weaning. *Obstetrics and Gynecology*.

Thomsen, A. C., T. Espersen, and S. Maigaard, 1984. Course and treatment of milk stasis, non-infectious inflammation of the breast and infectious mastitis in nursing women. *American Journal of Obstetrics and Gynecology*.

Tovarud, S. V., and A. Boass, 1979. Hormonal control of calcium metabolism in lactation. *Vitamins and Hormones: Advances in Research and Applications*.

Virtanen, S. M., L. Rasanen, A. Aro, et al., 1991. Infant feeding in Finnish children <7 year of age with newly diagnosed IDDM. *Diabetes Care*.

Walker, M., 1993. A fresh look at the risks of artificial infant feeding, *Journal of Human Lactation*.

Woolridge, M. W., 1986. Aetiology of sore nipples. *Midwifery*.

Woolridge, M. W., and Chloe Fisher, 1988. Colic, "overfeeding," and symptoms of lactose malabsorption in the breast-fed baby: a possible artifact of feed management? *Lancet*.

Woolridge, M. W., et al., 1990. Do changes in pattern of breast usage alter the baby's nutrient intake? *Lancet*.

Worthington-Roberts, B., J. Vermeersch, and S. R. Williams, 1985. *Nutrition in Pregnancy and Lactation*. Times Mirror/Mosby, St. Louis.

Chapter 3: Human Milk

Acheson, E., and S. Truelove, 1961. Early weaning in the aetiology of ulcerative colitis. *British Medical Journal*.

American Academy of Pediatric Committee on Drugs, 1989. Transfer of drugs and other chemicals into human milk. *Pediatrics*.

Auerbach, K. G., and L. M. Gartner, 1987. Breastfeeding and human milk: their association with jaundice in the neonate. *Clinics in Perinatology.*

Barger, J., and P. Bull, 1986. A comparison of the bacterial composition of breast milk stored at room temperature and stored in the refrigerator. *International Journal of Childbirth Education.*

Bartmess, J. E., 1988. The risk of polychlorinated dibenzodioxins in human milk. *Journal of Human Lactation.*

Belec, L., et al., 1990. Antibodies to human immunodeficiency virus in the breast milk of healthy, seropositive women. *Pediatrics.*

Bounous, G., P. A. Konshavn, A. Taveroff, and P. Gold, 1988. Evolutionary traits in human milk proteins (review article). *Medical Hypotheses.*

Britton, J. R., 1986. Discordance of milk protein production between right and left mammary glands. *Journal of Pediatric Gastroenterology and Nutrition.*

Carvalho, M. D., M. Hall, and D. Harvey, 1981. Effects of water supplementation on physiological jaundice in breastfed infants. *Archives of Diseases in Childhood.*

Carvalho, M. D., J. H. Klaus, and R. B. Merkatz, 1982. Frequency of breastfeeding and serum bilirubin concentration. *American Journal of Diseases in Childhood.*

Chaney, M. E., et al., 1988. Cocaine convulsions in a breast-feeding baby. *Journal of Pediatrics.*

Chen, Y., S. Yu, and W. X. Li, 1988. Artificial feeding and hospitalization in the first 18 months of life. *Pediatrics.*

Clare, D. A., 2003. Biodefense properties of milk: the role of antimicrobial proteins and peptides. *Current Pharmaceutical Design,* June.

Cunningham, A. S., 1979. Morbidity in breast-fed and artificially fed infants. *Journal of Pediatrics.*

Cunningham, A. S., 1988. Breastfeeding, bottle-feeding, and illness: an annotated bibliography, 1986. In: *Programmes to Promote Breastfeeding.* D. B. Jelliffe, and E.F.P. Jelliffe, eds., Oxford University Press.

Cunningham, A. S., D. B. Jelliffe, and E.F.P. Jelliffe, 1991. Breastfeeding and health in the 1980's: a global epidemiologic review. *Journal of Pediatrics.*

Davis, J. K., et al., 1988. Infant feeding and childhood cancer. *Lancet.*

Dolan, S. A., et al., 1986. Antimicrobial activity of human milk against pediatric pathogens. *Journal of Infectious Diseases.*

Drake, T. G., 1930. Infant feeding in England and in France from 1750–1800. *American Journal of Diseases in Childhood.*

Estrada, B., 2003. Human milk and the prevention of infection, *Infections in Medicine.*

Fulton, B., and L. Moore, 1990. Radiopharmaceuticals and lactation. *Journal of Human Lactation.*

Garza, C., R. J. Schanler, N. F. Butte, and K. J. Motil, 1987. Special properties of human milk. *Clinics in Perinatology.*

Goldman, A. S., 1993. The immune system of human milk: antimicrobial, antiinflammatory and immunomodulating properties. *Pediatric Infectious Disease Journal,* August.

Goldman, A. S., 2002. Evolution of the mammary gland defense system and the ontogeny of the immune system. *Journal of Mammary Gland Biology and Neoplasia,* July.

Goldman, A. S., S. A. Atkinson, and L. A. Hanson, eds., 1987. *Human Lactation, Vol. 3: The Effects of Human Milk on the Recipient Infant.* Plenum Press, New York.

Goldman, A. S., C. Garza, et al., 1982. Immunologic factors in human milk during the first year of lactation. *Journal of Pediatrics.*

Goldman, A. S., C. Garza, et al., 1990. Molecular forms of lactoferrin in stool and urine from infants fed human milk. *Pediatric Research.*

Goldman, A. S., R. M. Goldblum, and C. Garza, 1983. Immunologic components in human milk during the second year of lactation. *Acta Paed. Scand.*

Goldman, A. S., L. W. Thorpe, et al., 1986. Anti-inflammatory properties of human milk. *Acta Paed. Scand.*

Grummer-Strawn, L. M., and Z. Mei, 2004. Does breastfeeding protect against pediatric overweight? Analysis of longitudinal data from the centers for disease control and prevention pediatric nutrition surveillance system. *Pediatrics.*

Gyorgy, P., 1960. The late effects of early nutrition. *American Journal of Clinical Nutrition*.

Hambidge, J. K., 1977. The role of zinc and other trace metals in pediatric nutrition. *Pediatric Clinics of North America*.

Hamosh, M., and A. S. Goldman, eds., 1986. *Human Lactation, Vol. 2: Maternal and Environmental Factors*. Plenum Press, New York.

Hancock, J. T., et al., 2002. Antimicrobial properties of milk: dependence on presence of xanthine oxidase and nitrite. *Antimicrobial Agents and Chemotherapy*, October.

Hanson, L. S., S. Ahlstedt, B. Anderson, et al., 1984. Protective factors in milk and the development of the immune system. *Pediatrics*.

Hartman, P. E., S.E.G. Morgan, and P. G. Arthur, 1986. Milk letdown and the concentration of fat in breast milk. In: *Human Lactation, Vol. 2: Maternal and Environmental Factors*. M. Hamosh and A. S. Goldman, eds., Plenum Press, New York.

Heird, W. C., 1986. Potentially harmful effects of human milk upon the recipient infant. In: *Human Lactation, Vol. 3: The Effects of Human Milk on the Recipient Infant*. A. S. Goldman, S. A. Atkinson, and L. A. Hanson, eds., Plenum Press, New York.

Hendrixson, D. R., et al., 2003. Human milk lactoferrin is a serine protease that cleaves Haemophilus surface proteins at arginine-rich sites. *Molecular Microbiology*, February.

Heymann, S. J., 1990. Modeling the impact of breast-feeding by HIV-infected women on child survival. *American Journal of Public Health*.

Heymann, S. J., and P. Vo, 1999. The breast-feeding dilemma and its impact on HIV-infected women and their children. *AIDS*.

Hide, D. W., and B. U. Guyer, 1985. Clinical manifestations of allergy related to breast- and cow's milk-feeding. *Pediatrics* 75.

Host, A., S. Husby, and O. Osterballe, 1986. A prospective study of cow's milk allergy in exclusively breast-fed infants. *Acta Paed. Scand.*

Hytten, F. E., and A. M. Thomson, 1961. Nutrition of the lactating woman. In: *Milk, the Mammary Gland and Its Secretion, Vol. II*. S. K. Kon and A. T. Cowie, eds., Academic Press, New York.

Insull, W., Jr., J. Hirsch, A. T. James, and E. H. Ahrens, Jr., 1959. The fatty acids of human milk II: alterations produced by manipulation of caloric balance and exchange of dietary fats. *Journal of Clinical Investigations*.

Jelliffe, D. B., 1955. *Infant Nutrition in the Subtropics and Tropics*. World Health Organization, Geneva.

Jensen, A. A., 1987. PCBs, PCDDs and PCDFs in human milk, blood, and adipose tissue. *Science of Total Environment*.

Kasdan, Sara, 1956. *Love and Knishes*. Vanguard Press, New York.

Koletzko, B., and M. Rodriguez-Palmero, 1999. Polyunsaturated fatty acids in human milk and their role in early infant development. *Journal of Mammary Gland Biology and Neoplasia*, July.

Kramer, J. S., 1981. Do breast-feeding and delayed introduction of solid foods protect against subsequent obesity? *Journal of Pediatrics*.

Labbok, J. H., and G. E. Hendershot, 1987. Does breast-feeding protect against malocclusion? *American Journal of Preventive Medicine*.

Lawrence, R. M., and R. A. Lawrence, 2001. Given the benefits of breast-feeding, what contraindications exist? *Pediatric Clinics of North America*, February.

Liepke, C., et al., 2001. Purification of novel peptide antibiotics from human milk. *Journal of Chromatography B: Biomedical Science Applications*.

Lifschitz, C. H., et al., 1988. Anaphylactic shock due to cow's milk protein hypersensitivity in a breastfed infant. *Journal of Pediatric Gastroenterology and Nutrition*.

Macie, I. C., and H. J. Kelly, 1961. Human milk and cows' milk in infant nutrition. In: *Milk, the Mammary Gland and Its Secretion, Vol. II*. S. K. Kon and A. T. Cowie, eds., Academic Press, New York.

Mata, L., et al., 1988. Promotion of breastfeeding in Costa Rica: the Puriscal study. In: *Programmes to Promote Breastfeeding*. D. B. Jelliffe and E. F. P. Jelliffe, eds., Oxford University Press.

Mayer, E. J., R. F. Hamman, E. C. Gay, et al., 1988. Reduced risk of insulin-dependent diabetes mellitus (IDDM) among breast-fed children: The Colorado IDDM Registry. *Diabetes*.

Mellies, M. J., T. Ishikawa, P. Gartside, K. Burton, J. MacGee, K. Allen, P. Steiner, D. Brady, and C. Glueck, 1978. Effects of varying maternal dietary cholesterol and phytosterol in lactating women and their infants. *American Journal of Clinical Nutrition.*

Mestecky, J., et al., 1991. *Immunology of Milk and the Neonate.* Plenum Press, New York.

Minchin, M., 1989. *Breastfeeding Matters,* rev. ed. Allen & Unwin, Australia.

Neville, M. C., et al., 1986. Changes in milk composition after six months of lactation: the effects of duration of lactation and gradual weaning. In: *Human Lactation, Vol. 2: Maternal and Environmental Factors.* M. Hamosh and A. S. Goldman, eds., Plenum Press, New York.

Owen, C. G., et al., 2003. Infant feeding and blood cholesterol: a study in adolescents and a systematic review. *Pediatrics.*

Peterson, R. C., and W. A. Bowes, 1983. Drugs, toxins and environmental agents in breast milk. In: *Lactation: Physiology, Nutrition and Breast-Feeding,* M. C. Neville and M. Neifert, eds., Plenum Press, New York.

Rivera-Calimlim, L., 1987. The significance of drugs in breast milk: pharmacokinetic considerations. *Clinics in Perinatology.*

Rogan, W. J., 1986. Epidemiology of environmental chemical contaminants in breast milk. In: *Human Lactation, Vol. 2: Maternal and Environmental Factors.* M. Hamosh and A. S. Goldman, eds., Plenum Press, New York.

Romney, B. M., et al., 1986. Radiolnuclide administration to nursing mothers: mathematically derived guidelines. *Radiology.*

Schrago, L., 1987. Glucose water supplementation of the breastfed infant during the first three days of life. *Journal of Human Lactation.*

Schwartz, R. H., et al., 1987. Acute urticarial reactions to cow's milk in infants previously fed breast milk or soy milk. *Pediatric Asthma Allergy Immunology.*

Sheard, N., and W. A. Waler, 1988. The role of breast milk in the development of the gastrointestinal tract. *Nutrition Reviews.*

Slade, H. B., and S. A. Schwartz, 1987. Mucosal immunity: the immunology of breast milk. *Journal of Allergy and Clinical Immunology.*

Soisa, R., and L. Barness, 1987. Bacterial growth in refrigerated human milk. *American Journal of Diseases in Childhood.*

Specker, B. L., 1987. Sun and vitamin D: cyclical serum in breastfed babies. *Journal of Pediatrics*.

Specker, B. L., et al., 1987. Effect of vegetarian diets on Vit. D in breast-fed babies. *Obstetrics and Gynecology*.

Taguchi, S., and T. Yakushiji, 1988. Influence of termite treatment in the home on the chlordane concentration in human milk. *Archives Environmental Contaminants Toxicology*.

Takeda, S., Y. Kuwabara, and M. Mizuno, 1986. Concentrations and origin of oxytocin in breast milk. *Endocrinology Japan*.

Victoria, C. G., et al., 1987. Evidence for protection by breastfeeding against infant deaths from infectious diseases in Brazil. *Lancet*.

Wagner, V., and H. B. von Stockhausen, 1988. The effect of feeding human milk and adapted milk formulae on serum lipid and lipoprotein levels in young infants. *European Journal of Pediatrics*.

Williams, R. J., 1956. *Biochemical Individuality*. John Wiley & Sons, New York.

Chapter 4: How the Baby Functions: The Body

Anderson, J. W., et al., 1999. Breastfeeding and cognitive development: a meta-analysis. *American Journal of Clinical Nutrition*, October.

Angelsen, N. K., et al., 2001. Breastfeeding and cognitive development at age 1 and 5 years. *Archives of Diseases in Childhood*, September.

Aniansson, G., et al., 2002. Otitis media and feeding with breast milk of children with cleft palate. *Scandinavian Journal of Plastic Reconstructive Surgery and Hand Surgery*.

Auerbach, K., and L. M. Gartner, 1987. Breastfeeding and human milk: their association with jaundice in the neonate. *Clinics in Perinatology*.

Avoa, A., and P. R. Fischer, 1990. The influence of prenatal instruction about breast-feeding on neonatal weight loss. *Pediatrics*.

Ballard, J. L., C. E. Auer, and J. C. Khoury, 2002. Ankyloglossia: assessment, incidence, and effect of frenuloplasty on the breastfeeding dyad. *Pediatrics*, November.

Butte, N. F., et al., 1984. Human milk intake and growth in exclusively breastfed infants. *Journal of Pediatrics*.

Danner, S. C., and M. C. McBride, 1988. Sucking disorders in neurologically impaired infants. *Breastfeeding Abstracts*.

Dewey, K. G., 1992. Growth of breastfed and formula-fed infants from 0 to 18 months: the DARLING study. *Pediatrics*.

Dewey, K. G., 1998. Growth patterns of breastfed infants and the current status of growth charts for infants. *Journal of Human Lactation*, June.

Dewey, K. G., and B. Lonnerdal, 1986. Infant self-regulation of breast milk intake. *Acta Paed. Scand.*

Florey, C. D., et al., 1995. Infant feeding and mental and motor development at 18 months of age in first born singletons. *International Journal of Epidemiology*.

Forrest, F., 1991. Reported social alcohol consumption during pregnancy and infants' development at 18 months. *British Medical Journal*, July.

Garza, C., and M. De Onis, 1999. A new international growth reference for young children. *American Journal of Clinical Nutrition*, July.

Gomez-Sanchiz, M., 2003. Influence of breastfeeding on mental and psychomotor development. *Clinics in Pediatrics*, January/February.

Lennon, I., and B. R. Lewis, 1987. Effect of early complementary feeds on lactation failure. *Breastfeeding Review*.

Little, R. E., et al., 1989. Maternal alcohol use during breast-feeding and infant mental and motor development at one year. *New England Journal of Medicine*.

Lucas, A., et al., 1992. Breastmilk and subsequent intelligence quotient in children born preterm. *Lancet*, February.

McBride, J. C., and S. C. Danner, 1987. Sucking disorders in neurologically impaired infants: assessment and facilitation of breastfeeding. *Clinics in Perinatology*.

Matheny, R., and J. F. Picciano, 1986. Feeding and growth characteristics of human milk-fed infants. *Journal of the American Dietetic Association*.

Mathew, O. P., and J. Bhatia, 1989. Sucking and breathing patterns during breast- and bottle-feeding in term neonates. *American Journal of Diseases in Childhood.*

Meier, P. P., 1988. Bottle- and breast-feeding: effects on transcutaneous oxygen pressure and temperature in preterm infants. *Nursing Research.*

Meier, P. P., and E. J. Pugh, 1985. Breast feeding behavior in small preterm infants. *American Journal of Maternal Child Nursing.*

Meier, P. P., and G. C. Anderson, 1987. Responses of small pre-term infants to bottle- and breast-feeding. *American Journal of Maternal Child Nursing.*

Morley, R., et al., 2004. Neurodevelopment in children born small for gestational age: a randomized trial of nutrient-enriched versus standard formula and comparison with a reference breastfed group. *Pediatrics*, March.

Minchin, M. K., 1989. Positioning for breastfeeding. *Birth.* 16:67-80.

Newman, T. B., and M. J. Maisels, 2002. Evaluation and treatment of jaundice in the term newborn: a kinder, gentler approach. *American Family Physician*, February.

Paine, B. J., et al., 1999. Duration of breastfeeding and Bayley's Mental Development Index at 1 year of age. *Journal of Paediatrics and Child Health*, February.

Paradise, J. L., B. A. Elster, and L. Tan, 1994. Evidence in infants with cleft palate that breast milk protects against otitis media. *Pediatrics*, December.

Pinelli, J., et al., 2003. Effect of breastmilk consumption on neurodevelopmental outcomes at 6 and 12 month of age in VLBW infants. *Advances in Neonatal Care*, April.

Porter, M. L., and B. L. Dennis, 2000. Hyperbilirubinemia in the term newborn. *Acta Paediatrica*, October.

Steichen, J. J., et al., 1987. Breastfeeding the low birth weight pre-term infant. *Clinics in Perinatology.*

Temboury, M. C., et al., 1994. Influence of breastfeeding on the infant's intellecutal development. *Journal of Pediatric Gastroenterology and Nutrition*, January.

Weatherly-White, R.C.A., et al., 1987. Early repair and breast-feeding for infants with cleft lip. *Plastic and Reconstructive Surgery.*

Whitehead, R. G., A. A. Paul, and E. A. Ahmed, 1986. Weaning practices in the United Kingdom and variations in anthropometric development. *Acta Paed. Scand.*

Wilson-Clay, B., and K. Hoover. *The Breastfeeding Atlas*, 2nd ed. Lact-News Press.

Woolridge. J., 1986. The "anatomy" of infant sucking. *Midwifery*.

Young, H. B., et al., 1982. Milk and lactation: some social and developmental correlates among 1,000 infants, *Pediatrics*, February.

Chapter 5: How the Baby Functions: Behavior

American Academy of Pediatrics, Work Group on Breastfeeding, 1997. Breastfeeding and the use of human milk, policy statement. *Pediatrics*, December.

Barr, R. G., and M. F. Elias, 1988. Nursing interval and maternal responsivity: effect on early infant crying. *Pediatrics*.

Bell, R. Q., 1974. Contributions of human infants to caregiving and social interaction. In: *The Effect of the Infant on Its Caregiver*, L. M. and L. A. Rosenblum, eds., John Wiley & Sons, New York.

Berham, J. C., G. R. Pereira, J. B. Watkins, and G. J. Peckham, 1983. Nonnutritive sucking during gavage feeding enhances growth and maturation in premature infants. *Pediatrics*.

Blauvelt, H., 1956. Neonate-mother relationships in goat and man. In: *Group Processes, Transactions of the Second Conference*. Josiah Macy, Jr. Foundation.

Brazelton, T. B., et al., 1966. Visual responses in the newborn. *Pediatrics*.

Condon, W. S., and L. W. Sander, 1974. Neonate movement is synchronized with adult speech: interactional participation and language acquisition. *Science*.

DeCasper, A. J., and W. P. Fifer, 1980. Of human bonding: Newborns prefer their mothers' voices. *Science*.

Dodd, V., and C. Chalmers, 2003. Comparing the use of hydrogel dressings to lanolin ointment with lactating mothers. *Journal of Obstetrics, Gynecology, and Neonatal Nursing*. July/August.

Eliot, Lise, Ph.D., 1999. *What's Going On in There? How the Brain and Mind Develop in the First Five Years of Life*. Bantam Books, New York.

Ferguson, D. M., et al., 1987. Breastfeeding and subsequent social adjustment in six- to eight-year-old children. *Journal of Child Psychology, Psychiatry, and Allied Disciplines*.

Field, T. M., R. Woodson, R. Greenberg, and D. Cohen, 1982. Discrimination and imitation of facial expressions by neonates. *Science*.

Gerber, S., et al., 2004. The effect of skin-to-skin contact (kangaroo care) shortly after birth on the neurobehavioral responses of the term newborn: a randomized, controlled trial. *Pediatrics*, April.

Goren, C., et al., 1975. Visual following and pattern discrimination of facelike stimuli by newborn infants. *Pediatrics*.

Goubet, N., C. Rattaz, et al., 2003. Olfactory experience mediates response to pain in preterm newborns. *Developmental Psychobiology*, March.

Haith, M. M., T. Bergman, and M. J. Morre, 1977. Eye contact and face scanning in early infancy. *Science*.

Herbinet, E., and M. C. Busnel, eds., 1981. *L'Aube des Sens: Ouvrage collectif sur les perceptions sensorielles foetales et neonateles*. Stock, Paris.

Klaus, M. J., and P. H. Klaus, 1988. *The Amazing Newborn*. Addison Wesley, Boston.

Lipsitt, L. P., 1977. The study of sensory and learning processes of the newborn. *Clinics in Perinatology*.

Marmet, C., and E. Shell, 1984. Training neonates to suck correctly. *Maternal Child Nursing*.

Morley, R., et al., 2004. Neurodevelopment in children born small for gestational age: a randomized trial of nutrient-enriched versus standard formula and comparison with a reference breastfed group. *Pediatrics*, March.

Newman, J., and B. Wilmott, 1990. Breast rejection: a little-appreciated cause of lactation failure. *Canadian Family Physician*.

O'Connor, D. L., et al., 2003. Growth and development of premature infants fed predominantly human milk, predominantly premature infant formula, or a combination of human milk and premature formula. *Journal of Pediatric Gastroenterology and Nutrition*, October.

Retsinas, G., June 1, 2003. The Marketing of a Superbaby Formula. *The New York Times*.

Rohde, J. E., 1988. Breastfeeding beyond twelve months (letter). *Lancet*.

Salk, I., 1960. Effects of normal heartbeat sound on behavior of newborn infant: implications for mental health. *World Mental Health*.

Trainor, L. J., and R. N. Desjardins, 2002. Pitch characteristics of infant-directed speech affect infants' ability to discriminate vowels. *Psychology Bulletin Review*, June.

Wakschlag, L. S., and S. L. Hans, 1999. Relation of maternal responsiveness during infancy to the development of behavior problems in high-risk youths, *Developmental Psychology*, March.

Witters-Green, R., 2003. Increasing breastfeeding rates in working mothers. *Families, Systems, & Health*.

Chapter 6: Parents and Innate Behavior

Bottorff, J. L., 1990. Persistence in breastfeeding: a phenomenological investigation. *Journal of Advanced Nursing*.

Brazelton, T. B., 1983. *Infants and Mothers*, rev. ed. Delacorte Press, New York.

Cohen, S. P. 1987. High tech—soft touch: breastfeeding issues. *Clinics in Perinatology*.

Eibl-Eibesfeldt, I., 1989. *Human Ethology*. Aldine de Gruyter, New York.

Elander, G., and T. Lindberg, 1984. Short mother-infant separation during first week of life influences the duration of breast-feeding. *Acta Paed. Scand.*

Goodine, L. A., and P. A. Fried, 1984. Infant feeding practices: pre- and post-natal factors, affective choice of method and the duration of breastfeeding. *Canadian Journal of Public Health*.

Jelliffe, D. B., and E. F. Jelliffe, eds., 1978. *Human Milk in the Modern World*. Oxford University Press.

Jimenez, M., and N. Newton, 1979. Activity and work during pregnancy and the postpartum: a cross-cultural study of two hundred and two societies. *American Journal of Obstetrics and Gynecology*.

Kemper, K., B. Forsyth, and P. McCarthy, 1989. Jaundice, terminating breast-feeding, and the vulnerable child. *Pediatrics*.

Kemper, K., B. Forsyth, and P. McCarthy, 1990. Persistent perceptions of vulnerability following neonatal jaundice. *American Journal of Diseases in Childhood*.

Kennel, J. H., and M. H. Klaus, 1971. Care of the mother of the high-risk infant. *Clinics in Obstetrics and Gynecology*.

Klaus, M. H., and J. H. Kennell, 1982. *Parent-Infant Bonding*. C. V. Mosby, St. Louis.

Klaus, M. H., J. H. Kennell, and N. Plumb, 1980. Human maternal behavior at the first contact with her young. *Pediatrics*.

Millard, A. V., 1990. The place of the clock in pediatric advice: rationales, cultural themes, and impediments to breastfeeding. *Social Science Medicine*.

Modahl, C., and N. Newton, 1979. Mood state difference between breast and bottle-feeding mothers. In: *Emotion and Reproduction: Proceedings of the Serano Symposia, Vol. 20B*. L. Carenza and L. Zinchella, eds., Academic Press, New York.

Mori, M., et al., 1990. Oxytocin is the major prolactin releasing factor in the posterior pituitary. *Endocrinology*.

Newton, N., 1955. *Maternal Emotions*. Hoeber, New York.

Newton, N., 1978. The role of the oxytocin reflexes in three interpersonal reproductive acts: coitus, birth, and breast-feeding. In: *Clinical Psychoneuroendocrinology in Reproduction: Proceedings of the Serano Symposia*. L. Carenza, P. Panceri, and L. Zichella, eds., Academic Press, New York.

Newton, N., D. Foshee, and M. Newton, 1966. Experimental inhibition of labor through environmental disturbance. *Obstetrics and Gynecology*.

Newton, N., and C. Modahl, 1989. Oxytocin—psychoactive hormone of love and breast feeding. In: *The Free Woman: Women's Health in the 1990's*. E. V. van Hall, and W. Everaerd, eds., Parthenon Publishing Group, Park Ridge, N.J.

Parke, R. D., 1979. Perspectives on father-infant interactions. In: *The Handbook of Infant Development*. J. D. Osofsky, ed., John Wiley & Sons, New York.

Pruett, K. D., 1987. *The Nurturing Father.* Warner Books, New York.

Taylor, P. M., et al., 1986. Early suckling and prolonged breastfeeding. *American Journal of Diseases in Childhood.*

Wakschlag, L. S., and S. L. Hans, 1999. Relation of maternal responsiveness during infancy to the development of behavior problems in high-risk youths. *Developmental Psychology,* March.

Waletzky, L. R., 1979. Breastfeeding and weaning: some psychological considerations. *Primary Care.*

Weisenfeld, A., et al., 1985. Psychophysiological response of breast and bottle-feeding mothers to their infants' signals. *Psychophysiology.*

Whitehead, R. G., 1985. The human weaning process. *Pediatrics.*

Chapter 7: Helpers and Hinderers: How Breastfeeding Was Saved, and Why the Job Is Not Yet Done

American Academy of Pediatrics Committee on Nutrition, 1980. Human milk banking. *Pediatrics.*

American Academy of Pediatrics Committee on Nutrition, 1982. The promotion of breast feeding: policy statement based on task force report. *Pediatrics.*

Asquith, M. T., P. W. Pedrotti, D. K. Stevenson, and P. Sunshine, 1987. Clinical uses, collection, and banking of human milk. *Clinics in Perinatology.*

Auerbach, K. G., 1990. Breastfeeding fallacies: their relationship to understanding lactation. *Birth.*

Bauchner, H., J. M. Leventhal, and E. D. Shapiro, 1986. Studies of breast-feeding and infections. How good is the evidence? *J.A.M.A.* ("The Yale Study").

Baum, J. D., 1979. Raw breast milk for babies on neonatal units. *Lancet.*

Bergevin, Y., C. Dougherty, and M. S. Kramer, 1983. Do infant formula samples shorten the duration of breastfeeding? *Lancet.*

Carballo, M., 1988. The World Health Organization's work in the area of infant and young child feeding and nutrition. In: *Programmes to Promote*

Breastfeeding. D. B. Jelliffe and E.F.P. Jelliffe, eds., Oxford University Press.

Clement, D., 1988. Commerciogenic malnutrition in the 1980s. In: *Programmes to Promote Breastfeeding*. D. B. Jelliffe and E.F.P. Jelliffe, eds., Oxford University Press.

Cunningham, A. S., 1981. Breastfeeding and morbidity in industrialized countries: an update. In: *Advances in International Maternal and Child Health, Vol. I*. D. B. Jelliffe and E.F.P. Jelliffe, eds., Oxford University Press.

Cunningham, A. S., 1988. An historical overview of breastfeeding promotion in Western Europe and North America. In: *Programmes to Promote Breastfeeding*. D. B. Jelliffe and E.F.P. Jelliffe, eds., Oxford University Press.

Cunningham, A. S., 1988. Studies of breastfeeding and infections. How good is the evidence? A critique of the answer from Yale. *Journal of Human Lactation*.

Cunningham, A. S., D. B. Jelliffe, and E.F.P. Jelliffe, 1991. Breastfeeding and health in the 1980s: a global epidemiological review. *Journal of Pediatrics*.

Edwards, G., 1985. The lactation consultant: a new profession. *Birth*.

Frantz, K., P. Fleiss, and R. Lawrence, 1978. Management of the slow-gaining breastfed baby. *Resources in Human Nurturing Monograph*.

Habicht, J. P., J. DaVanzo, and W. P. Buitz, 1986. Does breastfeeding really save lives, or are apparent benefits due to biases? *American Journal of Epidemiology*.

Jelliffe, D. B., and E.F.P. Jelliffe, eds., 1988. *Programmes to Promote Breastfeeding*. Oxford University Press.

Jelliffe, E.F.P., 1988. Breastfeeding modules for integration into the curriculum of health professionals. In: *Programmes to Promote Breastfeeding*. D. B. Jelliffe and E.F.P. Jelliffe, eds., Oxford University Press.

Johnstone, H. A., and J. F. Marcinak, 1990. Candidiasis in the breastfeeding mother and infant. *Journal of Obstetric and Gynecologic Nursing*.

Kemper, K., et al., 1989. Jaundice, terminating breastfeeding, and the vulnerable child syndrome. *Pediatrics*.

Koop, C. E., and M. E. Brannon, 1984. Breast-feeding—the community norm. Report of a workshop. *Public Health Reports.*

Kramer, M. S., 1988. Infant feeding, infection, and public health. *Pediatrics.*

Lumley, J., 1987. Does it work? Obstacles to breastfeeding research. *Pediatrics.*

McKinney, W. P., D. L. Schiedermayer, et al., 1990. Attitudes of internal medicine faculty and residents toward professional interaction with pharmaceutical sales representatives. *J.A.M.A.*

Meara, H., 1976. La Leche League in the United States: a key to successful breastfeeding in a non-supportive culture. *Journal of Nurse Midwifery.*

Minchin, M., 1985. *Breastfeeding Matters: What We Need to Know About Breastfeeding.* Allen & Unwin, Australia.

Minchin, M., 1987. Infant formulas: a mass uncontrolled trial in perinatal care. *Birth.*

Naylor, A. J., and R. A. Wester, 1988. Health professional education: a key to successful breastfeeding promotion programmes. In: *Programmes to Promote Breastfeeding.* D. B. Jelliffe and E.F.P. Jelliffe, eds., Oxford University Press.

Naylor, A. J., and R. A. Wester, 1988. Providing professional lactation management consultation. *Clinics in Perinatology.*

Neifert, M., S. DeMarzo, J. Seachat, et al., 1990. The influence of breast surgery, breast appearance, and pregnancy-induced breast changes on lactation sufficiency as measured by infant weight gain. *Birth.*

Palmer, G., 1988. *The Politics of Breastfeeding.* Pandora, London.

Popkin, B. M., M. E. Fernandez, and J. L. Avila, 1990. Infant formula promotion and the health sector in the Philippines, *American Journal of Public Health.*

Reiff, M. I., and S. M. Essock-Vitale, 1985. Hospital influences on early infant-feeding practices. *Pediatrics.*

Ruowei, L., et al., 2005, Breastfeeding rates in the United States by characteristics of the child, mother, or family. *Pediatrics.*

Stokamer, C. L., 1990. Breastfeeding promotion efforts: why some do not work. *International Journal of Obstetrics and Gynecology.*

Winikoff, B., V. H. Laukaran, D. Myers, and R. Stone, 1986. Dynamics of infant feeding: mothers, professionals, and the institutional context in a large urban hospital. *Pediatrics*.

World Health Organization, 1981. *Contemporary Patterns in Breastfeeding: report on the WHO collaborative study on breastfeeding*. World Health Organization, Geneva.

World Health Organization, 1981. *International Code of Marketing of Breastmilk Substitutes*. World Health Organization, Geneva.

Young, S. A., and M. Kaufman, 1988. Promoting breastfeeding at a migrant health center. *American Journal of Public Health*.

PART II

Chapter 8: Before the Baby Comes

Marshall, H., and M. D. Klaus. 2002. *The Doula Book: How a Trained Labor Companion Can Help You Have a Shorter, Easier, and Healthier Birth*. Perseus Books Group, Philadelphia.

Noble, E., 1988. *Essential Exercises for the Childbearing Year*, 3rd ed. Houghton Mifflin, Boston.

Sears, W., and M. Sears. *The Pregnancy Book: Everything You Need to Know to Have a Safe and Satisfying Birth*. Little, Brown, Boston.

Simkin, Penny. *Pregnancy, Childbirth and the Newborn: The Complete Guide*. Meadowbrook Press, Minnetonka, MN.

Chapter 9: In the Hospital

Ehrenkranz, R. A., and B. A. Ackerman, 1986. Metoclopramide effect on faltering milk production by mothers of premature infants. *Pediatrics*.

Frantz, K., 1980. Techniques of successfully managing nipple problems and the reluctant nurser in the early postpartum period. In: *Human Milk: Its Biological and Social Value*. Excerpta Medica, Amsterdam.

Frantz, K., 1988. Recent knowledge concerning practical management. In: *Programmes to Promote Breastfeeding*. D. B. Jelliffe and E.F.P. Jelliffe, eds., Oxford University Press.

Lauwers, J., and D. Shinskie. 2000. *Counseling the Nursing Mother: A Lactation Consultant's Guide*, 3rd ed. Jones and Bartlett. Boston.

Sears, W., and M. Sears. 1994. *The Birth Book: Everything You Need to Know to Have a Safe and Satisfying Birth*. Little, Brown, Boston.

Sears, W., and M. Sears. 2001. *The Attachment Parenting Book: A Commonsense Guide to Understanding and Nurturing Your Baby*. Little, Brown, Boston.

Walker, M., and J. W. Driscoll, 1989. Sore nipples: the new mother's nemesis. *Maternal Child Nursing*.

Chapter 10: One to Six Weeks: The Learning Period

American Academy of Pediatrics. 1998. *Caring for Your Baby and Young Child: Birth to Age 5*, Bantam, New York.

American Academy of Pediatrics, 1998, Your Baby's First Year, Bantam, New York.

Feldman, R., et al., 2004. Mother-child touch patterns in infant feeding disorders: relation to maternal, child, and environmental factors. *Journal of the American Academy of Child and Adolescent Psychiatry*.

Hautman, M. A., 1979. Folk health and illness beliefs. *Nurse Practitioner*.

Kitzinger, Sheila, 1989. *Breastfeeding Your Baby*. Alfred A. Knopf, New York.

La Leche League International, 1987. *The Womanly Art of Breastfeeding*, 4th rev. ed. New American Library, New York.

Lim, R. 2001. *After the Baby's Birth: A Woman's Way to Wellness: A Complete Guide for Postpartum Women*. Ten Speed Press, Berkeley.

Morse, J. M., and J. L. Bottorff, 1989. Leaking: a problem of lactation. *Journal of Nurse Midwifery*.

Spector, R. E., 1979. *Cultural Diversity in Health and Illness*. Appleton Century Croft, New York.

Chapter 11: The Reward Period Begins

American Academy of Pediatrics, 1997. Does bedsharing affect the risk of SIDS? *Pediatrics*.

Ladas, A. K., 1972. Information and social support as factors in the outcome of breastfeeding. *Journal of Applied Behavioral Sociology*.

McKenna, J., and S. Mosko, 1993. Evolution and infant sleep: an experimental study of infant-parent co-sleeping and its implications for SIDS. *Acta Paediatrica* (supplement).

McKenna, J., 2000. Cultural influences on infant and childhood sleep biology, and the science that studies it: toward a more inclusive paradigm. In *Sleep and Breathing in Children: A Developmental Approach*. J. Loughlin, J. Carroll, and C. Marcus, Eds., Marcel Dakker, New York.

National Mental Health Association, 2003. *Recognizing Postpartum Depression*, Strengthening Families Fact Sheet, http://www.nmha.org/children/ppd.pdf

Sears, J., M. Sears, R. Sears, and W. Sears. 2003. *The Baby Book: Everything You Need to Know About Your Baby from Birth to Age Two*, rev. and updated. Little, Brown, Boston.

Small, M. E., 1998. *Our Babies, Ourselves*. Doubleday, New York.

Woolridge, M. W., 1995. Baby-controlled breastfeeding: biocultural implications. In *Breastfeeding: Biocultural Perspectives*. P. Stuart-Macadam, and K. A. Dettwyler, eds., Aldine de Gruyter, New York.

Chapter 12: The Working Mother: How Breastfeeding Can Help

Auerbach, K. G., and E. Guss, 1984. Maternal employment and breastfeeding: a study of 567 women's experiences. *American Journal of Diseases of Childhood*.

Broome, M. E., 1981. Breastfeeding and the working mother. *Journal of Gynecologic Nursing*, May/June.

Cohen, Rona, RN, MN, FP NP, 1995. Comparison of maternal absenteeism and infant illness rates among breast-feeding and formula-feeding women in two corporations. *American Journal of Health Promotion.*

Frederick, I. B., and K. G. Auerbach, 1985. Maternal-infant separation and breast-feeding: the return to work or school. *Journal of Reproductive Medicine.*

Katcher, A. L., and M. G. Lanese, 1985. Breast-feeding by employed mothers: a reasonable accommodation in the work place. *Pediatrics.*

La Leche League International, 1985. *Manual Expression of Breast Milk: The Marmet Technique.* Reprint No. 27. La Leche League International.

Pryor, G., 1997. *Working Mother, Nursing Mother: The Essential Guide to Breastfeeding and Staying Close to Your Baby After You Return to Work.* Harvard Common Press.

Reifsnider, E., and S. T. Myers, 1985. Employed mothers can breast-feed, too! *American Journal of Maternal Child Nursing.*

Shepherd, S. C., and R. E. Yarrow, 1982. Breastfeeding and the working mother. *Journal of Nurse Midwifery.*

United States Department of Labor, Bureau of Labor Statistics: NEWS, Washington, D.C., USDL 87-345.

Chapter 13: Nursing Your Older Baby

Family Health International, 1988. Consensus statement: breastfeeding as a family planned method. *Lancet,* November.

Gerrard, J. W., 1982. Untoward effects of weaning. *Canadian Medical Association Journal.*

Pryor, K, 1998. *Don't Shoot the Dog: The New Art of Teaching and Training,* 2nd ed. Pocket Books, New York.

Rempel, L. A., 2004. Factors influencing the breastfeeding decisions of long-term breastfeedings. *Journal of Human Lactation,* August.

Waletzky, L., 1977. Weaning from the breast. *World Journal of Psychosynthesis*.

Waletzky, L., 1979. Breast feeding and weaning. *Primary Care*.

West, C., 1980. Factors influencing the duration of breastfeeding. *Journal of Biosocial Science*.

Whitehead, R. G., 1985. The human weaning process. *Pediatrics*.

Resources:
Sources of Breastfeeding Information and Supplies

FOR FAST HELP WITH BREASTFEEDING PROBLEMS

1. Stay in touch with the patient education service at your hospitals. Many hospitals maintain a breastfeeding hot line for new mothers. Often the lactation consultant who first helped you in the hospital remains available by phone for as long as you need her.
2. Call La Leche League's toll-free number, 1-800-LA LECHE, main number (847) 519-7730, or go to their Web site, http://www.laleche league.org/leaderinfo.html for a directory of LLL groups in your area. The league offers telephone counseling and can put you in touch with the La Leche League leader who lives nearest you, usually within twenty-four hours.
3. Locate a certified lactation consultant in your area. Go to the Web site of the International Lactation Consultant Association, http://www.ilca.org/, and key in your zip code for a directory of LCs in your area.

ORGANIZATIONS

International Lactation Consultants Association: An organization of board-certified professional lactation counselors.

International Lactation Consultants Association
1500 Sunday Drive, Suite 102

Raleigh, North Carolina 27607, USA
Telephone: (919) 861-5577
Fax: (919) 787-4916
E-mail: info@ilca.org

La Leche League International: The international association for nursing mothers organizes a four-month series of meetings for expecting and new mothers to introduce them to the basics of breastfeeding and to provide warm and informed support as their babies grow. LLLI sells recommended books, videos, and supplies for breastfeeding mothers.

La Leche League International
P.O. Box 4079
Schaumburg, IL 60168-4079
Telephone: (847) 519-7730
Fax: (847) 519-0035
Order department: (847) 519-9585

Promotion of Mother's Milk, Inc.: Promotion of Mother's Milk, Inc. (Pro-MoM), is a nonprofit organization dedicated to increasing public awareness and public acceptance of breastfeeding. http://www.promom.org

Breastfeeding supplies, from electric breast pumps to pads and bras, can be found in some hospitals and pharmacies. The most complete and convenient sources these days, however, can be found online. Here are a few of the many sites that offer a selection of excellent supplies, clothing, and information on how and when to use them:

Breastfeeding Essentials: http://www.breastfeed-essentials.com
The Breast Site: http://www.thebreastsite.com/breastfeeding/breastfeeding
    supplies.aspx
Breastfeeding.com: http://www.breastfeeding.com
Medela, Inc.: http://www.medela.com
Lact-Aid, Inc.: http://www.lact-aid.com/

Nursing Mother Supplies: http://www.nursingmothersupplies.com

Mother's Milkmate (milk storage system): http://www.mothersmilk
mate.com

Motherwear (clothing for nursing mothers):
http://www.motherwear.com/main.asp

PUBLICATIONS

Magazines and journals about breastfeeding

Breastfeeding Abstracts: Quarterly publications for health professionals; abstracts and reviews of current publications in the area of human lactation, La Leche League International

New Beginnings: La Leche League's bimonthly journal about breastfeeding; personal stories, photos, research updates; free with annual membership

Mothering magazine: a monthly magazine and Web site oriented to the noncommercial, nonsexist, environmentally sound view of motherhood and family life, with emphasis on breastfeeding. http://www.mother-ing.com

The Journal of Human Lactation: The official journal of the International Lactation Consultant Association, *JHL* publishes peer-reviewed scientific articles on breastfeeding, as well as essays and commentary, book reviews, and a monthly overview of recent publications in the medical literature. Subscribe at http://www.sagepub.com

Books about breastfeeding

See the references section for Part 2 of this book for a list of valuable books on general infant care. Even the biggest bookstores can carry only a fraction of the books that are published each year, so you shouldn't be surprised if a book you want is not on the shelves of bookstores in your neighborhood. However, most bookstores will be glad to order any title you ask for, if they can find it in *Books in Print*, a catalog that lists the publisher and price of every current book. Often a shop can obtain the book you want in a few days, by mail or through local wholesalers. Any book can also ordered online at Amazon.com and other Internet-based booksellers. La Leche League International operates a mail-order store offering many books, including their classic *The Womanly Art of Breastfeeding*, and pamphlets about breastfeeding and child care. Visit their Web site to order their catalog.

Working Mothers

The corporate world and other employers are gradually coming around to the realization that keeping good employees healthy and on the job includes supporting nursing mothers. If your employer needs help understanding the benefits of giving new mothers the time and space to pump and store their breast milk, drop a letter based on the model below into your boss's in box or at the human resources department.

A PROPOSAL FOR PUMPING SPACE

To: Human Resources [and/or the principals of your workplace]
Fr: [Your name, and/or the names of all the nursing and expecting mothers in your workplace]
Re: Proposal for an onsite "lactation room"

Helping employees balance the demands of work and family results more productive workplace. One step that offers enormous support to many new parents of staff is to establish a lactation room for nursing mothers. This simple accommodation can make an employee's transition back to work successful and enduring. In fact, meeting the needs of nursing mothers has been shown to be so effective at retaining valued employees that more than 80% of the 100 Best Companies for Working Mothers offer this benefit.

Providing employees with a private, convenient lactation room has been shown to increase the rate of breastfeeding among employees and decrease the rate of absenteeism due to illness of dependent children. A study has shown that companies with onsite lactation rooms recorded 27% fewer maternal days off and 36% fewer illnesses among infants of employees. Breastfeeding has also been shown to improve the health of mothers, including a 40% reduction in the risk of breast cancer if they breastfeed for a lifetime total of at least two years. Mothers who nurse are also less likely to develop ovarian cancer and osteoporosis.

A lactation room is a private, sanitary location in which employees who are nursing mothers may pump and store their milk each day. Nursing mothers usually require 10–15 minutes twice a day to pump sufficient milk for their babies' needs. The space in which they pump that milk must have:

- a small room with a door that can be latched or locked from the inside;
- a comfortable chair and a small table on which a breast pump and other equipment or reading materials can be placed;
- an electrical outlet within a few feet of the chair and table.

Additional items will enhance the convenience of the space, including:

- a small refrigerator in which milk containers can be stored until the end of the workday;
- a sink for rinsing pump attachments;
- cabinets or shelving on which pumping equipment can be stored;

- a telephone for employees who would like to make or receive business calls while pumping.

Restrooms are inappropriate for these purposes as they are not sanitary and rarely provide sufficient privacy. Employee locker rooms are also unlikely to provide sufficient privacy. Borrowed private offices are not ideal as their use for pumping may inconvenience the primary occupants. Conference rooms may not be available for regular, timely use, and may not be sufficiently private. Only a dedicated space will meet all the needs of nursing mothers.

Thank you for your attention to this important proposal.

Note to California Residents: In 2002, the California Legislature passed the Lactation Accommodation law requiring all California employers to provide "A reasonable amount of break time and make a reasonable effort to provide a private space, other than a toilet stall, close to the employee's work area, to accommodate an employee desiring to express breastmilk for her baby." If you live in California and your employer does not provide a dedicated lactation space, bring this law to their attention.

Index